Orthodontic Concepts and Strategies

Orthodontic Concepts

and Strategies

Frans P.G.M. van der Linden

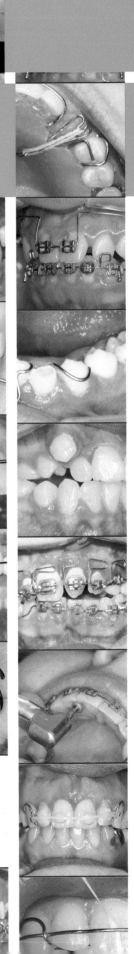

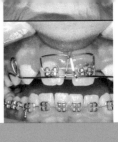

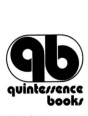

Quintessence Publishing Co, Ltd
London, Barcelona, Berlin, Chicago, Copenhagen,
Istanbul, Milan, Moscow, New Delhi, Paris, Prague,
São Paulo, Tokyo, and Warsaw

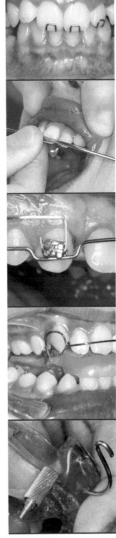

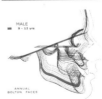

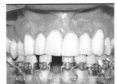

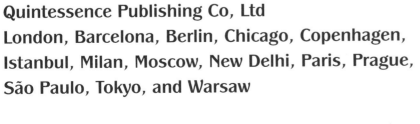

British Library Cataloging-in-Publication Data

Orthodontic concepts and strategies

ISBN 1-85097-094-7

Editor: Lisa Bywaters

Production: Ina Steinbrück

ISBN 1-85097-094-7

Printed in Germany

Contents

Contents

Preface

In previous textbooks by the author, emphasis was placed on the theoretical basis of orthodontics, which is so essential for diagnosis and treatment planning.[212-216, 221] Treatment procedures were covered only superficially, because the variation in methods and techniques is so great. In addition, techniques are improving continuously, and new materials and methods are introduced regularly.

The purpose of this volume is to provide clinically relevant information. How appliances should be used and what can be achieved with them are described and illustrated in detail, mainly with schematic drawings and clinical photographs. Practical aspects and tips for attaining the best results are provided. Clinical procedures are presented in such a way that the reader can apply them directly.

Furthermore, the contents are well suited for providing information to patients. The text is limited and directly related to the realization of the illustrated techniques. How a problem should be approached, where pitfalls can be expected, and how such dangers can be avoided are indicated. In addition, some long-standing myths and misconceptions are refuted.

Successful orthodontic treatment depends on many, often seemingly minor factors. If certain aspects are overlooked, the desired result cannot be attained, or the situation can even worsen. Detection of these elements is emphasized.

Orthodontic Concepts and Strategies

Acknowledgments

This book has come to fruition thanks to the outstanding photographs taken by J. L. M. van de Kamp and H. A. W. Bongaarts over a period of more than 30 years. Credit is also due to J. J. W. Siepermann and B. F. Bouwman for constructing or supervising the fabrication of dental casts and removable appliances. The chairside assistants, radiographers, and secretarial staff offered much support and help. The author is greatly indebted to all these people for their dedication, zeal, expertise, and constructive and pleasant cooperation.

Special thanks go to M. J. Th. Cillessen-van Hoek, who took care of the typing of the manuscript.

Dr H. Boersma, with whom the author worked for more than a third of a century, contributed again in many ways to the contents of this book.

Furthermore, the author wishes to recognize the contribution of Dr H. van Beek to chapter 7, which discusses headgear-activator combinations.

Dr J. Daskalogiannakis, the author of the respected Glossary of Orthodontic Terms, provided advice on the correct usage of terminology.

Finally, the editing by Lisa C. Bywaters contributed substantially to the quality of the text.

Orthodontic Concepts and Strategies

Complications During the Transition of Incisors

Primary teeth emerge with sufficient space in the dental arches. In contrast to the permanent anterior teeth, the primary incisors and canines have sufficient space within the jaws prior to their emergence in positions corresponding to the arrangement after eruption is completed. This space is provided by substantial growth of the jaws during the first 6 months after birth.[210,225] Nevertheless, great variation exists in the size of the primary teeth and the space available for them in the dental arches.[139] Some children have large diastemata in the primary dentition; others do not. In the presence of large diastemata, the transition proceeds unimpeded. Without diastemata, premature loss occurs and crowding of the permanent teeth results. Between these two situations lies the condition in which space in the dental arches is initially insufficient for the permanent incisors but is increased during the transitional period by displacement of primary teeth.

The ways in which orthodontic appliances can disrupt this increase in space are demonstrated in this chapter. Not only the detrimental effects but also the techniques used to repair the damage are shown.

First the chapter explains how the available space in the maxillary dental arch can increase during the transitional period and what happens if that increase cannot occur because space is extremely deficient. Subsequently, the discussion covers both developmental processes in the mandible. The simultaneous increase in space in the maxillary and mandibular dental arches is illustrated. In addition, the increase in space is demonstrated by a series of dental casts.

Furthermore, the position of the permanent teeth after emergence is discussed, because it depends not only on the available space but also on the occlusal contacts and the influence of the tongue and lips. The different effects of these factors in Class II and Class I situations are explained.

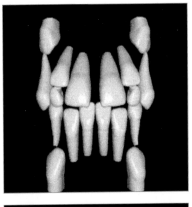
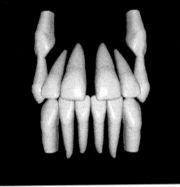
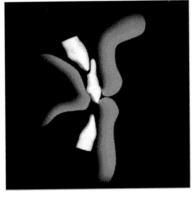
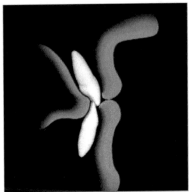

Orthodontic Concepts and Strategies

1

FIGURE 1-1

FIGURE 1-1

In the maxilla, the permanent central incisors are formed more cranially than are the lateral incisors. Their incisal edges are located apically to those of the lateral incisors (A). The central incisors start to erupt first and pass the lateral incisors (B). The roots of their predecessors resorb gradually. This resorption conforms in speed, extent, and shape to the movement and morphology of their successors. The primary incisors resorb from the palatal side, resulting in a thin labial section. The roots are resorbed almost completely by the time the primary incisors are shed (C). The permanent central incisors erupt alongside the primary lateral incisors, which migrate distally (D). After the primary lateral incisors have established contact with the primary canines, these pairs of teeth will migrate together distally; the canines will also move buccally. Through this process, sufficient space becomes available for the permanent central incisors to emerge (E). Subsequently, the permanent lateral incisors descend and emerge unimpeded without contacting the permanent central incisors (F). In accordance with the initial locations where formation started, the apices of the permanent lateral incisors are situated more palatally and occlusally than are those of the central incisors (G). The permanent incisors are tipped distally, and a large central diastema is present (H).[227] (Figs 1-1 to 1-6, 1-8, 1-9 and 1-12 are printed with permission from Dynamics of Orthodontics.[226])

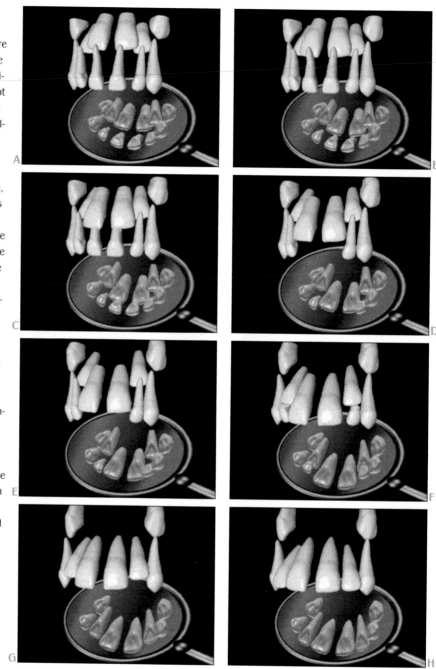

The transition can proceed without problems when abundant space is available within the jaws prior to emergence. The crowns of the central and lateral permanent incisors overlap each other only slightly, and the teeth emerge without interfering with the adjacent primary teeth.

An important difference between the two jaws is that the maxilla has a median suture, whereas the mandible does not. Consequently, the maxillary central incisors cannot approximate closely. Prior to emergence, the available space is used in an optimal way as the maxillary permanent central incisors are formed with their mesial surfaces parallel to and close to the median suture.[57, 223]

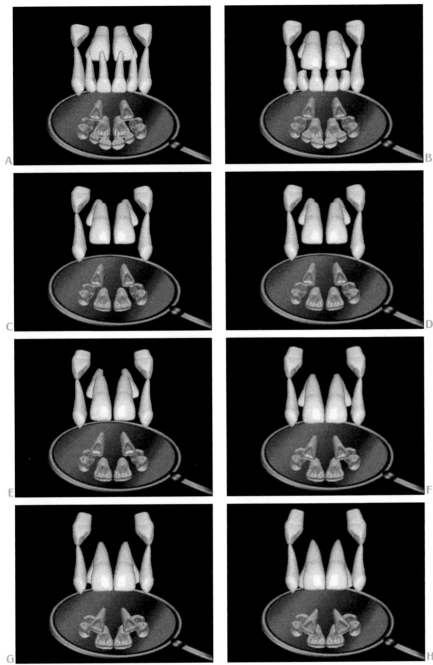

FIGURE 1-2

A primary dentition with small or no diastemata in the anterior region is an indication of insufficient space within the jaws for an undisturbed transition of the incisors. The intercanine distance is too small (A). This dimension is related to the width of the piriform aperture, next to which the forming parts of the permanent canines are situated. The incisal edges of the permanent central incisors are located close to not only the primary central incisors but also the lateral incisors (B). First the primary central incisors are shed (C) and shortly thereafter the lateral incisors (D). The permanent central incisors descend further without moving the primary canines distally or buccally, and the space in the dental arch does not enlarge (E). The permanent lateral incisors do not start to descend before the central incisors have emerged. Because space is insufficient, the lateral incisors cannot move labially, and emerge palatally to the permanent central incisors and primary canines (F). This palatal position of the lateral incisors involves the risk that they will end up in a crossbite with the mandibular incisors (G). Marked crowding is the result, partly because of the initial lack of space and partly because the primary canines were not moved (H). Both are the result of a discrepancy between the size of the maxilla and the tooth dimensions.[228]

The permanent maxillary central incisors erupt in distal angulation as teeth move in the direction in which they have been formed. Only when they meet an obstacle is the direction of eruption changed.

As already indicated, the most favorable condition for an undisturbed transition exists when excess space is available in the jaws. This ideal development is not illustrated or discussed here. However, after the incisors are fully erupted, diastemata in the maxillary anterior region will remain for some years until they disappear during adolescence.

The transition of the maxillary incisors associated with an increase in space in the dental arches is illustrated in Fig 1-1. Figure 1-2 shows the transition that results from premature loss of primary teeth and crowding.

FIGURE 1-3

In the mandible, the permanent central incisors are positioned initially more occlusally than are the lateral incisors. Furthermore, there is no median structure that prevents the central incisors from being close together (A). In the mandible, as in the maxilla, the roots of the primary incisors become resorbed mainly from the lingual side (B). The permanent lateral incisors do not start to move occlusally until the primary central incisors are lost (C). The erupting central permanent incisors are at some distance from the primary lateral incisors (D). The primary lateral incisors and canines are not moved. The roots of the primary lateral incisors resorb concomitantly with the eruption of their successors (E). This eruption of the permanent lateral incisors is associated with distobuccal movement of the primary canines (F). No or only small diastemata will remain after the permanent lateral incisors have reached the level of the occlusal plane (G). Conforming to their initial position, the root apices of the lateral incisors are more lingually positioned than are those of the central incisors. Accordingly, the lateral incisors are slightly more labially inclined than are the central incisors. The crowns of the lateral incisors are moved labially by the forces exerted by the tongue, leading to an aligned position in the dental arch (H).[227]

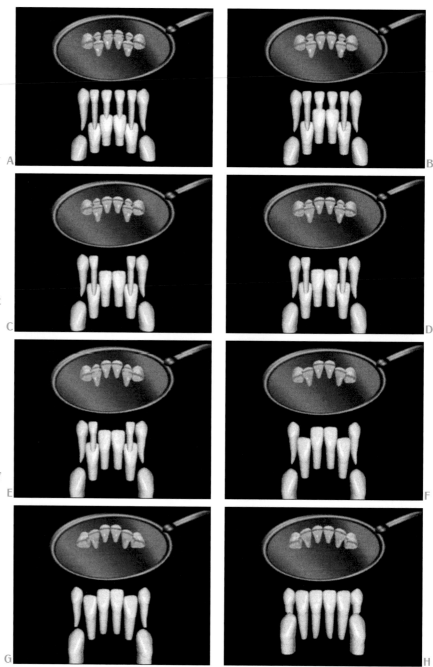

During early development, the mandible has a structure in the median plane that separates the left and right sides and contributes to the increase in jaw size before birth and some months thereafter. The potential for jaw widening is maintained in the maxilla until adulthood but is lost in the mandible on ossification of the symphysis prior to the emergence of the primary central incisors at about 6 months of age. After this ossification, the permanent mandibular central incisors can migrate mesially within the jaw and erupt later with little space between them.

The transition of the mandibular incisors associated with an increase in space in the dental arch is demonstrated in Fig 1-3; the transition resulting from premature loss and crowding is shown in Fig 1-4.

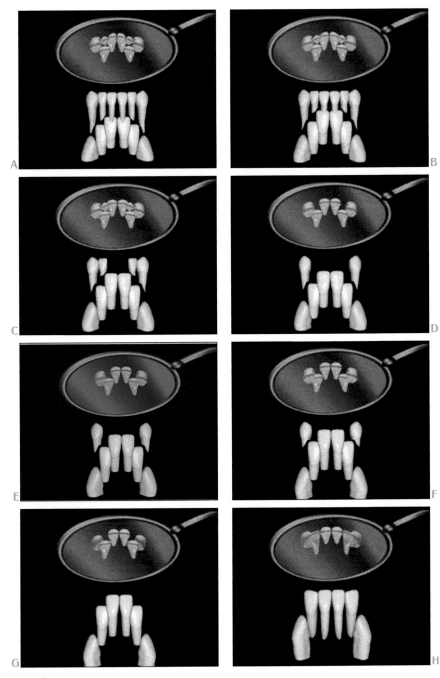

FIGURE 1-4

No or only small diastemata in the anterior region of the primary dentition are a sign of shortage of space in the mandible as well. Within the jaw, the permanent teeth overlap each other more than normal (A). With the eruption of the permanent central incisors, not only the roots of their predecessors but also the roots of the primary lateral incisors become resorbed (B). The primary central incisors are exfoliated first (C). Shortly thereafter, the primary lateral incisors follow (D). Not enough space remains for the permanent lateral incisors to erupt normally (E). With the eruption of the lateral incisors, the roots of the primary canines are resorbed prematurely (F). The canines are shed before the permanent lateral incisors emerge (G). Space becomes available in the dental arch for an improvement in position of the lateral incisors, to the detriment of the space remaining for the permanent canines, which subsequently will erupt buccally (H). In Fig 1-4, as in Figs 1-1 to 1-3, the transition is illustrated symmetrically. However, that is seldom the case, particularly in the mandible, where teeth can move through the median plane. Commonly, only one primary canine is lost prematurely, and the situation illustrated occurs on one side only.[228]

In the maxilla, the transition of the incisors occurs more or less independently on the left and right sides. That is less the case in the mandible, particularly in crowded situations. In the mandible, teeth can cross the median plane prior to or after emergence, and migration and tipping are not hindered by a structure in the median plane. Crowding can become concentrated on one side, and the midline of the dental arch may be displaced accordingly. Consequently, the primary canine will resorb prematurely only on that side. If subsequently the primary canine on the other side is extracted early, the incisors can migrate back, and the asymmetric positioning of the anterior teeth can be corrected. However, premature loss of primary canines can lead to other problems, such as an increase in crowding, lingual tipping of the incisors, and a deep bite.

FIGURE 1-5

The first maxillary anterior teeth to emerge, the central incisors, are not located nearest to the occlusal plane initially. Indeed, in both arches, the incisors with the smallest crowns are formed closest to the occlusal plane (A). The transition in the mandible begins before the transition in the maxilla. The process starts with the eruption of the permanent mandibular central incisors and the resorption of their predecessors (B). After the permanent mandibular central incisors have emerged, the lateral incisors and the permanent maxillary central incisors start to erupt (C). Subsequently, these teeth approach the primary teeth that are located distally to them (D) and migrate distally and buccally. This process occurs at about the same time in both arches (E). The transition of the incisors is completed as the permanent maxillary lateral incisors reach the occlusal plane (F). A few years later, the permanent mandibular canines start to erupt and their predecessors resorb and are shed (G). The maxillary canines are the last teeth to be replaced (H). Until that happens, the central diastema in the maxilla will not close, and the four incisors remain distally inclined. The permanent mandibular central incisors are already close at the start of eruption and often reach contact soon after emergence. Permanent mandibular incisors do not undergo a change in angulation, as maxillary incisors do.[227]

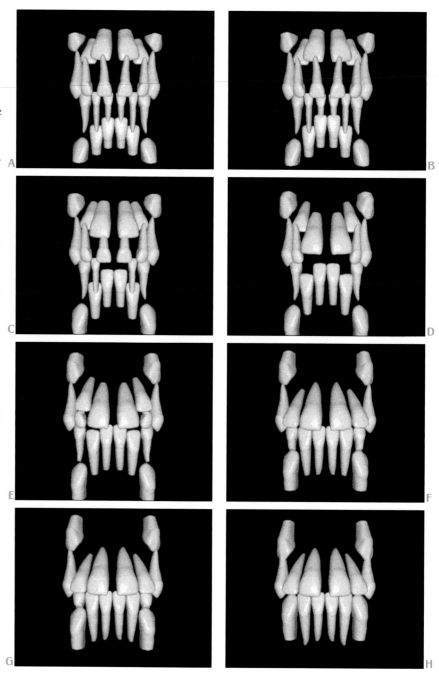

As a rule, the mandibular central incisors are the first anterior permanent teeth to emerge, at about 6 years of age; a year later they are followed by the mandibular lateral incisors, which appear in the mouth at about the same time as the permanent maxillary central incisors. This simultaneous emergence makes the increase in length of both dental arches coincide, as the movement of the primary teeth and the increase in available space in the dental arches are associated with the emergence of the permanent maxillary central incisor and the mandibular lateral incisor. This simultaneous increase in space in the dental arches has led to the impression that the increase in space in the two dental arches is coordinated. However, that is not true.

The limited space within the jaws lingual to the roots of the primary incisors is used in an optimal way for the housing of their successors. The permanent maxillary lateral incisor is located more occlusally than the central incisor, so the mesial portion of the lateral incisor crown can fit in the concavity on the palatal side of the central incisor crown.

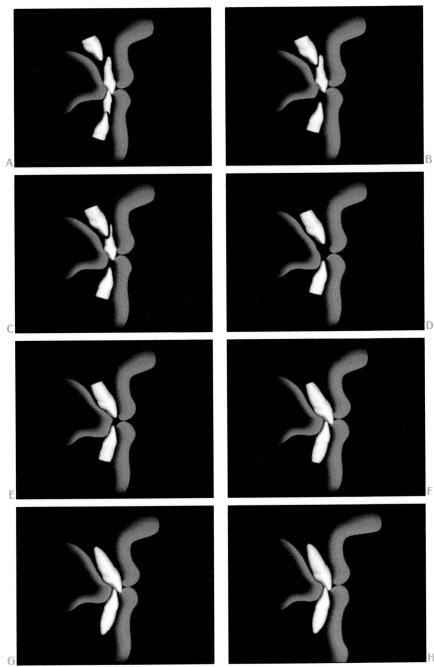

FIGURE 1-6

The upper lip covers the maxillary primary incisors, which are oriented about perpendicular to the occlusal plane, like the mandibular incisors. In both jaws, the crowns of the permanent incisors are apical and lingual to the roots of their predecessors. The lower lip covers not only the primary mandibular incisors but also the maxillary incisors slightly (A). The mandibular incisors are inclined somewhat labially (B). After emergence, their incisal edges will be located more labially than were the edges of their predecessors (C). This difference is greater in the maxilla, where the permanent incisors are inclined more labially before and after emergence than they are in the mandible. Their incisal edges also are positioned more labially than were their predecessors; this difference is more pronounced than in the mandible (D). After emergence, the maxillary incisors are affected by the pressure exerted by the tongue and lips (E). After contact between the opposing incisors has been established, the lower lip will support the maxillary incisors vertically (F). Root formation is completed after eruption is finished (G). With subsequent development of the face, the skeletal parts and the soft tissue structures enlarge, and the incisors will attain an upright position, more so in the maxilla than in the mandible (H).[227]

In a comparable way, the permanent mandibular central incisor is located more occlusally than the lateral incisor, and its smaller crown is situated close to the larger crown of the lateral incisor (Fig 1-5).

The space available for housing the not-yet-emerged permanent anterior teeth is relatively smaller in the maxilla than in the mandible. The crowns of the permanent maxillary anterior teeth are considerably larger than the crowns of the permanent mandibular anterior teeth. Before and after emergence, the maxillary incisors are more labially inclined than are the mandibular incisors (Fig 1-6). The anterior demarcation of the alveolar process at the level of the apices is located more posteriorly in the maxilla than in the mandible and more lingually in the canine region.

The root apices of the permanent lateral incisors, and subsequently those of the central incisors, cannot move distally before the roots of the permanent maxillary canines have descended to the level where their large crowns were located previously. With this change in angulation of the incisors from distal to mesial, the diastemata between them become smaller.

The transition of the maxillary anterior teeth is associated with typical features that deviate markedly from what is considered to be a harmonious arrangement of anterior teeth ("ugly duckling").[38]

FIGURE 1-7

This series of dental casts, from a girl with a Class II division 1 malocclusion, covers the period from 2 years 2 months to 7 years 6 months of age and shows the changes during the transition of the maxillary incisors. She had sucked her thumb until the emergence of the permanent maxillary central incisors and had an anterior open bite for many years. At the age of 4 years, the crown of the primary maxillary left incisor was fractured, and the tooth migrated distally and became discolored.

At the age of 2 years 2 months, large diastemata were present in the maxillary dental arch, and the tooth positioning on the left side was similar to the positioning on the right side (A, B). Three years later, little had changed on the right side. On the left side, where the trauma had occurred, both primary incisors had migrated, and the diastemata had closed (C, D). At the age of 6 years 1 month, the primary left central incisor was exfoliated; the right central incisor had moved distally and was in contact with the primary lateral incisor (E, F). Three months later, the situation had not changed (G, H). Two months after that, the permanent left central incisor had emerged. The primary right central incisor was shed in the process of impression making and saved to be incorporated in the plaster cast. The diastemata distal to the primary right lateral incisor and primary canine had decreased only slightly or not at all (I, J). One month later, these diastemata were closed, and the involved teeth had moved distally (K, L).

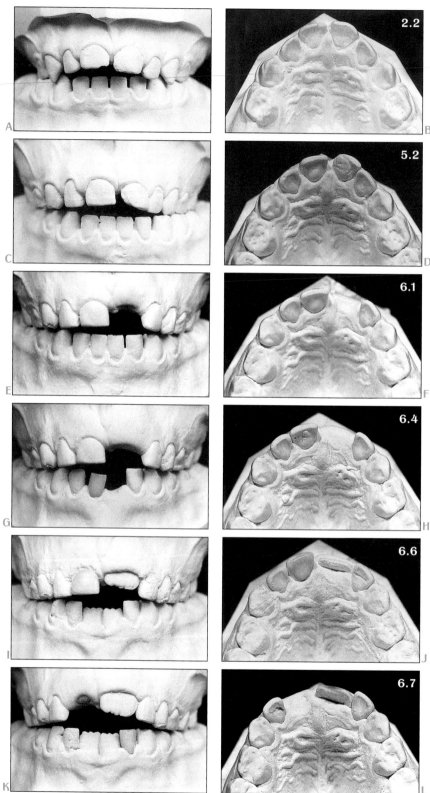

This phenomenon also occurs in the mandible, but less visibly and with a different presentation. Permanent mandibular central incisors can erupt parallel and close to each other. The permanent lateral incisors are situated lingually to the central incisors on emergence and often still have that orientation when they reach the level of the occlusal plane.

Subsequently, the crowns of the mandibular lateral incisors move labially and attain correct positions in the dental arch through pressure from the tongue when sufficient space is available. Their apices remain in a more lingual position than the apices of the permanent central incisors, as is the case in the maxilla.

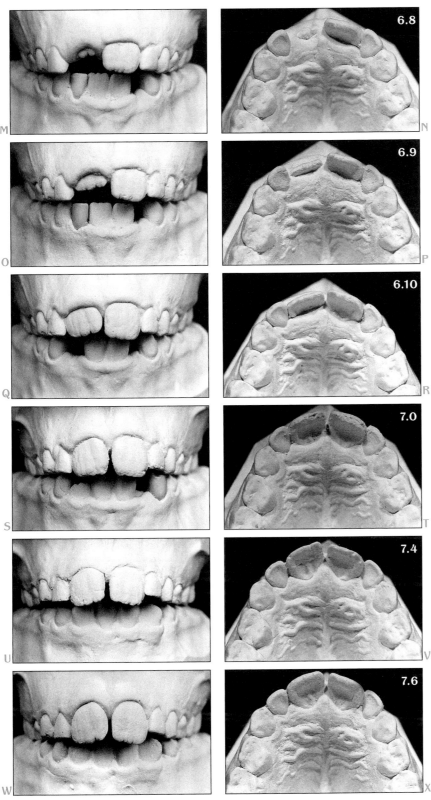

6.8

6.9

6.10

7.0

7.4

7.6

FIGURE 1-7 (CONTINUED)

One month later, the permanent right central incisor emerged with sufficient space, 2 months after its predecessor was shed (M, N). In the ensuing month, the permanent right central incisor erupted further and the space increased slightly because of the buccal movement of the primary canine (O, P). At the age of 6 years 9 months, the incisal edge of the permanent right central incisor, 3 months after its emergence, had reached almost the level of the incisal edge of the left central incisor (Q, R). In the 8 months following, few changes took place. The central diastema and the angulation of the incisors stayed more or less the same (S–X).

This series demonstrates that the gain in space needed for the larger permanent incisors, realized by the displacement of adjacent teeth, is a unilateral phenomenon related to the time of emergence of the largest of the two incisors on one side.

Almost all studies on the development of the dentition are based on annually collected records of dental casts, occasionally supported by radiographs.[13-15, 42, 50, 67, 92, 103, 119, 120, 143, 180] An exception in this field is the Nijmegen Growth Study, in which data were collected every 6 months and impressions were made every 3 months during the transitional periods.[211, 222] The information obtained from that study was an important resource for the descriptions and explanations presented in this chapter. Another source was the analysis of a large collection of human skulls encompassing all stages of development.[233]

The movement of the primary teeth associated with the eruption of the adjacent permanent incisors occurs in a much shorter period of time than had been assumed for many years. In the first half of the 1900s, the so-called development of physiologic diastemata was widely accepted.[107] The space available in the dental arches was assumed to increase gradually over a period of about 3 years.[13-15, 137, 138] This concept turned out to be incorrect. The needed increase in space occurs in a few months' time, is restricted locally, is associated with the eruption of the broadest incisor, and can occur asymmetrically (Fig 1-7).[212, 223]

FIGURE 1-8

This series of illustrations shows the development of a Class II division 1 malocclusion equivalent to the width of half a premolar crown. The sagittal relationship in the anterior region deviates in accordance with the disto-occlusion and results in an enlarged overjet. A deep bite in the primary dentition is rare. The eruption of the permanent central incisor has started in the mandible but not in the maxilla (A). After the mandibular central incisor has erupted, the process starts in the maxilla (B). In Class II division 1 malocclusions with normal dental arch conditions, the displacement of the primary teeth, associated with the eruption of the permanent maxillary central incisor and the permanent mandibular lateral incisor, takes place as it does in Class I situations (C). The second transitional period starts with the replacement of the mandibular canine (D). Subsequently, the primary maxillary first molar is replaced, at about the same time as the primary mandibular first molar (E). The first premolars end up in disto-occlusion (F). After the primary molars and canines are replaced, the excess space in the dental arches that becomes available during the second transitional period disappears, and a Class II intercuspation results (G). The outcome is a large overjet and overbite, a deep curve of Spee, and a relatively narrow maxillary dental arch (H).228

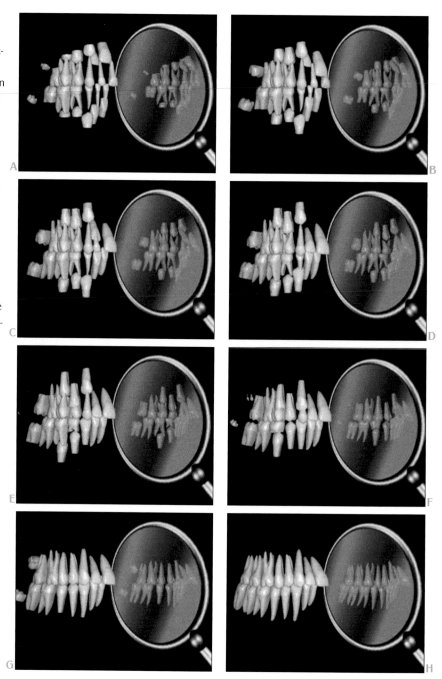

The changes previously described regarding the transition of the incisors in normal situations take place in a comparable way in Class II division 1 malocclusions as well as other malocclusions. However, the functional conditions after eruption vary with the kind of malocclusion and can affect the position of the permanent teeth unfavorably. Two types of condition can be distinguished in that respect: (1) those related to the occlusion and eruption and (2) those related to the position and behavior of the soft tissues. Examples of the first type in Class II division 1 malocclusions are the overeruption of mandibular incisors, the deepening of the curve of Spee, and the relatively too narrow maxillary dental arch (Fig 1-8). The same conditions occur in Class II division 2 malocclusions; in addition, the maxillary incisors and secondarily the mandibular incisors are tipped lingually by the pressure exerted by the lower lip on the maxillary incisors.

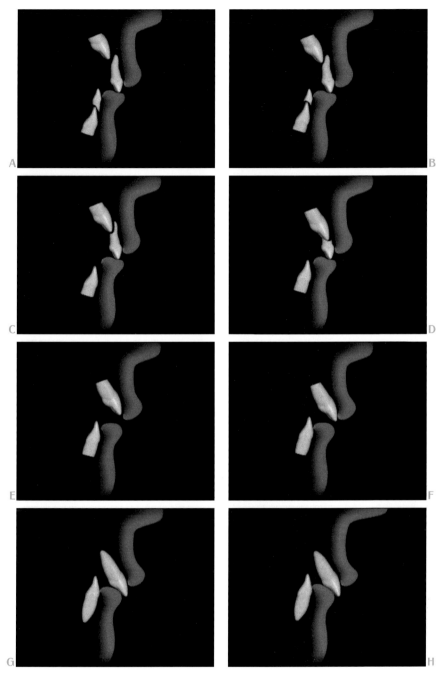

FIGURE 1-9

In the primary dentition of an individual with a severe Class II division 1 malocclusion, a large overjet exists; the lips are incompetent and not closed at rest (A). The transition proceeds normally otherwise (B). After the primary mandibular central incisor is lost, its successor will erupt more labially (C). That is also the case in the maxilla (D), where the position of the permanent central incisor is affected unfavorably by the lips. The lower lip can become positioned behind the maxillary incisor (E), with the result that the maxillary central incisor is not supported vertically by the lower lip or by the mandibular incisor. Consequently, the maxillary central and lateral incisors overerupt (F), as do the mandibular anterior teeth (G). Because of the positioning of the lower lip behind the maxillary incisor, this tooth will not upright with the maturation of the face. The mandibular incisor will be pushed lingually and become more upright than normal (H).

The tongue is not shown in these illustrations. If the tongue is positioned at rest within the dental arches, the mandibular incisors will continue to erupt until they reach the palate (not represented here). If the tongue rests on top of the mandibular incisors, vertical contact will not be reached, and a non-occlusion develops in the anterior region.[228]

The gradual lingual tipping of incisors in Class II division 2 malocclusions is caused by the second aspect of functional conditions, which includes the positioning of the lips. In Class II division 2 malocclusions, and Class I malocclusions with Class II division 2 characteristics (coverbites), the maxillary incisors are covered excessively by the lower lip, leading to the typical lingual inclinations. In Class II division 1 malocclusions, the lips have a different effect on the position of the incisors, particularly if the lower lip becomes "trapped" behind the maxillary incisors (Fig 1-9).

Figure 1-10 illustrates what can happen to a patient when treatment is started early and knowledge regarding the transition of incisors is inadequate.

FIGURE 1-10

A girl of 4 years 11 months had a Class II division 1 malocclusion with a large overjet. The dental arches were shaped well and showed few abnormalities. Diastemata were present in both anterior regions and distal of the primary maxillary canines (A–F). At 6 years 6 months of age, the permanent mandibular central incisors had emerged and attained a good position with adequate space (G). Few alterations had taken place in the maxilla during the previous 19 months (H). To improve the sagittal maxillomandibular relationship, a functional appliance—a type of open activator—was utilized. It contained a continuous labial arch with horizontal loops in contact with the maxillary primary incisors, canines, and first molars at the cervical level. A comparable labial arch was present at the incisal third of the crowns of the six mandibular anterior teeth (I, J). The appliance was worn during sleep and a few hours during the day. However, the processes involved in the transition of the incisors were not taken into account in the design and fabrication of the appliance, and a serious disturbance of the normal developmental course resulted. The labial arch had hindered the labially directed eruption of the permanent maxillary incisors. On emergence, the labial arch forced them in a palatal direction. Furthermore, the labial arch had interfered with the buccal displacement of the primary canines and the acrylic resin with their distal displacement. In addition, the labial bow had hindered the buccal movement of the primary maxillary molars. In the mandible, the labial bow had interfered with the labial movement of the permanent incisors and the buccal migration of the primary canines.

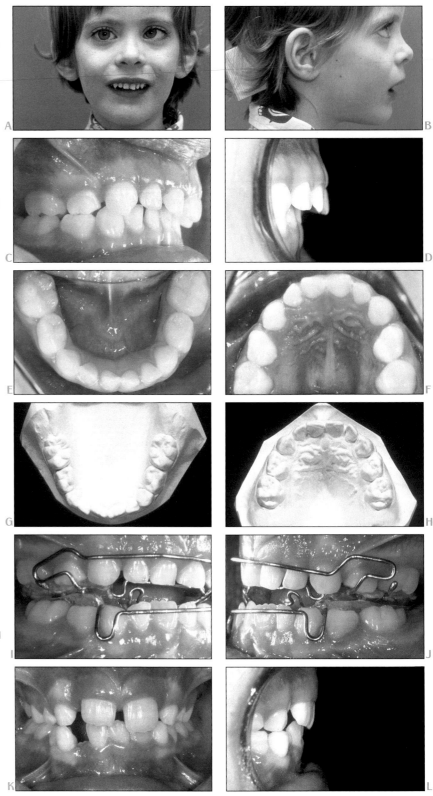

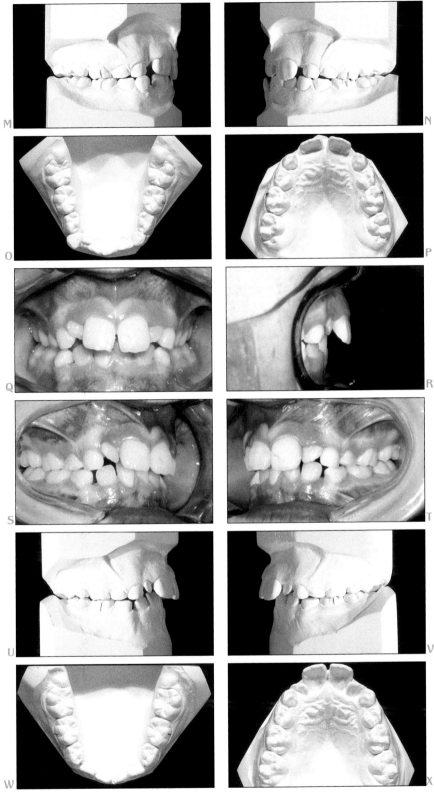

M · N · O · P · Q · R · S · T · U · V · W · X

FIGURE 1-10 (CONTINUED)

By the age of 7 years 7 months, the permanent maxillary central incisors had emerged and erupted in a direction almost perpendicular to the occlusal plane. The primary lateral incisors were lost prematurely. The space available for the eruption of their successors was inadequate. The permanent mandibular central incisors had tipped to the right side. The permanent right lateral incisor had emerged too far lingually, because of insufficient space. The midline in the mandibular dental arch deviated to the right side. The sagittal relationship between the dental arches had improved only slightly. The width of the maxillary dental arch was not adjusted to the improvement in sagittal relationship. The posterior teeth occluded in a transverse end-to-end position (K–P). The mandibular primary canines were extracted. The right canine was already very mobile, because its root had been resorbed to a large extent in association with the erupting permanent lateral incisor. No orthodontic appliance was placed. Nature was given a chance to correct the disturbed situation. More than 1 year later, at the age of 8 years 8 months, the mandibular incisors were aligned and tipped lingually, and little space remained for the permanent canines to erupt. However, the midline deviation was corrected. The permanent maxillary central incisors had proclined spontaneously. The permanent maxillary lateral incisors had erupted palatally. The dental arch relationship had changed to more of a disto-occlusion (Q–X).

FIGURE 1-11

At the age of 8 years 10 months, the primary maxillary canines were extracted so that the permanent lateral incisor could improve in position. Records were collected again at 9 years 8 months of age (A, B). Two months later, a removable plate with divided labial arches was placed in the maxilla to reduce the deep bite and control the space in the dental arch. A lip bumper was placed in the mandible in tubes attached to the primary second molars (C). After 1 year, sufficient space was gained in the mandible, and a lingual arch was placed to maintain the correction and prevent mesial migration of the permanent first molars (D). In the maxilla, bands with buccal tubes were cemented on the primary second molars, brackets were bonded on the anterior teeth, and a nickel-titanium archwire was inserted (E, F). At the age of 12 years 6 months, all four primary second molars were still present. Those in the mandible were sliced mesially, so that the first premolars could migrate distally (G). In the maxilla, bands with tubes were cemented on the permanent first molars, and a neutral (straight-pull) headgear and palatal bar were placed (H). In a later stage, the other permanent teeth were incorporated in the fixed appliances. At the age of 13 years 4 months, the treatment was almost completed (I, J).

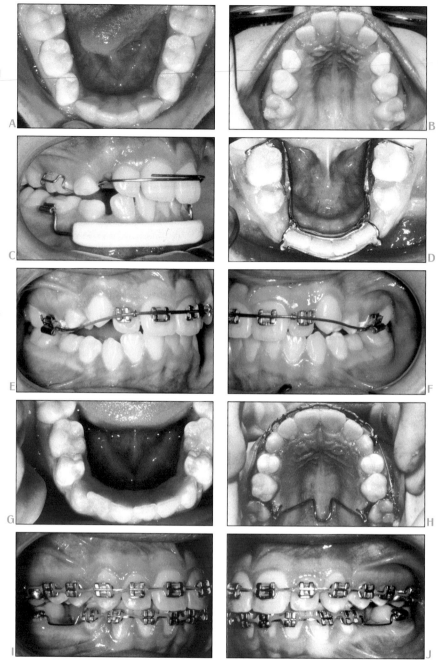

It took quite some time and effort to repair the damage caused by the early treatment. The overall treatment was more complicated and lasted longer than necessary. Nevertheless, a good and esthetically pleasant result was finally reached (Fig 1-11).

The course of treatment shown demonstrates that space lost in a dental arch can be regained and that an initially "missed" increase in arch length can still be obtained later. The restrictions that apply to the feasibility of achieving alignment of all permanent teeth in a balanced state are largely independent of the preceding development of the dentition. Indeed, the size and shape of the bony structures on which the alveolar processes are founded determine the range of variation in the length and form of the dental arches. In this context, the influence of the tissues should not be underestimated.

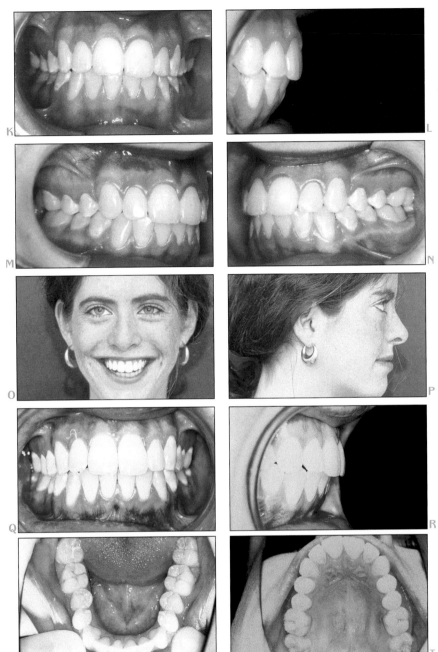

FIGURE 1-11 (CONTINUED)
However, the second premolars were rather late in erupting. Extraction of their predecessors had not resulted in an acceleration. Because of the late emergence of the mandibular second premolars, the active treatment could not be concluded until the age of 14 years 4 months, when an overall satisfactory result was obtained (K–N). The records collected at the age of 23 years 4 months showed a young woman with a beautiful face, a pleasant smile, and a good profile (O, P). The intraoral photographs demonstrated the proper alignment of teeth and the excellent occlusion (Q–T). Regrettably, the treatment of this patient took many years, mainly because of the negative sequelae of the early treatment. Most likely, the transition of the incisors would have proceeded without complication had the normal development of the dentition been allowed to proceed uninterrupted. The spontaneous corrections that occurred later neutralized some of the detrimental effects. Nevertheless, the role of the active treatment that was carried out to regain the lost space should not be underestimated. This case illustrates that thorough knowledge and understanding of the development of the dentition are essential to prevent the outcome from being, instead of the intended improvement, a deterioration of the conditions.

The length and form of the dental arches have a certain range of interindividual variation. That also applies to the morphology of the alveolar processes, the dimensions and configuration of which are determined by the teeth they contain. In some individuals the total width of the permanent teeth is relatively too large and exceeds the possibility of arriving at harmonious dental arches. Reduction of tooth material, either by extraction of teeth or by reduction in the width of crowns, is then a necessity.[184] Limitations in spatial conditions usually involve both jaws but sometimes only one, mostly the mandible.

FIGURE 1-12
In Class II division 1 malocclusions, the disto-occlusion is the primary factor, and the increased overjet, increased overbite, and deep curve of Spee are secondary effects (A). The same applies to the narrow maxillary dental arch, because its width depends on the occlusion with the mandibular dental arch (B).

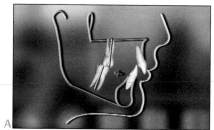 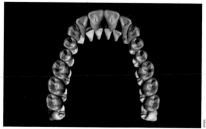

The primary factor in Class II division 1 malocclusions is the posterior positioning of the mandibular dental arch in relation to the maxillary arch. The other aspects, characteristic for Class II division 1 malocclusions, are secondary (Fig 1-12).

Facial orthopedics can influence the amount and direction of growth to some extent and have a favorable effect on the development of the dentition. Whether the resulting improvement in the maxillomandibular relationships is permanent or temporary depends on several factors, to be discussed in chapter 8.

The development of the dentition is characterized by great variation and not only in the relationship between jaw size and tooth size. Marked differences also exist in the size of corresponding primary and permanent teeth. Sometimes, small primary teeth are replaced by large permanent teeth. However, the reverse also occurs.[140] Large differences in that respect have more consequences for the anterior than the posterior teeth, because primary molars are broader than their successors. Normally, no extra space has to be gained for premolars. Problems in that region are the result of migration caused by crowding in the anterior region, so that the permanent canines tend to occupy the space intended for the premolars, or the result of crowding caused by mesial migration of the permanent first molars after premature loss of primary molars.

Use of Interceptive Orthodontic Procedures

The possibilities of preventing orthodontic anomalies are limited, because malocclusions are determined mainly genetically, and environmental factors play only a secondary role. Therefore, digit sucking has no permanent effect on the position of the teeth and morphology of the skeleton when the habit is stopped prior to the transition of the incisors.[162] That also is probably the case when the habit is stopped at a later stage. Nevertheless, it makes sense to intercept the habit before the permanent incisors emerge, particularly in Class II division 1 malocclusions. Specifically, the entrapment of the lower lip behind the maxillary incisors should be prevented to avoid an overeruption of the maxillary incisors that could result from lack of vertical support by the lower lip.

Normal functional conditions contribute to a favorable development of the dentition, which is one of the reasons to aim for a competent lip seal in individuals with an open mouth and to change mouth breathers into nose breathers. The term interceptive procedures in this context is meant to denote the guidance of the development of the dentition through intervention, without the use of appliances, with the aim of preventing, reducing, or correcting abnormal tooth positioning. Simple measures, such as the extraction of persisting primary teeth, which obstruct the eruption of their successors or their improvement in position after emergence, are not discussed in this chapter.

Four procedures are described and illustrated. The first technique involves reducing the crown size of primary teeth by grinding their mesial surfaces (slicing) to create more space for eruption and alignment of permanent teeth (Figs 2-1 to 2-4). The second procedure involves the simultaneous extraction approach: the removal in one session of primary first molars and their successors.[217] The advantages of this procedure are demonstrated on two patients (Figs 2-5 to 2-10). The third procedure is the serial extraction method, in which sequentially the primary canines, the primary first molars, and finally the first premolars are extracted, after they have emerged and further erupted (Fig 2-11). The fourth procedure encompasses measures for blocking migration of permanent teeth after premature loss of primary molars, again without the use of appliances (Fig 2-12).

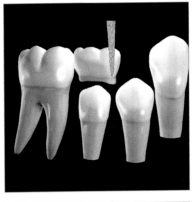

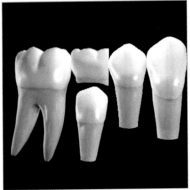

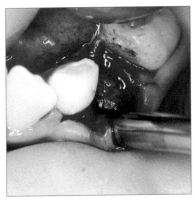

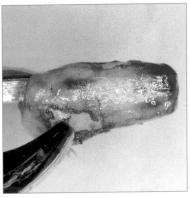

Orthodontic Concepts and Strategies

2

FIGURE 2-1

By appropriate grinding, at the right moment, of the mesial surfaces of the primary canines and molars, the difference in mesiodistal crown dimensions between primary molars and premolars can be utilized to improve the position of the anterior teeth and to prevent or reduce crowding. This procedure is known as slicing, a term dating from the time that thin, tapered diamond burs were not available yet and a disk was used to remove a slice. The advantage of long, thin diamond burs is that damage to the interdental papilla can be avoided. In addition, the mesial surface can be given a concave shape, according to the form of the tooth that has to move in that direction.

This series of illustrations presents the slicing procedure in the mandible. The mesial surface of the primary canine is removed with a thin, long, tapered diamond bur (A). The overlapping incisors receive the space to improve their position (B), because the lateral incisor can move distally (C). To provide more space for the permanent canine, the mesial side of the crown of the primary first molar is removed (D), resulting in sufficient space for the permanent canine (E), which can emerge in the correct position (F). At a later stage, the primary second molar is sliced (G). Especially when primary second molars are wide, which is often the case, significant space can be gained (H). The first premolar can erupt unimpeded (I). With the replacement of the reduced primary second molar by the second premolar, the permanent first molar will not migrate mesially or will migrate only slightly (J).

(Figs 2-1, 2-6, 2-7, and 2-11 to 2-13 are reprinted from Dynamics of Orthodontics.[226])

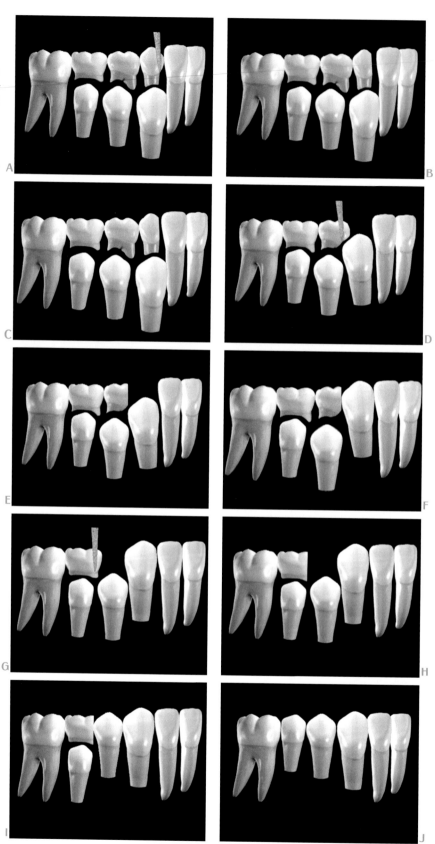

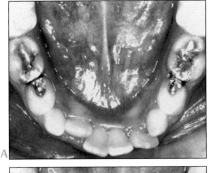

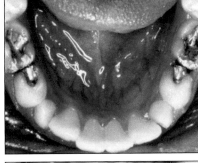

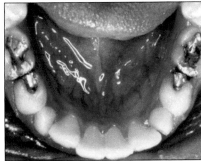

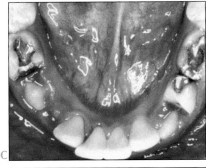

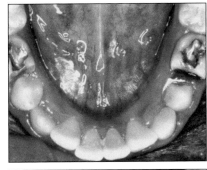

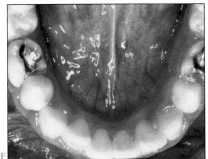

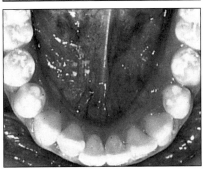

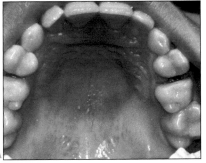

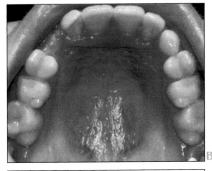

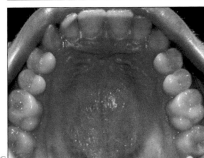

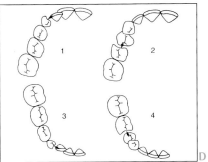

FIGURE 2-2

These illustrations demonstrate the beneficial effect of slicing the primary teeth in a patient with crowding in the mandible. Insufficient space was available in the dental arch for correct positioning of the lateral incisors (A); this was treated by slicing the mesial surfaces of the primary canines (B). On the right side, the primary second molar was sliced for the benefit of the erupting first premolar, which emerged before the canine. On the left side, the canine erupted first with sufficient space, because of the slicing of the primary first molar (C). On the right side, the erupting canine had moved the first premolar distally into the concavity of the primary second molar (D). On the left side, extra space was created by slicing the primary second molar (D), and the first premolar migrated distally (E). After the transition was completed, an ideal arrangement existed on the left side. On the right side, the lateral incisor was still positioned too far lingually (F). (Courtesy of Dr Marco Rosa, Trento, Italy.[171])

FIGURE 2-3

The leeway space is smaller in the maxilla than in the mandible. However, slicing in the maxilla can be effective as well. On both sides, the primary second molars were sliced with a diamond disk (A). The first premolars moved distally (B), and more space became available for the canines (C).

Concave grinding of canines results in a shape corresponding to the distal side of the lateral incisor, which allows maximal improvement (D1, D3). That also applies to primary molars, with the additional advantage that the pulp horns are not as easily exposed as when a disk is used (D2, D4).

FIGURE 2-4

Slicing of primary teeth becomes safer, simpler, and more effective when a piece of an interproximal strip is placed around the adjacent permanent tooth. That holds true especially for a permanent lateral incisor in contact with a primary canine. A thin, narrow strip with diamond grit only on one side is most suited for that purpose (A). A small piece of such a strip is inserted with a ligature-tying pliers on the lingual side and with the fingers on the buccal side (B). Subsequently, the strip is pressed and held. The strip prevents the lateral incisor from becoming damaged, and the side with the diamond grit counteracts slippage of the strip. In addition, the smooth surface offers guidance to the bur, resulting in the intended concave shape (C). The bur is introduced from the lingual side (D). Under abundant water cooling, the rotating bur is moved buccally, deep enough to avoid creation of a mesial step at the cervical level (E). If the bur is kept at the appropriate height, and the tooth is sliced more deeply in the middle, such a step and damage to the gingiva can be avoided (F). Subsequently, the sharp labial edge is rounded (G). The same is done occlusally and lingually (H). The procedure takes only a few minutes, is almost painless, and delivers good results. (Note: Situations in which water spray was used (E–H) did not photograph clearly.)

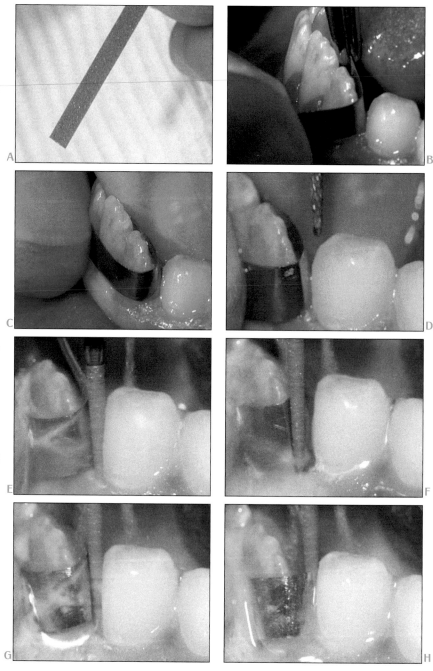

Indeed, with orthodontic appliances, the leeway space can be maintained by preventing the permanent first molars from migrating mesially to allow for the alignment of anterior teeth. A passive lingual arch, attached to bands on the permanent first molars and in contact with the lingual surfaces of the mandibular incisors, can serve that purpose. A disadvantage of this method is that the incisors cannot improve in position prior to the loss of the primary canines. Furthermore, the erupting permanent canines will hinder the spontaneous correction of incisors. It is questionable if this method is more effective than slicing, even without considering the involved inconveniences, risks of decalcifications and caries, and treatment time and costs. When a lingual arch is used, primary teeth are not sliced or extracted, and the transition proceeds without controlled guidance.

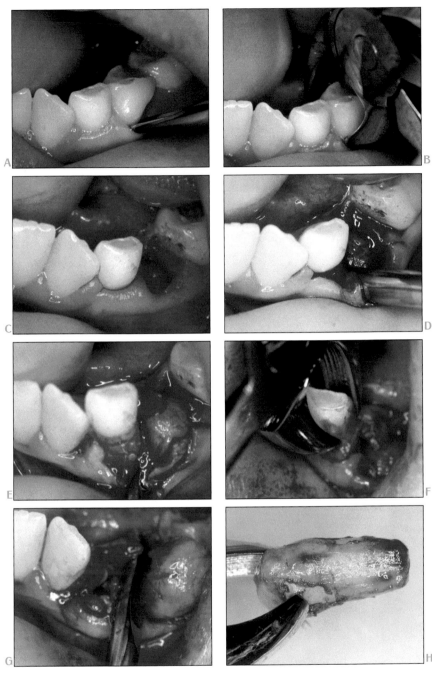

Figure 2-5

The simultaneous removal of a primary first molar and the underlying premolar starts with the loosening of the gingiva around the primary molar (A). In this patient, not only the primary first molar, but also the primary canine, was mobile. Initially, the primary canine was to be spared. Therefore, only the primary first molar was extracted (B). The follicle that surrounded the first premolar became visible (C). Prior to emergence, no direct connection exists between a tooth and the alveolar bone. The periodontal ligament develops after emergence; before that time, the follicle surrounds the tooth completely. Removal of a submerged tooth, therefore, is rather simple. If a straight, broad elevator is placed between the bone and the follicle, the first premolar can be removed through the opening that results from the extraction of the primary molar, without damaging the alveolar process (D). In this patient, the mobile primary canine interfered with the treatment (E) and was removed (F). Subsequently, the premolar could be approached from the mesial side and elevated (G). The follicle still covered the tooth to a large extent (H). Finally, a pair of anatomic tweezers should be used to determine if remnants of the follicle remain in the socket; such remnants must be removed. If pieces of the follicle are left behind, a cyst can develop. Suturing of the gingiva completes the treatment.

On the other hand, slicing has as its goals improvement in the positioning of the permanent incisors at an early stage and creation of extra space for the emerging permanent canines and premolars to allow them to erupt in a more proper position. The aim is to prevent these teeth from rotating on emergence or from moving lingually or buccally. Furthermore, slicing does not interfere with the pressures exerted on the dental arch by the tongue, lips, and cheeks. These pressures add to the spontaneous improvement of malalignments, particularly for the incisors. However, rotations are less likely to be corrected than are labiolingual displacements.

The extraction of primary first molars and first premolars in one session—the simultaneous extraction procedure—has specific advantages.[233] However, the buccal plate of the alveolar process should not be removed, as has been suggested in the past.[95, 200] Indeed, this procedure can be performed without damaging the alveolar process (Figs 2-5 and 2-6).

FIGURE 2-6

This series presents an overview of the removal of the primary first molars and the first premolars in one session and the associated favorable sequelae. The main indication for this procedure is extreme crowding, in which it is clear that permanent teeth have to be sacrificed (A). After the primary first molar has become mobile, and it has been confirmed radiographically that the first premolar is in close proximity to its predecessor and no teeth are missing, the two teeth can be removed (B). Prior to emergence, the permanent canine can move distally toward the space created by the enucleation (C). The same criteria and conditions apply to the maxilla (D). There also, extra space becomes available for displacement within the arch (E). In both arches, the permanent canines move distally prior to emergence (F). If the mandibular primary canine has not yet been shed, it should be extracted (G, H). The same applies to the maxilla (I, J). In situations with crowding in the anterior region, the primary canines should be extracted at an earlier stage, so that the permanent incisors can attain a better position soon after emergence. With severe crowding, the roots of the primary canines are resorbed prematurely, and these teeth are shed early when the permanent lateral incisors erupt. In a maxilla with severe crowding, the primary lateral incisors are lost prematurely on emergence of the permanent central incisors. With severe crowding, permanent lateral incisors often tend to emerge on the palatal side. This can be avoided by early extraction of the primary canines.

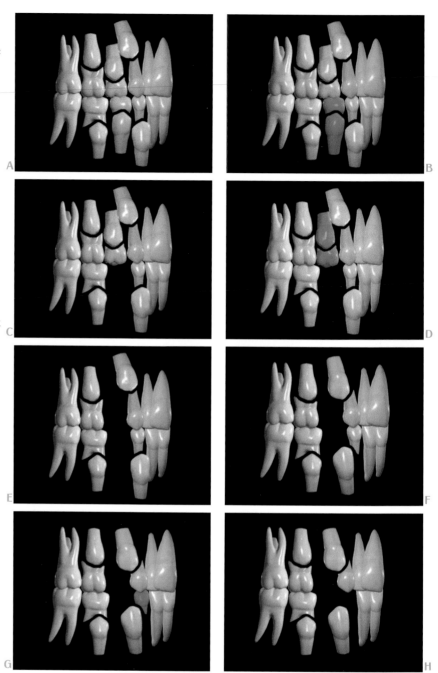

Simultaneous extraction can simplify the treatment of Class II division 1 malocclusions with extensive crowding (Figs 2-7 and 2-8). In Class II division 1 malocclusions with little or no crowding in the mandibular dental arch, the procedure can be performed in the maxilla only; a disto-occlusion of the molars and two sacrificed maxillary first premolars are the end result. The procedure is also suitable for Class II division 1 malocclusions with excessive crowding in both dental arches. However, undesirable migrations must be prevented and active therapy started in due time to correct the disto-occlusion and large overjet. That holds particularly true when the indication for extraction is based not on crowding but on bimaxillary protrusion (Figs 2-9 and 2-10).

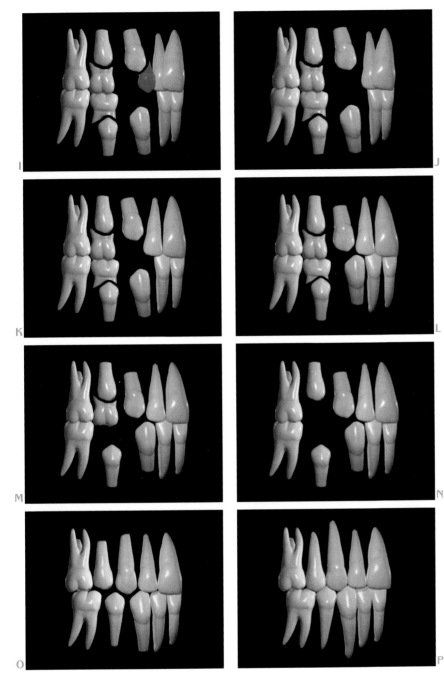

FIGURE 2-6 (CONTINUED)

Also in the maxilla, extraction of primary canines often is not needed, because they are lost prematurely. With further eruption of the permanent canines, space becomes available for the distal movement of the apices of the permanent lateral incisors (K). With simultaneous extraction, the permanent canine can move to the spaces where the crowns of the first premolars were located previously.[174] This leads to a favorable orientation for eruption. Particularly in the maxilla, simultaneous extraction can lead to results that require little or no additional mechanotherapy to improve tooth positioning. In normal situations, but certainly in crowded conditions, the crowns of the unerupted premolars and permanent canines are close together in the maxilla. That is not or is less the case in the mandible. In the maxilla, the crowns of the permanent canines often are positioned cranial to the first premolars and only slightly mesial to them. With simultaneous extraction, the permanent canine migrates to the large space that becomes available. Even when the permanent canines are located too far mesially and overlap the roots of the permanent lateral incisors, they will move distally over a large distance prior to emergence. The favorable displacement of the canines provides space for the uprighting of the lateral incisors (L). After some time, the primary second molars will be shed (M, N). After emergence of the second premolars, a good intercuspation develops (O). The mandibular canine is not angulated properly (P).

Simultaneous extraction should not be carried out when some doubt exists regarding the necessity of sacrificing permanent teeth. In such cases it is better to begin with the serial extraction method, extracting only the primary first molars and postponing the decision whether or not to extract the first premolars until these teeth have erupted (Fig 2-11). However, the advantage of simultaneous extraction is then lost. When the extraction of the first premolars is postponed until they have emerged, the space where the crowns were located prior to emergence is filled in by newly formed bone. With the extraction of a fully erupted premolar, only the space occupied by the narrow roots becomes available.

FIGURE 2-7

In a girl aged 10 years 6 months, who had a Class I malocclusion and severe crowding in the mandible and maxilla (arch length discrepancy –10 and –9 mm, respectively), the maxillary primary canines were lost prematurely. The permanent maxillary canines were located too far mesially, positioned labial to the lateral incisors. The four maxillary incisors were aligned. In the mandible, the lateral incisors were situated too far lingually, particularly the left lateral incisor, which also was rotated (A–D). The simultaneous extraction procedure was carried out. At the age of 10 years 8 months, the mandibular primary canines and all four primary molars and first premolars were removed. After that, the permanent canines moved distally within the jaws, and the mandibular incisors attained better positions. Eleven months after the extractions, all four canines had emerged and erupted distal to the lateral incisors. The maxillary dental arch was shaped well, and the position of the mandibular teeth had improved considerably. Only the left lateral incisor was still somewhat rotated and lingually located. The overbite had increased (E–H). One year later, at 12 years 7 months of age, the second premolars had emerged and almost had reached occlusion on the left side. The maxillary right premolar was still not fully erupted (I, J). Three months later, the right second premolars were near to reaching occlusion. A good intercuspation existed on the left side, and the diastemata were closed. On the right side, the canines occluded well, but the second premolars and first molars were in a disto-occlusion of one-quarter premolar crown width. Prior to the intervention, the occlusion was the same on both sides, and the dental midlines were coincident. The latter did not change after the extractions.

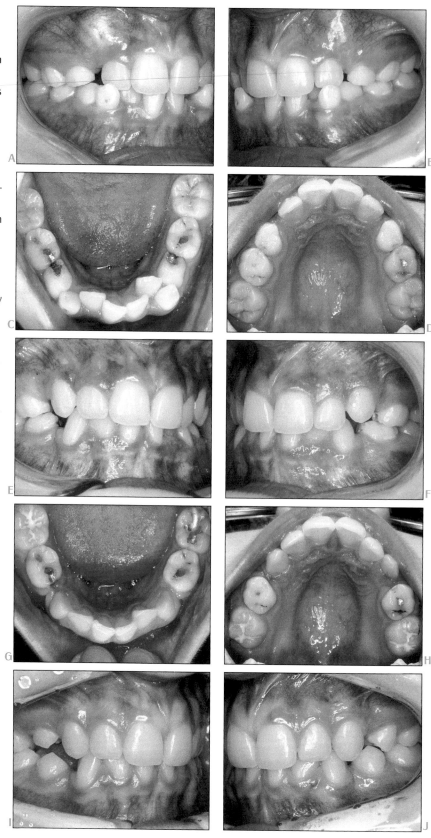

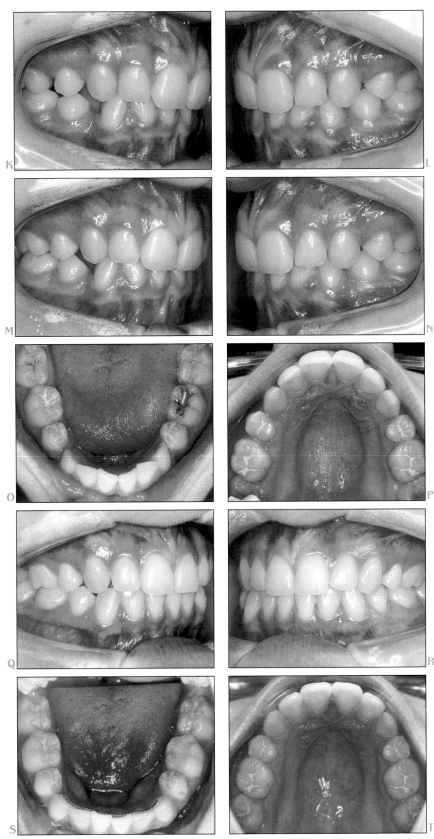

FIGURE 2-7 (CONTINUED)
The neutro-occlusion on the left side was maintained, but on the right side the mandibular first molar had not migrated as far mesially as the maxillary first molar, with the result that the neutro-occlusion changed into a disto-occlusion of one-quarter premolar crown width (K, L). Subsequently, the mandibular right posterior teeth moved slightly mesially, but the diastema distal of the canine was not closed, and some disto-occlusion remained. This less favorable course developed in the mandibular right posterior region because overeruption of the primary maxillary second molar blocked the mesial migration of the permanent mandibular first molar. Had this tooth been sliced to remove the hindrance, a more favorable situation could have developed on the right side. At the age of 13 years 8 months, 3 years after the extractions, a bite plate was placed in the maxilla as the first orthodontic appliance (M–P). This appliance reduced the overbite, leveled the curve of Spee, and facilitated the correction of the tooth positions in the mandible with the edgewise appliance. After 6 months, when the mandibular teeth were positioned well, fixed orthodontic appliances were placed on the maxillary teeth, and the bite plate was discarded. Four months later, at the age of 14 years 8 months, after 12 months of active treatment, all appliances were removed. A retention plate was placed in the maxilla, and a lingually bonded dead-soft braided wire was placed in the mandibular anterior region. Two years later, 1 year after the end of retention in the maxilla, the result was quite satisfactory (Q–T).

FIGURE 2-8

This series shows sections of lateral cephalograms and corresponding panoramic radiographs of the girl in Fig 2-7 at various ages. On the radiographs prior to treatment, taken at the age of 10 years 6 months, it was evident that the maxillary canines were located not cranial but mesial to the first premolars. A comparable situation existed in the mandible (A, B). The radiographs taken 6 months after the extractions indicated that in both jaws the canines had moved distally with no or only slight alterations in angulation (C, D). At the age of 11 years 7 months, the canines had emerged with a slightly distal angulation in the mandible and a good angulation in the maxilla. The primary second molars were still present (E, F). One year later, at the age of 12 years 7 months, the second premolars had emerged. The angulation of the mandibular canines had improved slightly on the left side, but not on the right side, where a diastema still existed (G, H). The radiographs taken at the age of 13 years 7 months, shortly before the start of active treatment, showed that the simultaneous extraction procedure had achieved satisfactory results in the maxilla without additional treatment. Prior to emergence, the canines had moved distally over a great distance without much alteration in angulation. That change did not occur to the same extent in the mandible. The angulation of the mandibular canines was not optimal (I, J). Additional correction with fixed appliances was required to reduce the overbite, level the curve of Spee, and arrive at an acceptable occlusion on the right side.

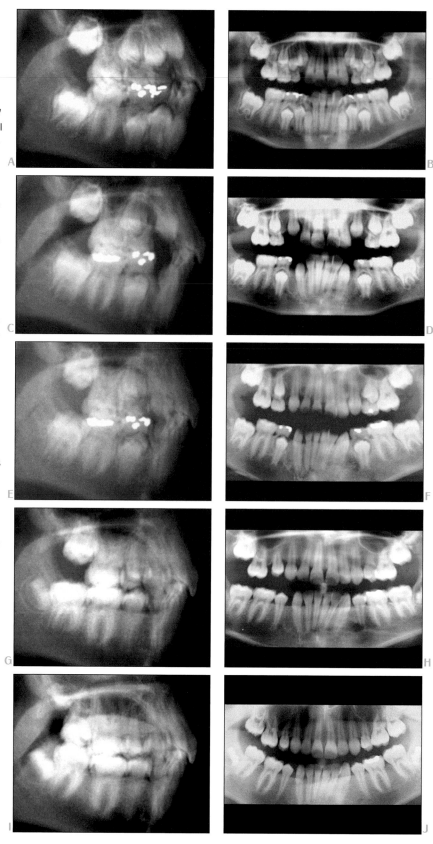

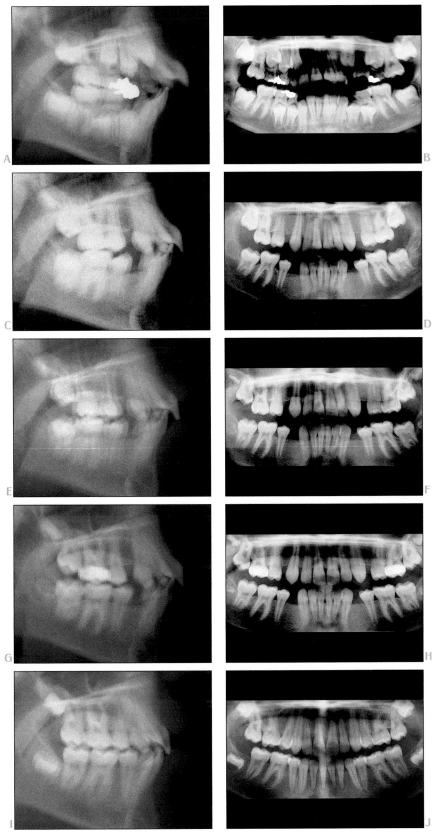

FIGURE 2-9

These are radiographs of a girl with a Class II division 1 malocclusion, presented on the two following pages (Fig 2-10). In her case, the indication to extract four first premolars was based not on crowding but on bimaxillary dentoalveolar protrusion. On the radiographs taken at 9 years 7 months, the severe labioversion of the mandibular and maxillary incisors was obvious. The permanent maxillary canines were located close to the first premolars and overlapped them vertically. They were not located over the lateral incisors, as in the patient in Figs 2-7 and 2-8, but over the primary canines. The primary first molars were still quite firm. Their roots had not resorbed enough yet to extract them. In addition, the premolars had to erupt further (A, B). For a successful simultaneous extraction procedure, the first premolar follicle should be visible on removal of the primary first molar and close enough to the occlusal plane for easy elevation. At the age of 10 years 3 months, the involved mandibular teeth were removed; the procedure was repeated 1 month later in the maxilla. The radiographs taken at 11 years 6 months showed that the maxillary incisors had been retroclined and the disto-occlusion had been corrected. These improvements were realized with a combined headgear-activator (Van Beek appliance). The canines in both arches had moved distally (C, D). The radiographs taken at 11 years 9 months of age (E, F) and 12 years 3 months of age (G, H) showed the further development. Fixed appliances were needed to obtain a satisfactory final result (I, J).

FIGURE 2-10

This girl of 9 years 7 months had a Class II division 1 malocclusion with a 14-mm overjet. She was an intensive thumb sucker, and no deep bite existed. The maxillary incisors had not overerupted but were positioned labially and proclined. Although adequate space was available in the maxilla (arch length discrepancy +2 mm) and only slight crowding existed in the mandible (–4 mm), the marked bimaxillary dentoalveolar protrusion necessitated the extraction of one tooth in each quadrant (A–F). It was decided to apply the simultaneous extraction procedure and to start active treatment immediately, because the correction of the disto-occlusion could be realized in the meantime. In addition, it was essential to prevent the mesial migration of the permanent first molars, because the space created by the extractions had to be used maximally for the retraction of the anterior teeth. Therefore, 3 months after the extractions were carried out, at the age of 10 years 7 months, a Van Beek combined headgear-activator was placed (G, H; SEE ALSO CHAPTER 7). After 14 months, the disto-occlusion was corrected, the maxillary incisors were partly retracted and uprighted, and occlusal contact had been realized in the anterior region. The diastemata distal to the canines were only slightly reduced, because the activator was trimmed and shaped in such a way that the posterior teeth were blocked in their mesial migration. In view of the goal to retrude the anterior teeth rather far, anchorage should be lost only minimally (I–L).

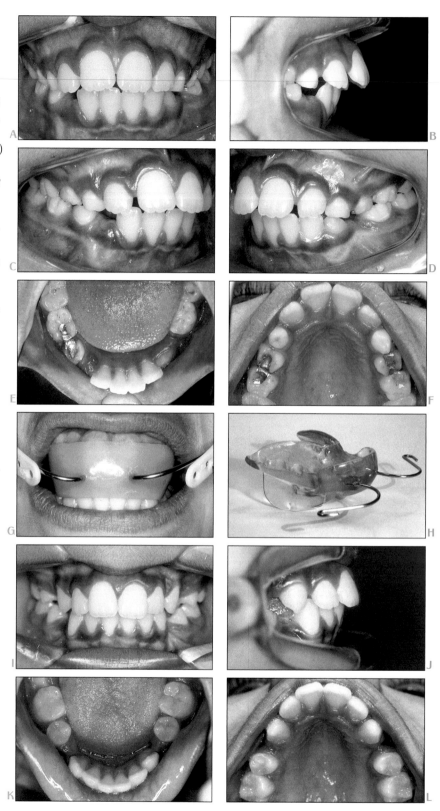

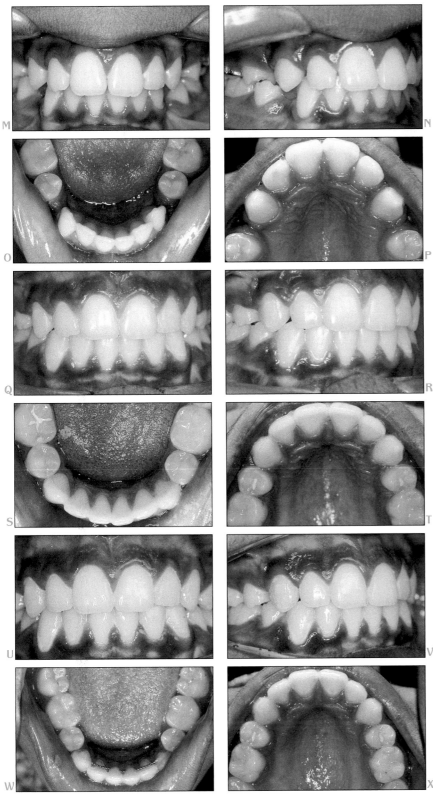

FIGURE 2-10 (CONTINUED)

Prior to the placement of fixed appliances at the age of 10 years 10 months, the permanent maxillary first molars were banded, and a cervical headgear was placed to prevent further mesial migration of the molars. Four months later, the position of the mandibular anterior teeth had improved, and the maxillary canines had moved distally (M–P). An edgewise appliance was placed at the age of 12 years 4 months in the mandible and 2 months later in the maxilla. At 14 years 5 months, all appliances were removed, and an esthetic result was obtained (Q–T). A retention plate was used in the maxilla; it was worn full time for the first 6 months and only during sleeping hours for the following 6 months. In the mandible, a dead-soft braided wire was bonded lingual to the anterior teeth. Two years later, little had changed (U–X).

The Van Beek combined headgear-activator has the advantage that the acrylic resin in the posterior regions can control the mesial migration of the posterior teeth while the maxillary anterior teeth are being retracted. The parietal headgear traction retains the appliance against the maxillary dental arch, where the effect is optimal. The disto-occlusion was corrected with this appliance, and the maxillary second premolars arrived at a neutro-occlusion on emergence. In addition, the maxillary anterior teeth were retracted considerably, while sufficient space remained to retract these teeth further and reach the desired result.

FIGURE 2-11

Serial extraction is, like simultaneous extraction, an interceptive procedure for dental arches with severe crowding. When the primary canines are not lost prematurely in these situations, the permanent incisors become malpositioned, overlap each other, and often are rotated (A). Serial extraction starts with the removal of the primary mandibular canines (B) and the maxillary canines (C), which provides space for the improvement in the positioning of the incisors (D). The crowns of the lateral incisors migrate distally (E). At a later stage, the primary first molars are extracted, as a rule first in the mandible (F) and later in the maxilla (G). When the primary first molars are extracted at the moment their roots have been resorbed to a large extent, the first premolars will erupt faster and emerge earlier. When the primary first molars are extracted too early, bone can be formed occlusal to the first premolars, resulting in a slowing of their eruption. Accelerated eruption of the first premolars is essential in serial extraction, because they should emerge prior to the canines. In the mandible, as a rule the canines emerge before the first premolars. Early extraction of the primary canine, as performed in serial extraction, results in reduction of available space in the dental arch and delayed emergence of the permanent canines, as is intended here (H).

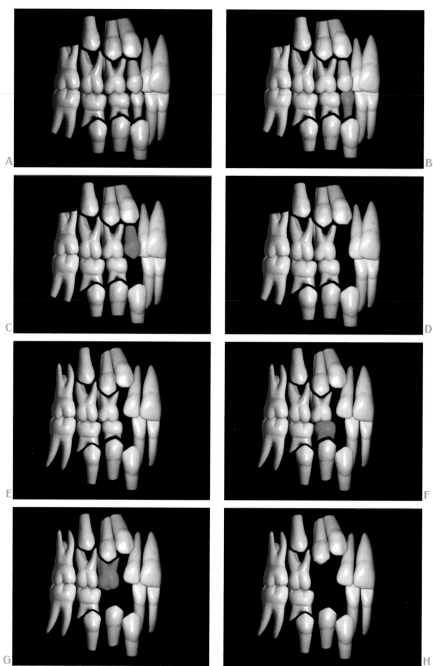

The serial extraction procedure is started with the extraction of the primary canines to allow alignment of the incisors. Prior to the eruption of the permanent canines, the primary first molars are removed, but not too early to prevent the formation of bone on top of the premolar crowns, which delays their eruption. As indicated already, the first premolars are extracted after emergence (Fig 2-11).[53, 90, 101, 240] Indeed, as explained before, the decision to extract the premolars can still be reconsidered. Sometimes more space becomes available within the dental arches than was estimated initially. If, in the meantime, an incisor is exfoliated by an accident, mesial movement of the posterior teeth to close the resulting diastema is still an option.

A disadvantage of both serial extraction and simultaneous extraction is the associated palatal tipping of the maxillary incisors and increase in overbite. As a rule, fixed appliance treatment is indicated to correct these shortcomings.

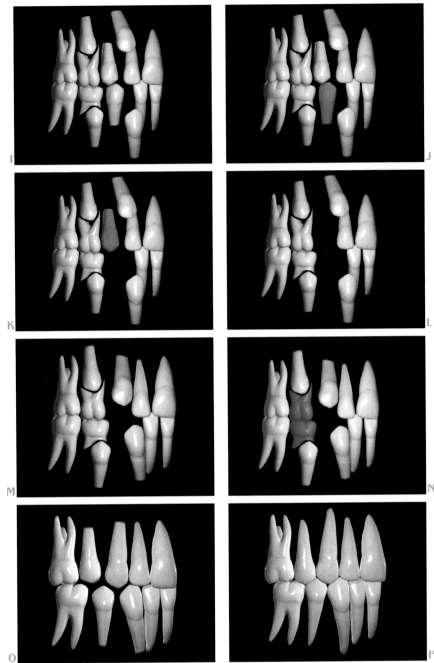

FIGURE 2-11 (CONTINUED)

The first premolars have to be extracted soon after their emergence (I), in most cases, first in the mandible (J) and then in the maxilla (K). After removal of the first premolars, space becomes available for the canines to move distally. In that respect, the conditions are less favorable than in simultaneous extraction, because the space that becomes available in the jaw is smaller. The socket reflects the size and form of the narrow and tapering roots. With simultaneous extraction, the space is much larger, because it reflects the large crown and the partly formed roots (L). The permanent canines move occlusally and distally. As long as the crowns have not emerged, the roots of the lateral incisors cannot move distally (M). During further eruption, the canines tip distally (N). After the primary second molars are lost and their successors have emerged, occlusion in the posterior region becomes established (O). Under favorable circumstances, a good intercuspation develops when a neutro-occlusion existed initially. However, the canines are tipped distally, more so in the mandible than in the maxilla. Furthermore, the mandibular second premolars are tipped mesially in most cases (P). Fixed appliances are needed to obtain an ideal result. However, the treatment time can be short because of the benefits of serial extraction.

The idea that premature loss of primary molars always leads to problems is a persistent misconception.[35, 36, 49, 87, 114, 122] Problems seldom arise in dental arches with sufficient space, because permanent molars can migrate mesially without negative sequelae, especially when the primary second molars have a large mesiodistal crown dimension. In situations without an excess of space, the story is different, because crowding may increase or develop. However, that often concerns situations for which orthodontic therapy is indicated anyway.

Whether and how far permanent molars will migrate mesially depends mainly on the occlusion. In a neutro-occlusion, with broad primary mandibular second molars that are lost prematurely, the opposing teeth can overerupt and block the mesial migration of the permanent mandibular first molars (Fig 2-12, A and B). However, loss of the primary maxillary second molar allows undesirable migration in most instances (Fig 2-12 C and D).[212]

FIGURE 2-12

When a primary mandibular second molar is lost prematurely in a neutro-occlusion, the opposing primary maxillary second molar can overerupt and block the mesial migration of the permanent mandibular first molar (A, B). That does not occur when a primary maxillary second molar is lost prematurely (C, D). However, a mandibular primary second molar can overerupt after a piece of its mesial occlusal side is ground away and act subsequently as a block for mesial migration of the permanent maxillary first molar (E). A comparable result is obtained when a block of resin composite is bonded on the occlusal surface of the primary mandibular second molar (F). In deviating sagittal occlusions, the grinding away of tooth material or building of a resin composite block has to be done at different places, but the principle stays the same. Of course, these procedures will not work in patients with a posterior open bite or nonocclusion. Primary teeth will erupt, as permanent teeth do, until occlusal contacts or other factors impede their eruption. Strategic use of this mechanism offers the possibility of preventing undesirable migration and eliminating the need for space-maintaining appliances.

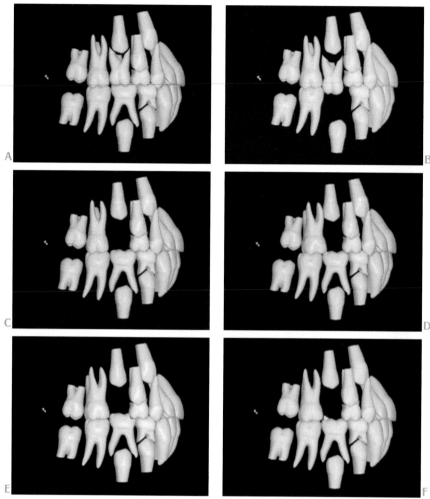

When the occlusion does not allow the overeruption of a primary molar, grinding away the interfering part of that tooth is an adequate solution (Fig 2-12, C and E). Building up the occlusal surface with a resin composite block also can prevent undesirable migration (Fig 2-12, F). These simple interceptive procedures eliminate the need for placement of space maintainers, which are often placed unnecessarily, because in the long run no negative sequelae of the premature loss remain.

The effective execution of interceptive procedures without the use of orthodontic appliances requires conscientious observation of and insight into the normal and abnormal development of the dentition. If this development is guided after the transition of the incisors is completed, much can be gained in situations with limited or even excessive crowding. That also applies to the premature loss of primary molars.

Use of Removable Appliances

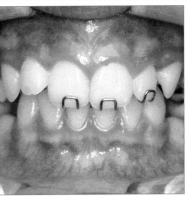

Removable appliances, made initially of rubber and later of acrylic resin, with metal parts for tooth movement and clasps for anchorage, have been developed and refined mainly in Europe.[31-33, 44, 147, 148]

It is assumed that the reader is familiar with the principles of removable appliances, so emphasis is placed on their clinical use. Special attention is given to the increase in the potential of removable appliances made possible through the introduction of resin composites to dentistry.

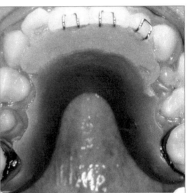

Removable appliances have their limitations. Parallel movements and torque movements are not possible, because forces cannot be combined with moments. Only fixed appliances offer three-dimensional control.

Good results can be obtained with removable appliances in the mixed dentition, prior to the use of fixed appliances and in combination with partial fixed appliances. However, in extraction cases, acceptable results are difficult to obtain without the use of fully fixed appliances, particularly in the mandible. Furthermore, successful use of removable appliances depends largely on the cooperation of the patient. The fact that the appliance can be removed may lead to less usage than prescribed. How frequently the appliance is worn depends partly on the information and motivation provided by the clinician but to a large extent on the discomfort associated with the wearing of the appliance.

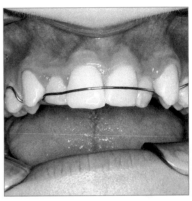

To ensure that patients wear the appliance as described, and that means always except during cleaning, its design and construction should be as comfortable and simple as possible.[181, 182] In addition, the treatment has to be explained well, and the insertion of the appliance must be performed with care.[34]

Attention will be paid to the potential for reducing the discomfort associated with wearing a removable appliance to an acceptable level.

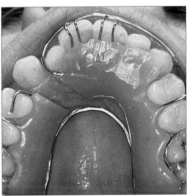

Orthodontic Concepts and Strategies

3

FIGURE 3-1

In normal functional conditions, the tongue is in contact with the palate and the lingual sides of the teeth. The other intraoral soft tissues are in contact with the teeth and alveolar processes (A). In the mandible, little space is available for a removable appliance (B).

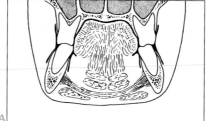
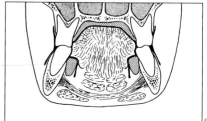

FIGURE 3-2

Undercuts are needed for the retention of clasps. Maxillary premolars and molars have a buccal undercut at the cervical region of the crowns; mandibular posterior teeth have no or only small buccal undercuts. In the mandible, the undercuts are located at the lingual surfaces of the crowns (A). The effect of the undercuts is increased by the inclination of the teeth in the maxilla, but decreased in the mandible (B). The plate can be kept thin in the maxilla but not in the mandible (C). In addition, the occlusion leaves more space for metal parts in the maxilla than in the mandible (D). A transverse bridge between the posterior parts is impossible in the mandible (E) but is standard in the maxilla (F).

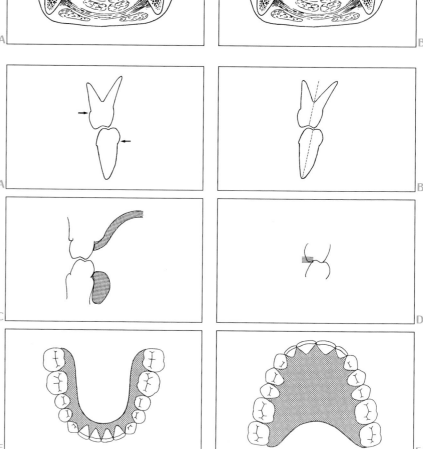

Removable appliances are mainly used in the maxilla. A thin plate that does not extend far posteriorly reduces the space for the tongue only slightly. After such a plate is worn for a few days, speech is not disturbed, and keeping it in the mouth during meals does not involve much discomfort (Fig 3-1).

In the mandible, a plate has to be thick to be sufficiently sturdy and to contain the extensions of the clasps and springs. In addition, the gingiva at the lingual side of the alveolar process is more sensitive than the palatal mucosa. Furthermore, the mylohyoid line can be located rather high and be prominent, which reduces the space available for a plate even more. The lingual side of the mandibular alveolar process posterior to the canines slopes lingually, which limits the area of contact for the acrylic resin. Furthermore, a large difference exists between the two arches regarding the availability of buccal undercuts at teeth for clasps, which are essential for the fixation of the plate and the handling of reaction forces. Removable plates can be applied effectively in the maxilla but not as easily in the mandible (Fig 3-2).

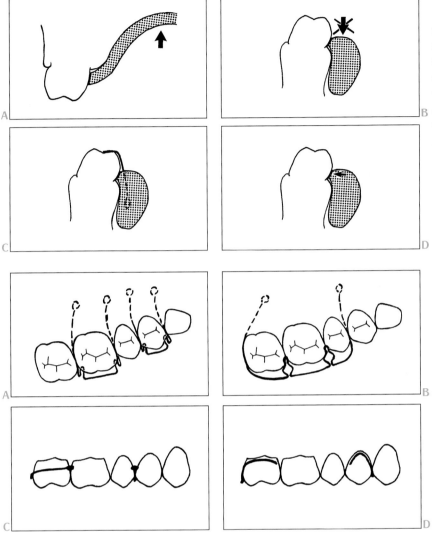

FIGURE 3-3
The palate provides resistance against the cranial movement of the plate (A). The mandible does not have such a natural vertical stop (B), and occlusal rests are needed to prevent downward movement (C). In the mandible, the undercuts at the lingual side of premolars and molars can contribute to the retention of the plate, although the available zone is small (D).

FIGURE 3-4
In the mandible, the buccal surfaces provide little or no retention for clasps. The Adams clasp makes use of the undercuts on the mesiobuccal and distobuccal corners (A). The arrow clasp of Schwarz (B) uses the embrasures for that purpose. The same applies to the ball clasp and the three-quarter ball clasp described by Booy,[33] which wraps around the most distally located tooth without touching its buccal surface but is in contact with the distal surface (C). Three-quarter clasps utilize the buccal undercuts and are, without additional aid, effective only in the maxilla (D).

A removable plate should stay in place; otherwise the active parts will not be effective and the plate will be uncomfortable to wear. Adequate resistance against reaction forces in the vertical, sagittal, and transverse directions is essential. In addition, the construction has to provide ample retention for the plate. In the maxilla, the palate offers sufficient vertical support; in the mandible, special provisions, such as occlusal rests, have to be incorporated (Fig 3-3).

The margins of the plate in contact mesially with the posterior teeth and the metal parts will resist a distal movement of teeth by reaction forces. Mesial movement is likewise restricted. In addition, the palate provides extra support, particularly when it has a steep anterior slope. In the transverse direction, the margins of the plate and the slope of the palate at the lingual side and the metal parts at the buccal side offer adequate resistance. Undercuts and clasps of various designs are used to obtain sufficient fixation (Fig 3-4).

FIGURE 3-5

In the maxilla, increase in the retention of clasps will seldom be needed, but sometimes the morphology and inclination of a premolar provide insufficient undercut (A). Particularly for the mandible, the buildup of resin composite undercuts is an important technique (B). With that approach, the clasp can be kept free of the cervical region. The resin composite undercut is bonded with the appliance in the mouth (C). However, the resin composite rim should not be too broad or too long, to avoid making removal of the appliance cumbersome (D). Otherwise, the clasp has to bend out too far, can become deformed, and loses its effectiveness (E). A small overhang of resin composite keeps the clasp in place (F).

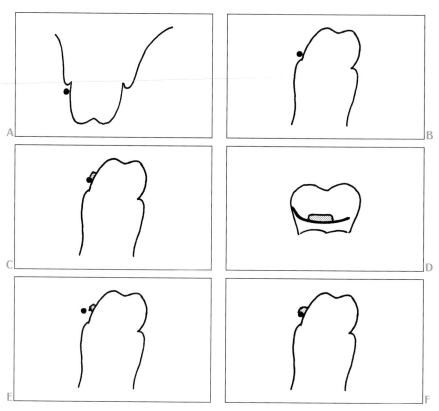

Arrow clasps and ball clasps take advantage of the embrasures between adjacent teeth. Their disadvantage is that they tend to move the teeth apart. Furthermore, arrow clasps extend far buccally, and ball clasps are stiff. Adams clasps make use of the undercuts on the mesiobuccal and distobuccal corners. To obtain adequate retention there, plaster has to be removed locally at the dental cast. Adams clasps provide effective fixation. However, they have the tendency to extrude teeth, especially when activated too much. In addition, they can cause periodontal damage. Arrow clasps, ball clasps, and Adams clasps cross the occlusal region, which in most instances leads to the patient's biting on wires. That will not be the case initially, when the mandibular incisors touch a bite plane. However, when the plate is worn correctly, the posterior teeth will erupt, and the patient may occlude on the metal. Occlusion on clasps can lead to their deformation. In addition, the plate becomes more uncomfortable for the patient to wear.

The aforementioned complications do not apply to three-quarter clasps (C-clasps) when they are placed around the most distally located tooth or when the part of the wire that crosses the occlusal region can be located so that it will not be touched by opposing teeth.

The introduction of resin composites in dentistry not only facilitated the use of fixed appliances but also increased the range of application of removable appliances and their potential. Artificial undercuts can be built up with resin composite, which substantially increases the possibility of arriving at sufficient fixation of the plate with clasps that do not interfere with the occlusion (Fig 3-5).

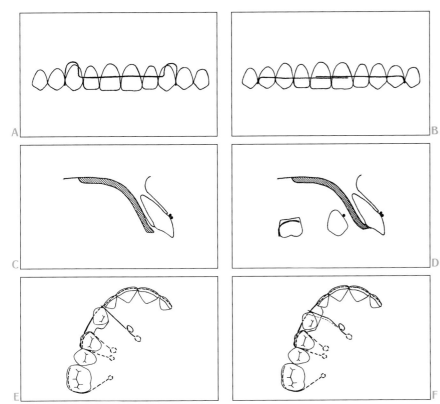

<figure>

FIGURE 3-6

The continuous labial arch with U-loops for activation is shown (A). The divided labial arches described by Booy[33] provide more control over tooth movements but less stability (B). Initially, the acrylic resin should lie against the palatal surfaces and the alveolar process. When teeth are to be retruded, the acrylic resin has to be trimmed in the palatal area as well as in the region where the alveolar process has to remodel (C). A pigtail spring can be used for mesial and distal movements and should be located cervical to the largest circumference of the crown (D). The movement is guided in the proper direction by the labial arch and the strategically trimmed acrylic resin margin (E). The spring should be activated only a few millimeters; the direction of the force can be adjusted by placing a kink in the straight section (F).

</figure>

Only a limited number of the active metal parts are described here. The possibilities for obtaining more precisely directed and controlled forces for movement of teeth will be elucidated.

Active metal parts placed cervically in contact with a tooth, or below an undercut because of the inclination, support the fixation of a plate. A good example of this is a labial arch used at labially inclined maxillary incisors. The traditional continuous labial arch with two U-loops allows the retrusion of maxillary incisors and some other movements. Booy[33] has introduced divided labial arches, which apply smaller and more controllable forces. However, divided labial arches deform easily and require careful handling by the patient.

Controlled movement of teeth depends on the application of the appropriate forces and on the potential for migration of the teeth. The latter requires strategic trimming of the acrylic resin, not only at the margin in contact with the crowns but also where the alveolar process has to remodel (Fig 3-6).

Screws have been used for many years to expand and compress dental arches. However, screws have several disadvantages: They increase the thickness of the plate, exert high and intermittent forces, have to be adjusted often, and are difficult to keep clean.

FIGURE 3-7

The direction of movement cannot be controlled when the object being pushed against is round. What happens then can be compared with the result of pushing against a chair with three swiveling wheels (A). In contrast, pulling at a round object offers control over not only the magnitude of force but also the direction of force, and the movement can be guided (B). The bonding of buttons (C) and cleats (D) is a simple procedure. Elastics can be hooked to these attachments and generate pulling forces, resulting in controlled tipping movements. In that way, canines can be moved distally and palatally (E) and molars can be moved mesially and rotated (F).

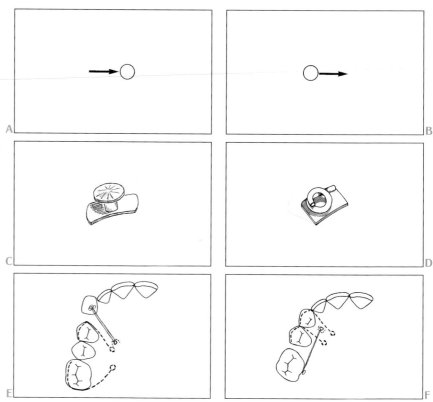

Expansion and compression of dental arches, as well as local increases and decreases in dental arch length, can be realized with heavy stainless steel springs, as is explained later in this chapter.

A force always evokes a reaction force in the opposite direction. Reaction forces have to be managed. Active metal parts cause reaction forces that tend to move the plate in the opposite direction. Labial arches for retrusion of incisors tend to move the plate in the anterior direction. A protrusion spring for the labial movement of a maxillary lateral incisor will evoke a reaction force that tends to move the plate away from the palate, resulting in an extra load on the anchorage teeth and often an improper positioning and mobility of the plate.

With an elastic, a simple force can be exerted at one specific point. However, as with springs used to push against teeth, no parallel movements are possible with elastics only. A tooth will tip with its rotation point about the midpoint of the length of the attached part of the root. However, with elastics, the desired forces of 30 to 50 g can be realized in a controlled way, and that is not the case with springs. Commercially available elastics vary in length, thickness, and material. However, only a small assortment is needed for use in conjunction with removable appliances.

The advantages associated with the use of elastics for pulling forces are clarified in Figs 3-7 and 3-8 and demonstrated in clinical examples in Figs 3-9 and 3-10.

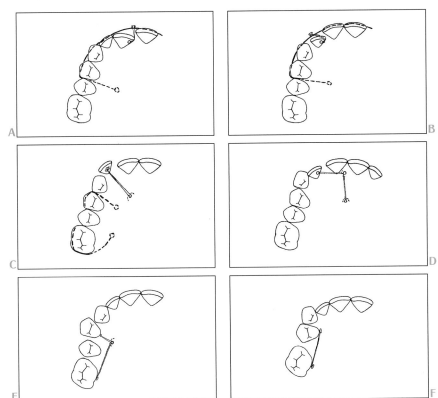

FIGURE 3-8

For labial movement of an anterior tooth, a button is placed at the palatal surface; when rotation is needed the button has to be located on the side where most movement has to occur (A). When the tooth also has to move in the mesial or distal direction, a hook at the continuous labial arch can be useful (B). Cleats in the acrylic resin of the plate are most suited for palatal movements (C). The direction of the force can be altered by the incorporation of a guiding hook (D). Controlled movement of two teeth with use of a guiding hook is shown (E). The reciprocal movement of two teeth with an elastic and two buttons is shown (F).

A certain distance between the two points of application is required for an effective use of elastics. That is not a problem in the palatal movement of maxillary teeth, because the palate provides sufficient space for a hook to be embedded in the acrylic resin far apart from the crown. The elastic can extend around the crown from a button at the labial surface to the hook, but a cleat at the palatal surface is more elegant and provides a better controlled force.

For labial movement, the elastic has to be placed around the crown and attached at the palatal surface, because otherwise the distance will be too small. For crown movement without rotation, the elastic can encircle the tooth. For rotations and combinations of labial and mesiodistal movements, the elastic should extend from the button to the hook directly (Fig 3-8).

The possibilities for applying pulling forces with elastics in conjunction with removable appliances are numerous. In the maxilla, tipping movements and rotations can be realized effectively with elastics and buttons or cleats. If needed, two buttons or cleats can be bonded to one crown to create a couple.

In this respect, the possibilities are fewer in the mandible than in the maxilla. Mandibular incisor crowns are small and difficult to handle. In addition, guiding hooks are often needed to provide sufficient distance for elastics.

A solitary elastic never may be placed around two adjacent teeth to close a diastema. The elastic will move in an apical direction, the patient will assume that the elastic is lost and put on a new one, and the result will be a bloodless extraction of two teeth.

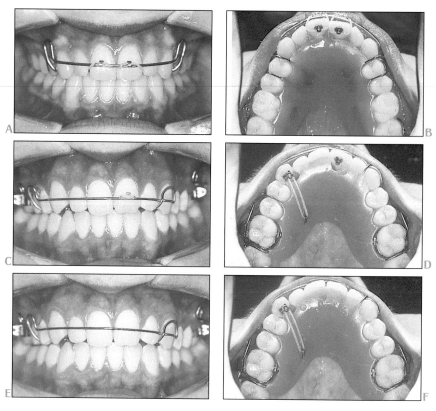

FIGURE 3-9

A continuous labial arch of 0.8-mm spring hard stainless steel wire will not bend when light elastics are attached for the labial movement of incisors, if the acrylic resin fits well against the adjacent teeth. The elastic was placed cervically of the button and traveled around the tooth to the hook on the labial arch (A, B). For palatal movement, a hook has to be placed in the acrylic resin, and its location will determine the direction of the force. At the same time, one tooth was moved palatally and another tooth labially (C, D). After the incisor attained its proper position, the button and hook were removed, and acrylic resin was added to provide a good palatal fit of the margin of the plate to the incisor (E, F).

Furthermore, with the use of elastics, excessive movement of teeth has to be prevented. A continuous labial arch can serve as a blockade at the labial side, just as the acrylic resin margin can at the palatal side.

Vertical movements can be carried out with elastics. The extrusion of a single tooth can be indicated (Fig 3-10); sometimes an intrusion is necessary. These movements can be realized with a continuous labial arch with a step in the wire at the involved tooth. Resin composite stops must be placed at the adjacent teeth to prevent dislodgment of the labial bow and to manage the reaction forces.

Vertical movements of teeth, particular extrusions, have a tendency to relapse, so adequate retention should be provided, for which a thin dead-soft braided wire (0.015 or 0.0175 inch) is most appropriate.

Concomitant with the intrusion or extrusion of a single tooth, the alveolar process is remodeled; as a consequence the gingival margin changes accordingly. In a patient with a high smile line and full presentation of the maxillary teeth, the appearance can become unacceptable. Gingivectomy and contouring of the crowns with resin composite can provide a harmonious gingival margin.

Although some patients are willing to wear clumsy appliances, in general, a negative correlation exists between the associated discomfort and the compliance. Hence, aiming for minimal discomfort is of the utmost importance.

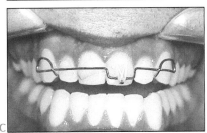
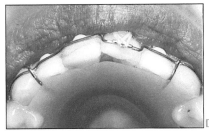

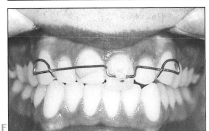
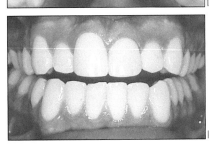

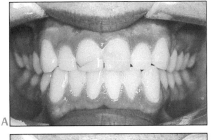
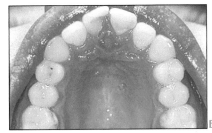

FIGURE 3-10

In this patient, both maxillary central incisors were fractured in an accident shortly after orthodontic treatment was finished. The fracture in the left incisor extended to the palatal side of the root, which made it difficult to restore the tooth without extruding it first (A, B). A continuous labial arch with claps functions at the canines, as preferred by the author for retention plates, was modified (SEE CHAPTER 18). The buttons were fabricated from resin composite and barely visible. Prior to the treatment, the cervical margins of the central incisors were at the same level (C, D). After the treatment, they differed markedly (E). That was also the case after the crowns were modified with resin composite (F). This irregularity was corrected with a gingivectomy later.

A plate that impinges on the mucosa or has extending metal parts that irritate the cheeks or lips is likely to be removed. A thick plate reduces the space for the tongue too much and makes speaking and eating more uncomfortable than necessary. Occluding on clasps or other metal parts is annoying to the patient. The same applies to protruding sharp wires. A plate that is anchored insufficiently or moves with speaking and swallowing is difficult to adapt to.

One cannot expect that an appliance that has these shortcomings will be used as prescribed, and even a motivated patient will have difficulties wearing the plate all the time. As emphasized several times, the continuous use of the plate is a prerequisite of adequate results. An appliance that is removed before eating is often not reinserted directly after the meal. Treatments will last longer than needed, which does not contribute to the patient's motivation.

One of the advantages of the use of elastics is that they pull the plate to the teeth, which increases the stability and prevents movement of the plate. With the use of elastics, clasps are less essential than when forces are produced by metal parts.

When forces are exerted through elastics, the plate can be simpler and thinner, making it easier to wear and keep in the mouth all the time. However, one has to be sure that the patient is able to handle the elastics and that he or she has an adequate supply of them.

FIGURE 3-11

When the incisors are tipped labially, a continuous labial arch, and to a lesser extent, divided labial arches, will provide resistance against caudal movement of a plate. The palatal surfaces of the anterior teeth offer support against cranial movement (A). Neither retentive aspect applies when the incisors are in upright positions (B). A vertical stop can be created with claws of 0.6-mm spring hard stainless steel wire (C). However, the claws will eventually deform because of the patient's occluding at the plate (D). Placement of a resin composite undercut inside the claws can prevent bending away of the claws and caudal movement of the plate (E). Good adaptation and a slight overhang of the resin composite keeps the claw in place (F).

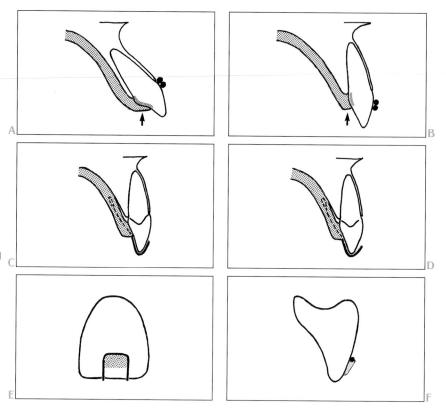

The first insertion of a plate by the clinician has to be done carefully and requires some time. Bubbles in the acrylic resin should be removed, because they can interfere with the adaptation to the teeth or compress the gingiva. The margin of the acrylic resin should be free of the cervical margins to avoid irritation of the gingiva. The easiest way to achieve this is to have the technician apply a small layer of wax at the cervical margins of the plaster cast prior to the addition of the acrylic resin. At the beginning, labial bows and springs should be activated only slightly to facilitate the adjustment to and acceptance of the appliance by the patient. After instructions are given, insertion and removal of the plate are practiced, and the patient is not allowed to leave the chair before knowing how to handle the appliance properly. Growing accustomed to the plate should take the patient only a short period of time; acceptance and habituation take only a few days when the plate is worn all the time except for cleaning. After 2 or 3 days, eating and speaking can be accomplished without problems.

At every appointment, the absence of hindrances to tooth movement must be confirmed. The same applies to occlusal interferences. In addition, the dentition must be examined to determine if the projected tooth movement has been realized. Furthermore, clasps and active parts have to be adjusted, hooks for elastics may be added or moved to another position, and acrylic resin may trimmed or added. The location of occlusal contacts in habitual occlusion should be determined. In addition, attention has to be paid to signs that indicate whether the plate is worn as prescribed. Indicative in that respect are the presence of impressions of the plate and wire parts in the gingiva, the dexterity of the patient in handling the appliance, and deposits and wear facets on the plate.

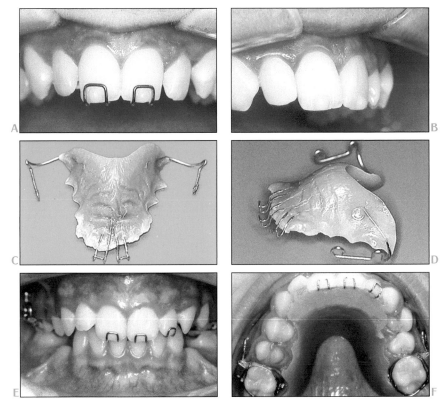

FIGURE 3-12
The claws cross the incisal edges and rest against the labial surfaces (A). Resin composite is placed within the claws (B). Together with the claws, the two clasps in the molar regions provide sufficient retention (C). Three or four claws offer even more stability (D). With this design, primary posterior teeth can be replaced by their successors. In addition, the width of the maxillary dental arch can be adjusted to the width of the mandibular dental arch. Claws also can be placed at lateral incisors (E, F).

A difference in the patient's speech when the plate is in place and when it is removed is proof that the patient is not wearing the appliance all the time. When there is doubt whether the patient is wearing the appliance during meals, the clinician can pose the trick question: "Do you sometimes forget to put the plate back after a meal?"

When the maxillary incisors are tipped palatally, as in Class II division 2 malocclusions, a specially designed plate is recommended. In these cases, the appliance can reduce the deep bite, stimulate the vertical development of the lower face, and remove the pressure of the lower lip at the labial surfaces of the inverted maxillary incisors. The problems of fixation, sagittal and vertical support, and deformation of wires can be solved with claw clasps and resin composite buildups at the incisors (Figs 3-11 and 3-12).

As already mentioned several times, the cooperation of the patient in continuous wear of the plate depends largely on the associated discomfort. In that respect, the firm fixation of the plate is most important. Claw clasps provide excellent retention.

The thickness of the plate also determines the acceptability of the appliance: the thinner, the better. That also applies to the complexity of the plate: the fewer metal parts, the simpler.

FIGURE 3-13

A bite block has to be sufficiently high to realize the desired movements of teeth in the anterior region as in this reversed overjet (A, B). After the goal is reached, the bite block has to be trimmed away.

In deep bites, the plate should be this palatal to the incisors (C, D). In the area where the mandibular anterior teeth touch, the acrylic resin should be trimmed away until the clearance between the opposing molars is not more than 1.0 to 1.5 mm. Subsequently, the plate should be modified until all mandibular anterior teeth are touching (E). The height of the bite plane should not be increased until the posterior teeth are fully in occlusion (F).

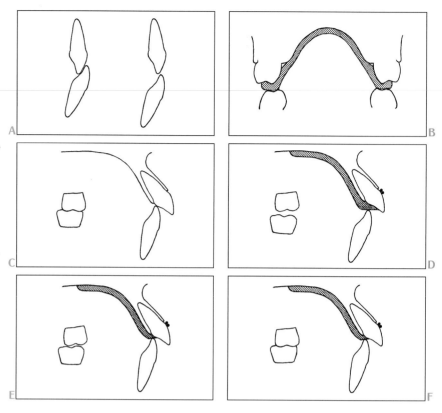

In addition to their ability to move teeth with their metal parts and elastics, removable appliances can correct occlusal disturbances and level the curve of Spee with their acrylic resin parts. A posterior bite block can be used to correct reverse overjets. Usually, such a bite block is added to a maxillary plate, which also contains active components. The acrylic resin covering of the occlusal surfaces is fabricated in the laboratory and should be kept thin, so that additional buildup can be performed in the mouth with quick-curing acrylic resin after the proper height has been established by local adjustment of the delivered plate. The patient occludes in habitual occlusion in the still soft acrylic resin to establish the overall proper height. Subsequently, excess has to be trimmed to allow smooth gliding in the transverse and sagittal directions. After the reverse overjet is corrected, the bite block can be eliminated (Fig 3-13, A and B). Working the other way around and trying to grind high posterior bite blocks down to the ideal height is more difficult, more time consuming, and less accurate than the aforementioned procedure.

A comparable approach is recommended for the anterior bite plane. Most technicians make the plate too thick palatally in the incisor region, and extensive trimming has to be performed at the chairside.

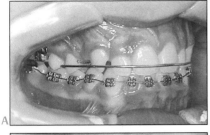
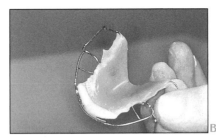

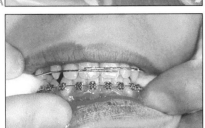
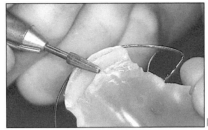

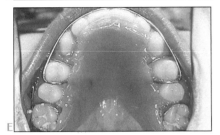
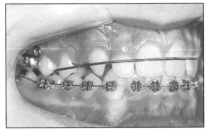

Figure 3-14

The height of the bite plane should not be increased before the premolars or primary and permanent molars occlude completely (A). For slight thickening of the bite plane, a small amount of quick-curing acrylic resin is added in the anterior region (B). The desired height can be easily determined by placing stretched out cotton rolls between the posterior teeth and having the patient occlude on them (C). After the acrylic resin has hardened, the smooth surface has to be trimmed to allow undisturbed sagittal and transverse movements (D, E). The bite plane is raised only slightly (F).

After the plate is inserted in the mouth, the position where the mandibular anterior teeth occlude can be marked on the acrylic resin by scratching with a sharp instrument along the labial surfaces. Subsequently, a groove is ground at the required height in which the mandibular anterior teeth occlude. The patient is asked to occlude into the groove after it has been filled with quick-curing acrylic resin. Outside the mouth, the built-up area is trimmed until only a slight indication of the contact with the teeth remains. In that way a flat surface that supports the six mandibular anterior teeth vertically is obtained.

In most instances, a plate prepared without the aforementioned procedure will allow contact with only one or two incisors, even if the plate is kept thin. Such a plate causes unnecessary discomfort. A plate that allows contact with four or six mandibular anterior teeth is more convenient and accepted more readily.

A high bite plane has to be avoided not only for the associated discomfort but also because it does not make sense. A high bite plane is needed only when the lower lip has to be kept away from the labial surfaces of the maxillary incisors, as is required in Class II division 2 malocclusions (see chapter 12). The presence of a large clearance between the opposing posterior teeth involves the risk of tongue interpositioning, which will hinder the eruption of the posterior teeth.

The height of the bite plane should not be increased before the posterior teeth have established contact and have had the time to adapt in inclination to the resulting intercuspation. This adaptation is particularly relevant when the sagittal relationship between the two dental arches has been improved in the meantime.

A bite plane can be used not only to reduce a deep bite (Figs 3-13, C to F, and 3-14) but also to facilitate the correction of a transverse disturbance in the occlusion of the posterior teeth.

FIGURE 3-15

The patient had severe crowding in the maxillary anterior region and a blocked out right canine (A). Space was created with a Crefcoeur appliance,[44] used first on the left side (B). Subsequently, the left separation was filled with acrylic resin, and the plate was sawed through on the right side, to create space there (C, D). On both sides of the separation, the teeth were firmly anchored (E). Resin composite undercuts at the lateral incisor and first premolars increased the retention (F).

In another patient, the use of a Crefcoeur appliance in combination with claws at the central incisors already had provided sufficient space. Although the heavy spring had been in contact with the palatal mucosa, irritations did not develop. The gingiva near the teeth also was not affected (G). The increase in width of the separation was an indication of the increase in dental arch length (H).

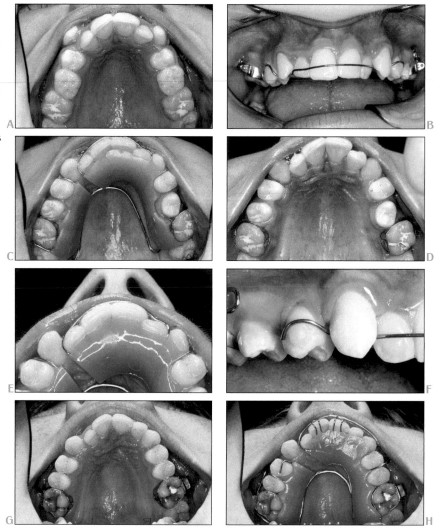

As already mentioned, besides screws, hard spring stainless steel wire of 1.2 mm in diameter can be used to expand or compress dental arches (Fig 3-15). These heavy springs have the advantage that they can expand or compress in a V shape. The first such spring was designed by Coffin,[43] who attached the spring in the anterior area of the two halves of the plate. In the design advocated by Crefcoeur,[44] the spring is fixated posteriorly, which allows increases and decreases in arch length not only in the median plane but also in other regions of the dental arch. Essential to this design is fixation with clasps and acrylic resin so that the plate stays in place, particularly adjacent to the separation. The plate is rather unstable because it is composed of two parts connected with only a spring that tends to move them apart or together (Figs 3-15 and 3-17).

The activation of such a spring is not simple. The wire is stiff and difficult to bend. Special attention and skill are required to keep the two parts in the same plane and to prevent deformation of the shape of the dental arch. The force of the spring is primarily exerted at the teeth adjacent to the separation, the location at which expansion is the goal.

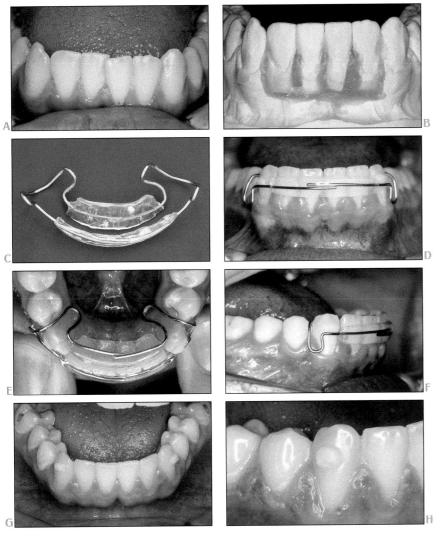

FIGURE 3-16

After loss of the bonded dead-soft braided wire retainer, crowding developed in the mandibular anterior region (A). The approximal surfaces of the incisors and the mesial sides of the canines were stripped prior to taking the impression. From a duplicate of the plaster cast, an ideal diagnostic setup was prepared (B). The spring retainer can be activated locally by adding or removing acrylic resin (C). The desired orthodontic movements were realized (D, E). With the narrow U-loops in combination with the resin composite undercuts at the canines, the spring retainer stayed in place, did not dislodge vertically, and was effective (F–H).

However, the force should be distributed over the other teeth in the dental arch segments. That requires firm retention by clasps and acrylic resin. In that respect, three-quarter clasps with resin composite undercuts are most effective and also have the advantage that they do not creep cervically.

The spring retainer introduced by Barrer[10] is a special form of a removable appliance intended to correct crowding in the mandibular anterior region in previously orthodontically treated patients. First, the mesiodistal dimensions of the mandibular anterior teeth have to be reduced, to provide space for the correction of the malpositioning. The original design has no clasp function and tends to dislodge, which makes the appliance less effective. The spring retainer presented here is a modification of the Barrer design and has narrow U-loops and resin composite undercuts at the canines. With this modification, the appliance does not dislodge and works well (Fig 3-16).

FIGURE 3-17
A patient in the mixed dentition stage had a scissors bite (crossbite) on the left side (A, B). The occlusion of the maxillary primary molars and permanent first molar was corrected with a Crefcoeur appliance.[44] With such an appliance, a dental arch can be compressed or expanded with a gradual continuous force. The extension on the Adams clasp kept the primary molars inclined palatally (C, D). The obtained result is shown (E, F).

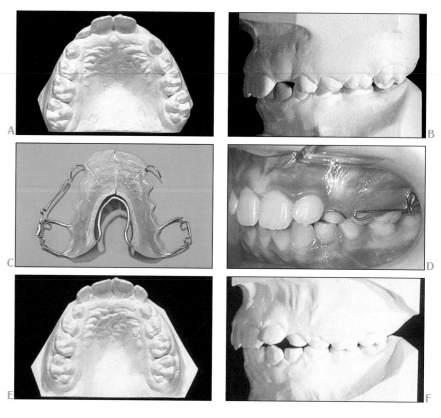

Effective use of removable appliances requires an eye for details and a good estimation of what is supposed to happen between two appointments. When the appliance is activated, the fact that the patient may not show up for the next appointment, and the fact that it could be quite some time before he or she appears again, should be considered.

As explained before, removable appliances can be used effectively in the maxilla but are quite cumbersome in the mandible. In addition, cooperation is difficult to obtain with mandibular removable appliances, because they cause considerably more discomfort than maxillary plates.

In short, the use of removable appliances is by no means simple; it requires much attention, careful handling, some mechanical insight, inventiveness, and a good relationship with patients.

Use of Headgears

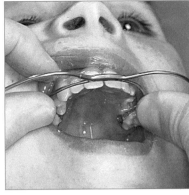

With a headgear, a force is applied to the dental arch, while the reaction force is absorbed outside the mouth. As a rule, the force is exerted on the permanent maxillary first molars and the reaction force is absorbed most often by the neck (cervical headgear) and less frequently by the head (parietal or high-pull headgear).

A headgear influences the maxillofacial skeletal growth. That applies not only to the direction of growth but also to the amount of growth that takes place during treatment. However, it never has been proved that facial orthopedic therapy that is concluded before the completion of facial growth alters the size and shape of the skeletal structures in the long term. On the other hand, the maxillomandibular relationship can be improved, facilitating the correction of a disto-occlusion. When a solid intercuspation of premolars and canines is achieved at the end of treatment, this improvement is not lost later. More information on this topic is provided in chapter 8. Headgears are also used to prevent permanent first molars from migrating mesially or to distalize first molars to gain space in the maxillary dental arch. The widening of dental arch associated with headgear treatment also contributes to the increase in dental arch length. Furthermore, the permanent maxillary first molars can be rotated distally, which provides additional space. In subsequent chapters, the possibilities for combining headgears with other appliances are discussed. Indeed, headgears can be used effectively with plates, activators, and partial or complete fixed appliances. The theoretical and practical aspects of headgears, especially those of cervical headgear, are explained. Recommendations for the fitting and formation of molar bands are given. In addition, a simple method of adapting, activating, and inspecting a cervical headgear is presented. Clinical examples illustrate the possibilities and limitations. Recommendations are given for the examinations to be carried out at control visits.

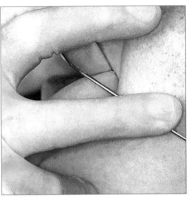

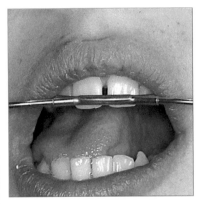

A headgear is a relatively simple appliance with few complications. A molar band can become loose, or the headgear can be deformed. The intervals between appointments can be long when the headgear is well adjusted and the applied force is not too great.

Considerable improvements can be realized with headgears in Class II division 1 malocclusions, particularly when crowding is present in the maxillary dental arch.

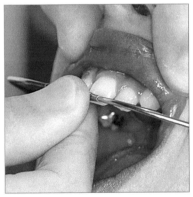

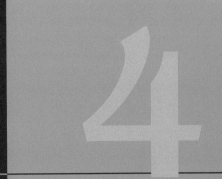

Orthodontic Concepts and Strategies

4

FIGURE 4-1

The growth sites of the facial skeleton, subdivided into three types, and their relative contributions in the vertical and sagittal directions are presented. The deposition and resorption of bone at surfaces is not included. Arrows and the relative sizes of the rectangular blocks are used to indicated the contributions of the spheno-occipital synchondrosis (blue), the mandibular condyle (red), and the sutures and the alveolar processes (green).

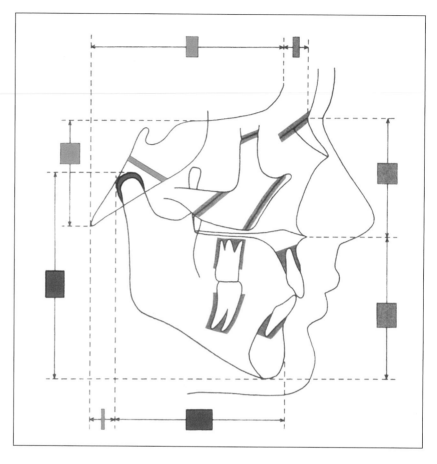

Preferably, the treatment of a Class II division 1 malocclusion should be started before the transition of the dentition is completed, to benefit from the growth potential that can be utilized for the correction of the deviating relationship of the dental arches. The same applies to the guidance of the development of the dentition, because intervention prior to the loss of the primary second molars presents the opportunity to make use of the extra space that becomes available through their replacement.

For both facial growth and development of the dentition, the phenomenon of adaptability also can be exploited. The adaptability of the dentition originates in the periodontium; that of the skeleton derives from the sutures and the condyles and to a smaller degree from the periosteum. The sutures and condyles lose their adaptability with aging.[213]

The condyles are the most important growth sites of the facial skeleton and have a large capacity for adaptation. Furthermore, their direction of growth can vary. In addition, the condyles can exhibit temporary growth accelerations, provoked by structures located outside the condyles. The sutures function as growth and adaptability sites. The periosteum also plays an essential role in adaptability and maintains its potential to absorb and deposit bone on surfaces until the end of life. The various growth sites are indicated in Fig 4-1.

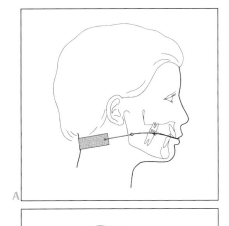

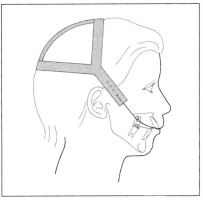

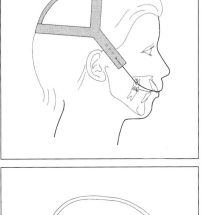

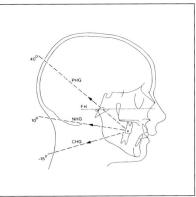

FIGURE 4-2
Various headgears differ in the direction of force applied to the permanent maxillary first molars: Cervical headgear (A); parietal (high-pull) headgear (B); neutral headgear with a traction parallel to the occlusal plane (C); directions of traction of the various headgears: parietal headgear (PHG); neutral headgear (NHG); cervical headgear (CHG)) in relation to Frankfort horizontal (FH) (D).

The spheno-occipital synchondrosis is important for the vertical growth of the posterior region of the face and contributes to the sagittal growth of the face adjacent to the cranium. It is assumed that the spheno-occipital synchondrosis has no capacity for adaptation and that its growth is not influenced by local factors.

The condyle can be considered as a combination of a cartilaginous growth site and an adaptability site. The condyle can deliver a large contribution in a short period of time, because cartilage can grow interstitially. By its orientation, the condyle contributes to the increase in posterior facial height, as well as to the sagittal increase in the length of the mandible. The vertical growth of the anterior region of the craniofacial skeleton depends on the increase in height of bony structures. The increase in height of the inferior region of the face is realized by the buildup of the alveolar processes associated with the formation and eruption of teeth. The increase in height of the superior region of the face is realized mainly by growth at the sutures, which by their orientation contribute to not only the vertical but also the sagittal development of the midface.

Facial orthopedic therapy with extraoral traction is frequently used in Class II malocclusions. Headgears can be used alone or in combination with plates, activators or other myofunctional appliances, and partial or complete fixed appliances. Headgears can be distinguished on the basis of the direction of their traction (Fig 4-2).

FIGURE 4-3

Schematic presentation of the relationships among skeleton, dentition, and function (including the soft tissues) in the form
of a system of the dentofacial complex.
Theoretically it can be stated that the
three entities have a certain variation in
their realization, of which the ranges are
indicated by thin lines. The range is smaller for the functional aspect than for the
other two factors. The thickness of the
arrows, which indicates the relationships,
suggests that the most important influence is supposed to be function, including
the soft tissues.[213]

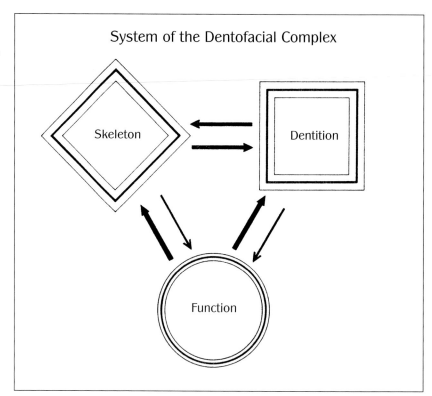

System of the Dentofacial Complex

Skeleton

Dentition

Function

FIGURE 4-4

The wearing of a cervical headgear by a
patient with a Class II malocclusions and a
normal vertical facial configuration leads
to an increase in the lower facial height
(A). After treatment, the mandible grows
primarily anteriorly and returns to its individual growth pattern (B).

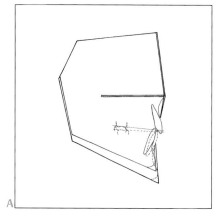

A

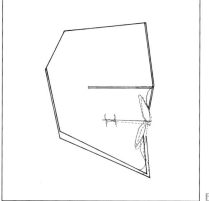

B

It is assumed that the genetic information for the growth of the face is mainly passed on through the information that determines the development of the neuromuscular system and soft tissues.[206, 230] This concept asserts
that the growth of the craniofacial skeleton is subordinate to, and largely dependent on, the development of the
neuromuscular system and the soft tissues. Although the amount of growth that can take place at the condyles is
probably genetically determined, the direction of condylar growth, and the periods in which this growth is accelerated, probably depend more on other factors than on genetic factors.

The relationship among skeleton, dentition, and function (including the soft tissues) can be expressed as a
system of the dentofacial complex (Fig 4-3). In this theory, it is assumed that the functional aspect can vary less
within one individual than can the two other factors.[213]

In addition, it is assumed that the influence of the function on the skeleton and dentition is greater than the
reverse. In a normally growing individual, the three factors will be in balance continuously, and each factor will be
within its own range of variation.

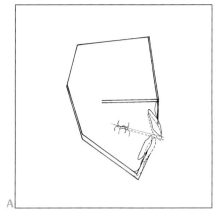
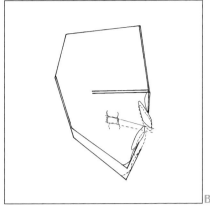

FIGURE 4-5

In a patient with a large anterior facial height, a parietal headgear can restrict the vertical development of the midface, the eruption of the maxillary molars, and the increase in lower facial height (A). After treatment, the length of the ramus and the height of the lower face increase markedly, while the maxillary molars erupt further (B).

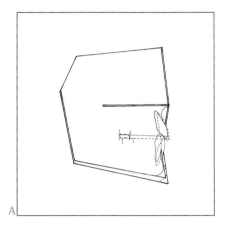
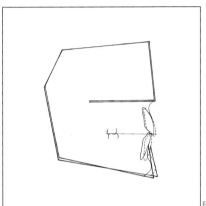

FIGURE 4-6

In a patient with a small anterior facial height, vertical development can be stimulated with a cervical headgear. The permanent maxillary first molars can be extruded, and extra growth of the ramus can be realized (A). After treatment, the alterations partially recede, and the individual growth pattern returns (B).

Without this range of variation, the maturation of the separate factors would have too little latitude for interaction among the three factors, each of which develops in its typical mode and tempo.[213]

A headgear restrains the anterior development of the maxilla. With cervical traction, an extruding force is exerted at the permanent maxillary first molars. It has been documented that with cervical headgear therapy the length of the mandibular ramus increases more than would have occurred otherwise.[16] After treatment, the face returns to its individual growth pattern and compensates for the change in direction caused, through the treatment, by a period of less vertical and more anterior growth (Fig 4-4).[89]

Indeed, in patients with a large anterior facial height, a parietal headgear can change the direction of facial growth and inhibit the vertical development. However, thereafter a substantial vertical increase occurs, and the individual growth pattern resumes (Fig 4-5).

A comparable and opposite course is observed in patients with a short anterior facial height after treatment with a cervical headgear; the evoked increase in lower facial height dissipates gradually (Fig 4-6).

When the internal and external functional components are in balance, growth will conform to the average growth pattern (A). When internal functional components dominate over the external functional components, growth will mainly be in the caudal direction, leading to an increase in space for the internal functional components. This development is often associated with tongue interpositioning, an anterior open bite, an open mouth, labial tipping of the incisors, and a receding chin (B).

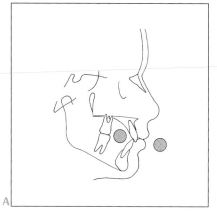
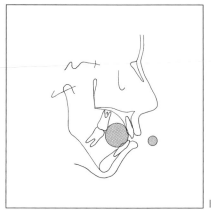

A   B

FIGURE 4-8

When external functional components dominate over the internal functional components, and more space is available for the latter than is needed, growth will occur mainly in the anterior direction, and the lower anterior facial height will increase only slightly or not at all. This type of development is found in Class II division 1 malocclusions with an excess of external functional components (A) and is typical of Class II division 2 malocclusions (B).

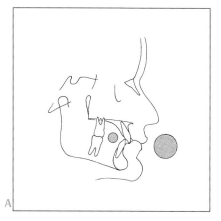
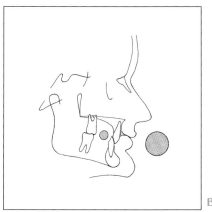

A   B

As explained, an important role in facial growth has to be assigned to functional aspects. It is assumed that the vertical development of the face, and particularly that of the lower region, is largely determined by the interaction between internal and external functional components. In a normal situation, an equilibrium exists between the two with a variation in expression within the range of acceptable norms.

When internal functional components dominate, excessive vertical facial growth will occur. A compromised nasal passage, a large tongue, and hypertrophic adenoids and tonsils can necessitate more space. Internal functional components comprise not only the oral but also the nasal and pharyngeal areas and spaces and the activities occurring there. The external functional components include the muscles and soft tissues at the external side of the facial skeleton and are likewise acting through their size and volume as well as their activities. It is hypothesized that not the incidental muscle contractions but the conditions at rest are essential in this respect. A large amount of soft tissues at the anterior side of a face with a competent lip seal will have a different effect than a thin, flabby covering with an open mouth. Furthermore, it is assumed that with dominance of the internal functional components, the face, and particularly its lower region, will grow primarily vertically (Fig 4-7). In the opposite situation, with dominance of the external functional components and an excess of internal space, the height of the lower anterior face will remain small (Fig 4-8).[219]

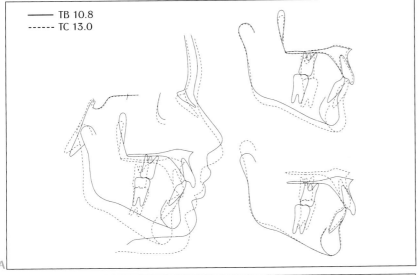

- TB 10.8
------ TC 13.0

A

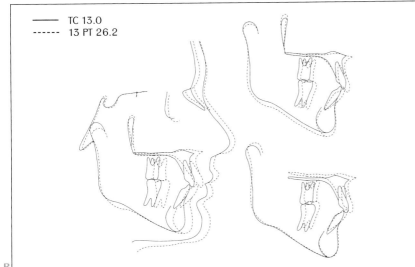

- TC 13.0
------ 13 PT 26.2

B

Figure 4-9

Tracings of the patient shown on page 63 in Fig 4-19. The effect of the treatment with the cervical headgear was favorable. The maxilla did not develop anteriorly, but the mandible did markedly. The extensive vertical development of the face is striking. The lower anterior facial height increased considerably, the maxillary molars erupted further, and the ramus became longer. However, the posterior section of the maxilla did not enlarge, and the space available for the second and third molars did not increase (A). After treatment, facial height did not increase, and the mandible and maxilla grew anteriorly. The inferior border of the mandible became more horizontal, and the chin attained a more anterior position (B).

(TB = treatment beginning;
TC = treatment completed;
13 PT = 13 years posttreatment)

The effect of a cervical headgear depends on the facial growth. With a favorable growth pattern and sufficient growth during treatment, a good result can be obtained with proper use of the headgear and good cooperation of the patient. With 14 hours' daily wear of a headgear, marked improvements can be obtained in a relatively short period of time (Fig 4-9).

More space can be created in the maxillary dental arch by a headgear, because the permanent first molars are prevented from migrating mesially, are distalized, or are rotated.[124] In addition, keeping the cheeks away from the teeth and alveolar processes leads to an increase of arch width, and the maxillary dental arch will widen as the mandibular dental arch will gradually occlude more anteriorly ("rail" mechanism).

The improvements that can be obtained with extraoral traction in Class II malocclusions are derived from skeletal and dental effects. In most patients, the dental alterations contribute more than the skeletal alterations. However, the distal movement of the permanent maxillary first molars can have a negative effect on the spatial conditions in the posterior section of the apical area. That applies especially to situations in which the posterior section of the apical area is small.[214, 215] In medium-sized posterior sections, the position of not-yet-emerged molars can change unfavorably.

FIGURE 4-10

When the posterior section of the apical area is small, a problem can arise; the space for the second and third molars will increase less than would have been the case without headgear therapy, and insufficient space remains for the third molar to emerge (A, B). When the posterior section of the apical area is medium sized, headgear therapy does not necessarily lead to negative sequelae for the third molar (C, D). When the posterior section of the apical area is large, sufficient space will be available for the second and third molars to attain positions in the dental arch (E, F).

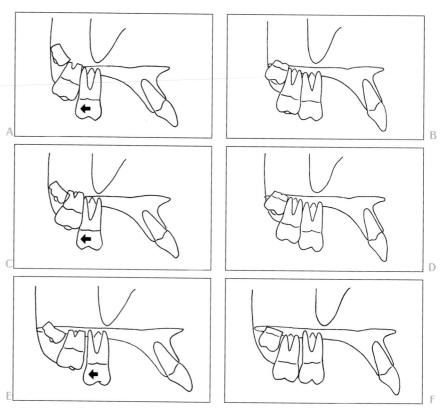

FIGURE 4-11

When the posterior section of the apical area is small, the permanent second molar will erupt late and be located partly cranial to the first molar (A). With the use of a headgear, the three molars can become positioned more on top of each other (B).

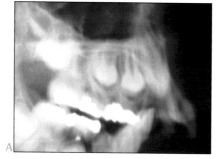
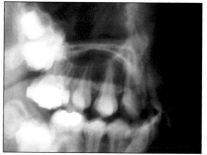

However, distalizing permanent maxillary first molars over a short distance will not lead to complications in patients in whom the posterior sections of the apical area are large. The second and third molars can emerge unimpeded and attain a good occlusion. If the posterior section of the apical area is too small, the second molar will erupt too far buccally and will be distally angulated. On emergence, the second molar can arrive in exo-occlusion, and that happens occasionally in headgear treatments. A comparable phenomenon can occur with the third molar later. In patients who have been treated with a headgear, the maxillary third molar can even emerge buccal to the second molar (Figs 4-10 and 4-11).

A reduction in the ultimate size of the posterior section of the maxillary apical area is probably also caused by a reduction in bone formation at the maxillary tuber. The more posterior position of the maxillary complex, caused by the headgear treatment, is the result of less anterior development of the maxilla than otherwise would have occurred. The resulting reduction in the ultimate size of the posterior section of the apical area can be clinically relevant.

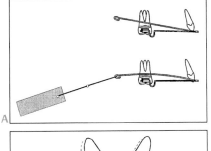

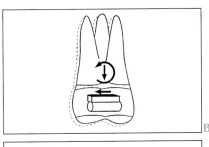

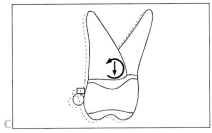

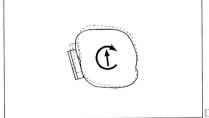

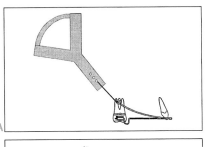

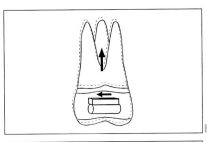

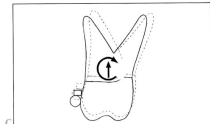

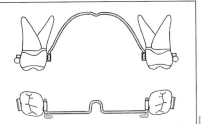

FIGURE 4-12

A cervical headgear has to be adjusted so that the line of force will run slightly cranial to the center of resistance of the molar. When the elastic is attached, the outer bow will bend and the centerpiece will be located slightly higher (A). The force and couple at the molar will lead to its movement (B). Because the point of application of force is on the buccal side, the extruding component will be combined with a couple that tends to move the root apices buccally (C). The eccentric application will add a couple to the distal force (D).

FIGURE 4-13

A parietal headgear has a short outer bow that extends about as far posteriorly as the inner bow (A). An intruding force is placed on the maxillary molar, with or without a couple in the sagittal plane, depending on the length of the outer bow and its angle with the occlusal plane (B). Because the point of application is on the buccal side, a couple that tends to move the root apices palatally will result (C). These shortcomings of a parietal headgear can be partially compensated for with a palatal bar (D).

The mechanical aspects and movements of the permanent maxillary first molars are illustrated in Figs 4-12 and 4-13. The inner bow of the headgear has a diameter of 0.045 inch (about 1.1 mm), and the outer bows have a diameter of 0.060 inch (about 1.5 mm). The large outer bows of the cervical headgear are bent when activated, so the forces and couple shown in Fig 4-12, B, are somewhat incorrect.

The molar will be moved in a parallel direction and not tipped when the line of force passes through the center of resistance, located slightly apical to the furcation. When the line of force passes cranial to that center, the root apices will tip distally. If the line passes caudal to the center of resistance, the crown will tip distally. The farther the line of force is from the center of resistance, the larger the couple.

Cervical headgears are less visible than are parietal headgears, do not disturb the hair style, and are accepted more readily. In addition, if cervical headgears are used properly, the maxillary molars remain in occlusion. Because the long-term skeletal effects of the two types of headgears do not seem to be different, the cervical headgear is preferred.

The inner bow of the headgear should run about parallel to the occlusal plane and be somewhat wider (± 2.0 mm) at the molar tubes, although a transverse passive headgear already has some expansion effect.

FIGURE 4-14

The proper size of the band is selected on the plaster cast and not in the mouth (A). In the mouth, the band should encircle the crown and, after some seating pressure, not dislodge. Subsequently, the cervical margin is festooned, and the band is shortened occlusally where needed (B, C). The modified band is placed around the crown and pushed through the contact points with a band setter (D1). With a flat amalgam plugger, placed lengthwise at the marginal edge, the band is seated further. Subsequently, the band is moved cervically with a band seater (D2) as the patient occludes first on the buccal side and then on the palatal side, while the buccal side of the band is held in place with a scaler B or an Ash 49 (Dentsply Ash, Surrey, England) (E, F). After the patient occludes on the palatally located seating lug, it is often necessary to place the band setter at the distopalatal edge of the band to seat it properly. If the clinician has both hands in contact with each other, the patient's occlusal force can be transmitted to the scaler or Ash 49, which helps the buccal side of the band to remain in place (G). The band should fit well all around (H).

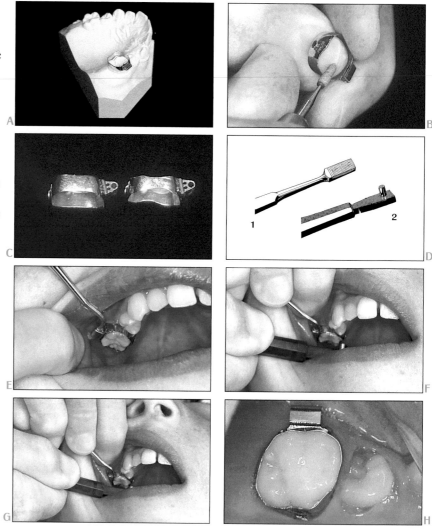

The fitting and placement of the molar bands requires special care. The bands should fit tightly and be located properly; their cervical margins should be located just below the gingival margin.[55] Most commercially available, preformed bands are insufficiently festooned. Hence, they have to be trimmed to a tapering margin on the mesial and distal aspects prior to placement in the mouth. Because of the festooning, the bands can be pushed further around the crowns before the contact points are reached. The fine tapering margins facilitate passing of the contacts points without deformation, and separation is not needed.

In most cases, the height of the band at the disto-occlusal margin and at the distopalatal cusp has to be reduced. When these modifications are carried out before the band is fitted and adapted to the shape of the crown, the band only has to be placed in the mouth one time before cementation. Repeated placement and removal of the band is annoying to the patient and results in a band that is too wide and unnecessarily hardened. First the band has to be seated on the buccal side, where the crown has its largest convexity. Subsequently, the palatal side is seated, and the patient strategically occludes on a band setter (Fig 4-14). With proper trimming, fitting, and cementation of a band in a patient with healthy gingiva, no bleeding should occur, and the band should not interfere with the occlusion.

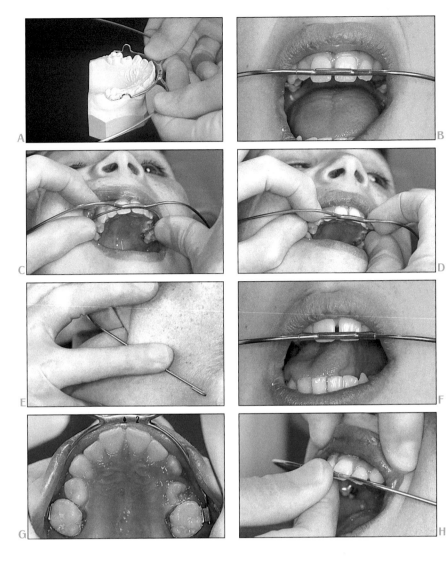

FIGURE 4-15
Headgears are available in five inner bow sizes. On the plaster cast, the proper size is selected, and the length and shape are adjusted (A). The headgear is inserted in the right tube, and the location where the left side of the inner bow ends is noted. Subsequently, the headgear is adjusted until both ends can be inserted easily in the tubes, the correct distance to the teeth has been reached all around, and the centerpiece is positioned slightly above the incisal edges of the central incisors (B). The thumbs are placed firmly against the U-loops (C), and the index fingers are placed on top of the inner bow to lower the location of the centerpiece (D). Subsequently, the ring fingers are used to bend the outer bows down parallel to each other (E). Before the elastic is attached, the lower side of the centerpiece should be at the level of the incisal edges. When the elastic is attached, the centerpiece moves up and the outer and inner bows have to be adjusted once more so that the centerpiece is located slightly above the incisal edges (F). This arrangement results in the desired small couples at the molars, which prevent their tipping. The headgear should be free of the teeth all around (G) and should not touch the incisors when firmly pushed against the centerpiece (H).

Preparatory measures, such as the selection and preparation of bands, the selection of the headgear size, and the subsequent adaptation of the headgear, have to be performed on the dental cast.

The inner bow should be located 3.0 mm from the posterior teeth and 2.0 mm from the anterior teeth. It is recommended that the same criteria always be used for fitting and adjusting headgears. That applies especially to the height of the centerpiece of the headgear before and after the elastic is attached to the hook (Fig 4-15). When the centerpiece is located slightly superior to the incisal edges of the maxillary central incisors, the piece is situated at the level where lips of normal length and positioning touch each other. In a patient with a short upper lip and open mouth posture, the proposed location will lead to stretching of the upper lip to reach the headgear. In Class II division 2 malocclusions, the lower lip will be kept away from the labial surface of the maxillary incisors.

When the same criteria are used consistently, control examinations can be carried out more effectively and more reliably. When the centerpiece has moved more than 3.0 mm cranially, the apices of the permanent first molars have tipped distally. If the centerpiece is positioned too low, then the crowns have tipped distally. A decrease in the distance between the centerpiece and the labial surfaces of the maxillary incisors is a sign of an increase in dental arch length.

As stated before, marked improvements can be realized with a headgear, which can be supported by a plate and/or partial fixed appliances if necessary (Figs 4-16 to 4-19).

FIGURE 4-16

A boy 12 years 6 months of age, with a Class II division 1 malocclusion, was treated with only a headgear. He had an asymmetric open bite caused by thumb sucking (A, B). He stopped this habit after the headgear was placed. After 2 years 6 months, a good occlusion in the posterior regions was obtained, and the treatment concluded (C, D). Five years later, at the age of 20 years 0 months, the bite was closed and the maxillary incisors were retruded further (E, F). Ten years after treatment concluded, at the age of 25 years 3 months, the face had matured, while few changes had taken place in the dentition (G, H).

Indeed, digit-suckers often stop the habit when an appliance is placed. However, in headgear treatment, subsequent spontaneous corrections are limited because the lips are kept away from the anterior teeth, which will not move sufficiently in the palatal direction without an additional appliance. Furthermore, blocked out canines do not move completely within the dental arch when sufficient space has become available. After the headgear treatment was concluded in this patient, the incisors moved further palatally, and the canines arrived at a good occlusion.

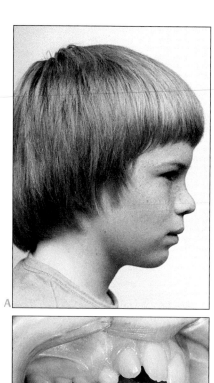
A

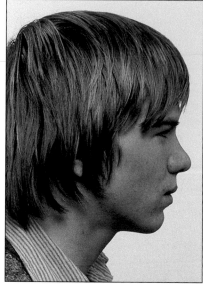
C

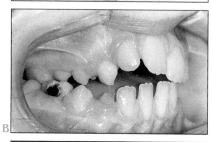
B

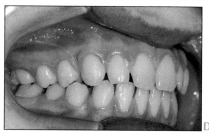
D

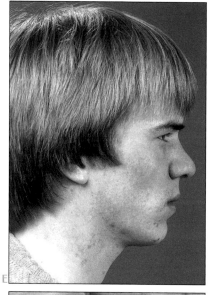
E

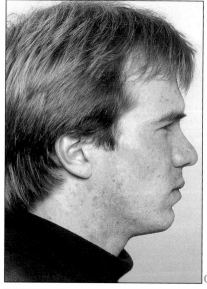
G

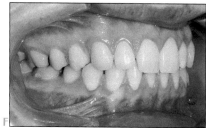
F

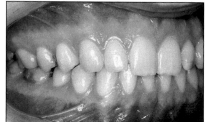
H

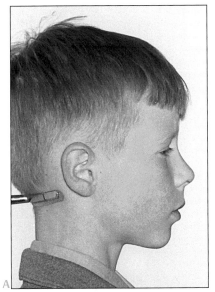

A

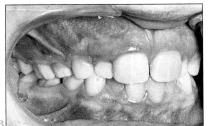

B

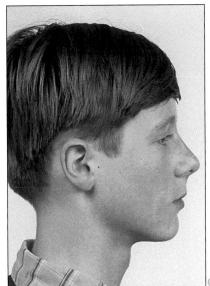

C

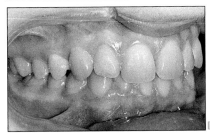

D

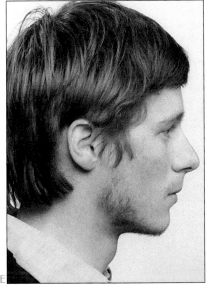

E

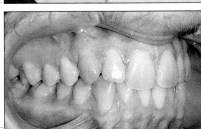

F

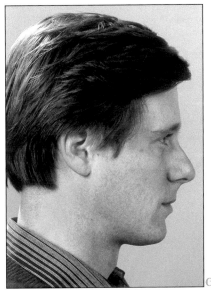

G

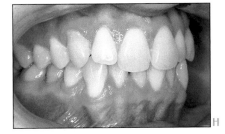

H

FIGURE 4-17

A boy 12 years 2 months of age had a moderate disto-occlusion and in the maxilla, mesially positioned posterior teeth and crowding in the canine region (A, B). After treatment of 2 years 6 months with only a cervical headgear, sufficient space for the maxillary canines was gained, and a good intercuspation of the posterior teeth was reached (C, D). After the treatment, the overbite decreased. Five years after treatment, at 20 years of age (E, F), and 15 years later, at 30 years of age (G, H), little had changed. In the meantime, the face had matured and the profile had straightened.

The overbite often decreases with headgear treatment, but that had not occurred in this patient. A plate could have corrected the deep bite. A plate is also suitable for correcting tooth positions and especially for retruding labially tipped incisors.

In this patient, good intercuspation in the posterior regions was attained, while the maxillary dental arch became wider. With the mesial movement of the mandibular dental arch, the maxillary premolars and molars are guided buccally (rail mechanism). This movement is facilitated because the headgear keeps the cheeks away from the posterior teeth. In addition, the tongue pressure contributes to the widening of the maxillary dental arch. A cervical headgear exerts a force on the molars that tends to extrude them, keeps them in occlusion, and moves their apices to the buccally. Furthermore, with the cervical headgear, the apices of the molars can be maintained or moved distally, which increases the intercuspation and ultimately the stability of the result.

FIGURE 4-18

In a girl with a Class II division 1 malocclusion, a headgear was placed at the age of 11 years 2 months (A, B). After 2 years 6 months, a good result was achieved, partly through the use of partial fixed appliances in the last phase of treatment. She only had brackets at the maxillary incisors to improve their position (C, D). At the age of 33 years, 20 years after the completion of treatment, few changes had occurred in the dentition (E, F). Initially, the patient had extensive crowding in the maxilla, where the primary right canine was lost prematurely (G). Sufficient space was created with the cervical headgear during the first 18 months of treatment (H). The dental cast made when she was 33 years of age revealed that the second molars could erupt undisturbed because the third molars were not formed (I). The distal rotation of the permanent first molars contributed substantially to the increase in maxillary dental arch length. With their rhomboid shape, mesially rotated maxillary permanent molars (G) occupy extra space (H). Their derotation can be carried out effectively with a cervical headgear. For that purpose, the end that fits in the molar tube has to be rotated slightly, so that the other end, when it is not inserted, extends 3.0 to 4.0 mm distal to the tube. If the other molar also has to be rotated, the same procedure applies. The insertion of the inner bow becomes easier by pushing from the buccal direction at the U-loops when the ends are placed in the openings of the tubes.

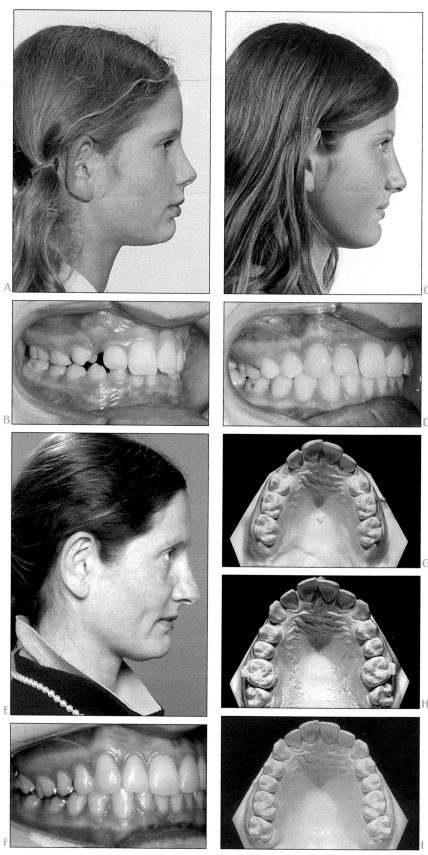

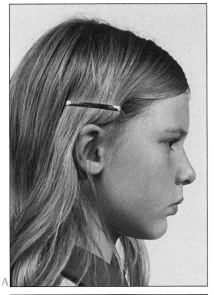

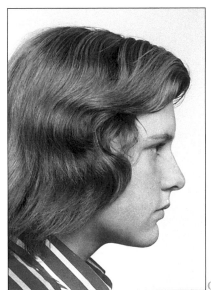

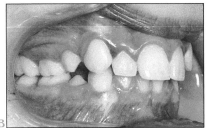

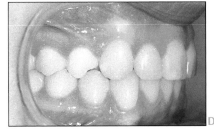

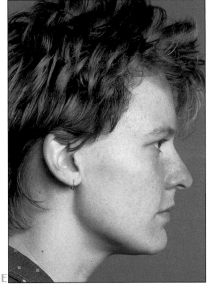

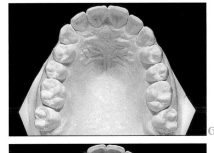

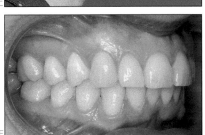

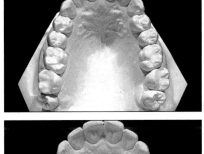

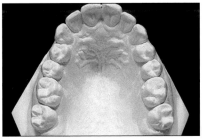

FIGURE 4-19

A girl aged 10 years 8 months, with a Class II division 1 malocclusion and crowding in the maxillary dental arch, had not yet lost her primary second molars (A, B). If that is the case, the difference in mesiodistal crown dimensions between these teeth and their successors can be utilized to relieve the crowding and to improve the molar occlusion. The cervical headgear preserved the extra space that became available with the transition, reducing the maxillary crowding and the disto-occlusion. In the mandible, the crowding in the anterior region disappeared, and the incisors aligned through only mesial slicing of the primary second molars. At 13 years 0 months of age, after a treatment of slightly more than 2 years, a good result was obtained; headgear treatment was supported by the use of partial fixed appliances with brackets at the maxillary incisors for a short period of time (C, D). Thirteen years later, at 26 years of age, the dentition had changed little (E, F). However, insufficient space had remained for the maxillary second and third molars, partly because of the use of the headgear. At 10 years 8 months of age, sufficient space for the permanent maxillary second molars was anticipated. However, after treatment, they were buccally tipped and distally inclined (G). At 26 years of age, the third molars had emerged but were malpositioned (H). After they had been extracted, the position of the second molars improved (I). As mentioned before and demonstrated in Fig 4-9, the increase in size of the posterior section of the apical area can be inhibited through the use of a headgear. The absence of third molars, as in the patient in Fig 4-18, furthers the correct positioning of second molars. However, early removal of maxillary third molars is not recommended.

In conclusion, some remarks are made regarding the instruction of patients, and the application and recall procedures in headgear treatments.

The patient has to be well informed and well motivated. The headgear must be worn 14 hours a day. Elementary school children are requested to wear the headgear during sleeping hours and in classes; older children are instructed to wear the appliance not at school but instead in the evenings. The headgear should be removed during meals and contact sports. Sometimes, the permanent maxillary first molars are sensitive to occluding in the morning. That is not abnormal; however, if it is painful, then a too great or incorrectly directed force has been used.

The headgear may never be removed with the elastic hooked on at both sides. In several countries, eye injuries have been reported when the headgear was removed with attached elastics.[1, 175, 176, 201] In addition, a headgear can become loose while the patient is sleeping and cause injury.[152] As a solution, elastic devices that release with a strong pull have been introduced.

At the start of the treatment, the headgear should be only slightly activated, and the elastic force should be kept small at about 200 g. At the next appointment, the activation can be increased, and the force of the elastic can be augmented to between 400 and 500 g.

After instruction, the patient has to learn how to insert and remove the headgear and hook on the elastic. If the elastic is fixed at the left side of the outer bow, the handling of the headgear becomes easier for the patient as well as for the right-handed clinician. The clinician has to examine several aspects when the patient returns for the next appointment, 6 to 8 weeks after delivery of the appliance. The height of the centerpiece is the most important of these factors. An excessive upward movement of the centerpiece is a sign that the outer bows had been positioned too high, causing the apices of the first molars to tip distally. The activation of the expansion and the rotation of the molars have to be checked and adjusted, and the fixation of the molar band must be confirmed. In addition, the dentition must be examined to ensure that the maxillary second molars are being well cleaned.

When the effects of the treatment are evaluated, attention has to be paid to the transverse occlusion of the permanent first molars and the sagittal improvement of the occlusion of the posterior and anterior teeth.

When it is obvious that the applied elastic force is satisfactory, it should not be increased. Furthermore, by bending the head backward, the force exerted by a cervical headgear increases. Sometimes it is assumed that a patient with a headgear should sleep on his or her back, but there is no need for that. During sleep, the position of the body changes so frequently that the headgear functions as intended.

Most of the time, headgear treatment alone will not deliver the desired result. In general, a deep bite will not be sufficiently reduced, and malalignments of incisors will be only partially corrected. With additional use of a maxillary plate and/or partial fixed appliances, these and other shortcomings can be corrected.

Combination of extraoral traction with an activator or other functional appliances increases the potential for improvement within a limited period of time, as will be explained in chapter 7.

Use of Headgear-Plate Combinations
With Herman Boersma

The potential to influence the facial growth and development of the dentition at an early age can be used in the treatment of Class II division 1 malocclusion. About half of the required correction can be realized, for example, with a headgear and the other half by tooth movements. As clarified in chapter 4, permanent maxillary first molars can be derotated and distalized. In addition, the space that becomes available when the primary molars are replaced by the narrower premolars can be utilized when the permanent first molars are restrained from migrating mesially.

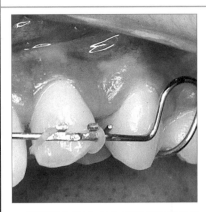

The tooth movement mesial to the permanent first molars can be carried out by a plate. With pigtail springs the premolars and canines can be distalized and with labial arches incisors retruded and improved in position. Prior to the movement of the incisors, the deep bite should have been corrected with the bite plane.

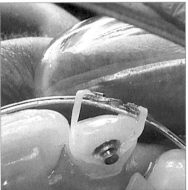

Good results can be obtained by the combination of a headgear and a plate. However, that does not apply to patients with a severely deviating sagittal jaw relationship and excessive space in the maxillary dental arch, to patients in whom the maxillary incisors are overerupted or positioned steeply, or to patients with a high lip line.

Well suited for such treatment are moderate Class II division 1 malocclusions with normal mandibular and maxillary dental arches and a favorable growth pattern. The combined approach works especially well for treatment of crowding in the maxilla. In that case, the plate should not be used before sufficient dental arch length has been gained.

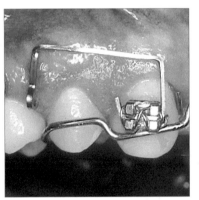

It is essential that the plate be worn all the time, except during cleaning of the dentition and the plate; otherwise the deep bite will not be corrected. The headgear should be worn 14 hours a day, no more and no less.

In the preceding two chapters, the use of plates and headgears was explained. Hence, the general aspects of handling these appliances will not be discussed in this chapter.

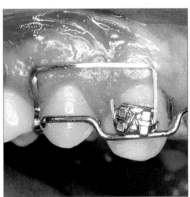

Orthodontic Concepts and Strategies

5

FIGURE 5-1

Buccally positioned canines can be moved palatally with an elastic placed on hooks attached for that purpose. The elastic should only touch the teeth to be moved (A). Similarly, maxillary incisors can be retruded and rotated with an elastic that extends from the connection between the inner and outer bows on one side to a hook placed on the other side (B).[215]

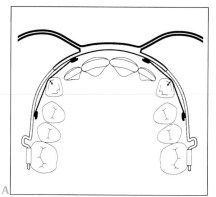
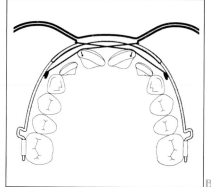

FIGURE 5-2

If one outer bow is shortened, and the other bow is bent away from the cheek, an asymmetric action can be realized (A). The smaller force is exerted at the side where the inner bow has been shortened. At the molar on the other side, the greater force is combined with a palatal component, which may lead to a palatal movement or even crossbite of the molar (B). This movement can be counteracted with a plate and through widening of the inner bow.

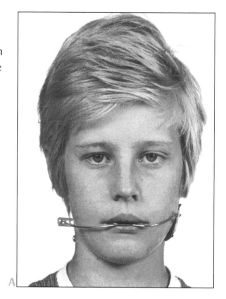
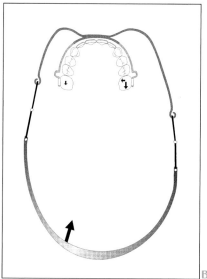

Buccally erupted maxillary canines will be pushed palatally when sufficient space for movement is available in the dental arch. As explained in chapter 4, headgear interferes with this spontaneous correction, because the cheeks and lips are kept away from the teeth. With elastics attached to the headgear, the canines can be moved palatally. In a comparable way, incisors can be retruded and rotated slightly (Fig 5-1).[215]

When later use of a plate is planned, the retraction of incisors with elastics on a headgear makes little sense, because movements can be better controlled with labial arches. Early palatal movement of buccally positioned maxillary canines through the use of elastics on the headgear is more meaningful, because the labial arches of the subsequently used plate will not have to extend as far.

With an asymmetric headgear, a differential force can be applied to the permanent maxillary first molars. In that approach, the reaction force is not absorbed at the center of the neck but more to the side, where the smallest force is applied (Fig 5-2). The undesirable palatally directed force at the first molar, at which the greatest force is applied, can be neutralized with a plate.

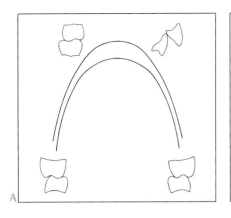
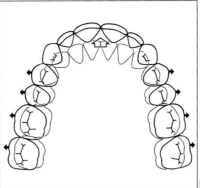

FIGURE 5-3

In a Class II division 1 malocclusion, the maxillary dental arch is too narrow, because its width is partly determined by the occlusion. In addition, the mandibular incisors overerupt (A). As the disto-occlusion becomes corrected, the parabolic shape of the dental arches will lead to a gradual widening of the maxillary dental arch through the interdigitation of the posterior teeth. This phenomenon is called the rail mechanism (B).

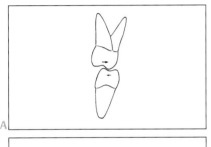
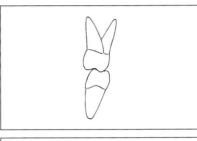
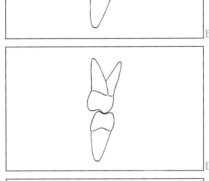
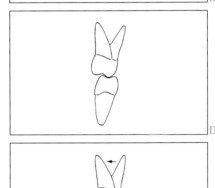

FIGURE 5-4

After emergence, posterior teeth are guided into occlusion through the cone-funnel mechanism, and an initially deviating relationship (A) will improve (B). When the bite is raised with a bite plane, while the disto-occlusion improves, the maxillary teeth will be stimulated to move buccally (C) through the functioning of the cone-funnel mechanism when occlusal contact is reached again (D). Before a solid intercuspation is attained, the apices will also move buccally (E). A cervical headgear stimulates this movement of the apices as it exerts an occlusally directed force on the buccal side of the crown (F).

As explained previously, the primary factor in Class II division 1 malocclusions is the disto-occlusion of the dental arches. In general, the width of the mandibular dental arch will be normal. However, the width of the maxillary dental arch will be adapted to the width of the mandibular dental arch through the occlusion. Consequently, the maxillary dental arch will be narrower than normal. When the mandibular dental arch attains a more anterior position, the maxillary dental arch will widen through the "rail" mechanism (Fig 5-3).

Therefore, when the transverse occlusion is maintained or established again, the adaptation in width in the maxilla will often consist of apposition of bone at the midpalatal suture. Furthermore, the maxillary alveolar process can remodel by apposition and resorption of bone; this is less the case in the mandible. With the use of a combination of a headgear and a plate, the position of the posterior teeth can improve spontaneously. Furthermore, the headgear can contribute to the widening of the maxillary dental arch and to the buccal movement of the apices of the maxillary first molars (Fig 5-4).

FIGURE 5-5

Interpositioning of the tongue in the posterior region interferes with adjustments ensuing from the occlusion of the maxillary teeth with the mandibular teeth (A). Depending on the extent of the tongue interpositioning, the teeth involved will have no contact at all or will make contact only at the buccal cusps (B). During orthodontic treatment, open bites can increase and displace.

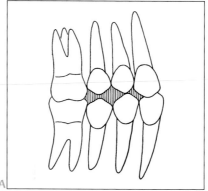

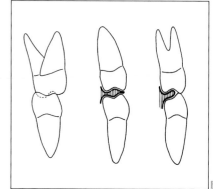

FIGURE 5-6

In a complete open bite and non-occlusion, contact between mandibular and maxillary teeth is nonexistent or incomplete (A). A lack of adjustment in the transverse and sagittal occlusion of all opposing teeth is an indication of a complete open bite and non-occlusion (B).

With aging, one third to one half of open bites and non-occlusions close spontaneously.

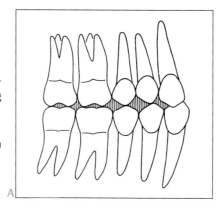

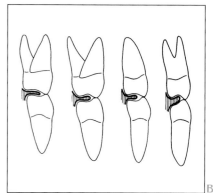

The absence of a solid intercuspation is usually the result of tongue interpositioning in the posterior regions. In such cases the maxillary dental arch will be too narrow, because the "cone-funnel" mechanism and the rail mechanism cannot function. The non-occluding premolars and molars are inclined buccally in the maxilla and less lingually in the mandible than they are when a solid transverse intercuspation exists. In the sagittal direction, the coordinating role of the occlusion is not satisfied.

The reaction to orthodontic treatment of Class II division 1 malocclusions with an open bite or non-occlusion in the posterior region differs from the reaction of malocclusions with a solid intercuspation. The narrow maxillary dental arch will not widen spontaneously. A complicating factor is the tendency for an increase in the open bite during treatment.

Most open bites and non-occlusions in the posterior region are incomplete and are limited to the premolars (Fig 5-5). When the molars are also involved in the interpositioning of the tongue, these teeth will not occlude fully (Fig 5-6). Although a headgear can guide the growth of the jaws, the treatment result will not be secured by the occlusion. Unfortunately, it is difficult to predict if an open bite will close spontaneously with aging and if a non-occlusion will resolve.

As explained earlier, in addition to the narrow maxillary dental arch, the increased overjet and overbite and increased curve of Spee have to be considered as secondary factors in a Class II division 1 malocclusion. With headgear treatment, the maxillary dental arch widens spontaneously, but the deep bite is insufficiently reduced in most cases. In general, the overjet will only partially improve, because the deep bite is a hindrance.

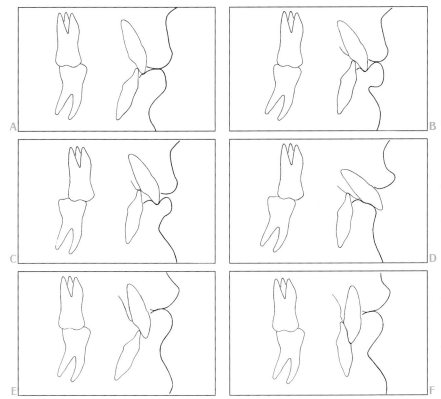

FIGURE 5-7

In normal occlusion, there is a small overjet and overbite, and the maxillary incisors are covered by the upper lip to a large extent (A). In a mild disto-occlusion, the overbite is increased, but the maxillary incisors are not overerupted because of the resistance provided by the lower lip (B). Lip resistance can also be present in a more severe disto-occlusion with a large overjet and overbite (C). However, when the lower lip is positioned palatal to the maxillary incisors, these teeth will overerupt (D). When the maxillary incisors are not intruded, or the anterior lower facial height is increased only slightly, the lower lip will cover the maxillary incisors excessively after treatment (E). Subsequently, the pressure from the lower lip will tip the maxillary incisor in the palatal direction, and a coverbite will develop. Secondarily, the mandibular incisors are tipped lingually (F).

In Class II division 1 malocclusions, the relationship between the incisors and the lips is of great importance. When the lower lip support the maxillary incisors vertically, these teeth will not overerupt. If lip support is inadequate, then the treatment becomes more complex (Fig 5-7). When the lower lip becomes positioned palatal to the maxillary incisors, early treatment is indicated to prevent the overeruption of these teeth and to reduce the risk of their fracturing.

Headgear treatment in patients in whom the lower lip is positioned palatal to the maxillary incisors will lead to an improvement in the posterior regions but not in the anterior region, and excessive spacing will develop in the maxillary dental arch. The lip interpositioning can be eliminated with a lip bumper in the mandible that keeps the lower lip positioned forward and allows the mandibular incisors to move labially.

A coverbite can develop, and maxillary incisors can overerupt after orthodontic treatment, when the lower lip covers too much of the labial surfaces of the maxillary incisors (Fig 5-7, E and F).[215] In extreme cases, the labial gingiva of the mandibular incisors can be stripped, and the palatal mucosa can be damaged.

In severe Class II division 1 malocclusions, an acceptable result cannot be reached with only a headgear and a plate. The deviating sagittal relationship and tooth positions will not be corrected as required. With the additional use of partial fixed appliances in the maxilla, various shortcomings can be corrected, as will be demonstrated later (see chapter 9). The same applies, as already mentioned, to combined headgear-activator treatment, which offers more possibilities to improve the maxillomandibular relationships than a headgear alone (see chapter 8).

FIGURE 5-8

The headgear is placed first to treat the disto-occlusion because it is the primary factor in the malocclusion and because this correction requires the longest treatment time (A). When the headgear is placed prior to the loss of the primary maxillary second molars, the mesial migration of the permanent first molars can be prevented (B). When sufficient space has been obtained in the maxillary dental arch, the plate is placed (C, D). The divided labial arches run adjacent to the mesial marginal ridges of the second premolars. After the first premolars have been moved against the second premolars, the pigtail spring continues to distalize both teeth. In that procedure, the section of the labial arch that runs between the premolars has to be adapted. After the plate is built up with quick-curing acrylic resin around the palatal side of the premolars and the ends of the springs are built in, the canines are activated. In the meantime, the height of the bite plane is increased stepwise. The incisors should not be retruded before the canines have been distalized and quick-curing acrylic resin has been placed around the ends of the springs and at the mesial and palatal surfaces of the canines (E). Only after that has been completed can the acrylic resin be trimmed away palatal to the incisors and at the anterior alveolar region (F).

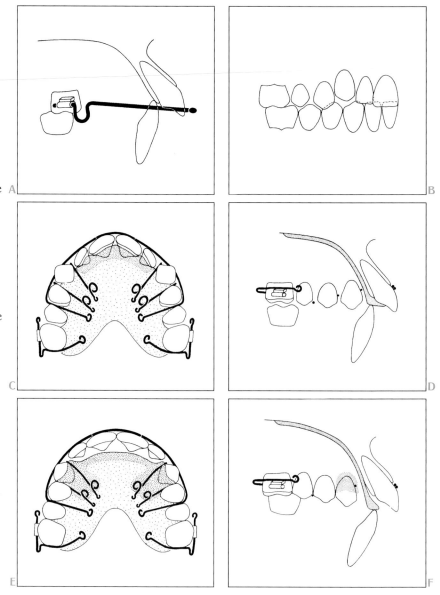

As a rule, sufficient space in the maxillary dental arch should have been gained before the plate is placed. However, sometimes earlier use is indicated, such as with a deep bite and contact in the anterior region. When sufficient space is already available at the start of treatment, the plate should be placed shortly after the headgear. That also applies to everted incisors with diastemata (Fig 5-8).

When the premolars are distalized, the labial arch should not be a hindrance and should not interfere with their spontaneous buccal movement. When a canine is distalized, the movement can be guided between the labial arch and the trimmed margin of the plate.

It is impossible to retrude the incisors and reduce the deep bite at the same time, because the plate will tip when the mandibular incisors occlude at the bite plane.

In an anterior open bite, the incisors should not be retruded before the premolars and canines have been moved distally; otherwise, the cumulative reaction forces will move the permanent first molars mesially, particularly if the headgear is not worn as prescribed.

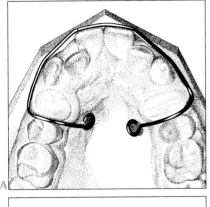

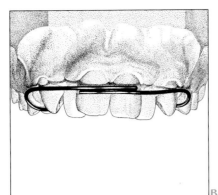

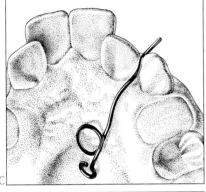

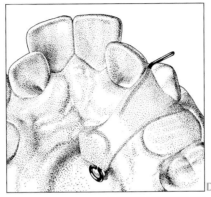

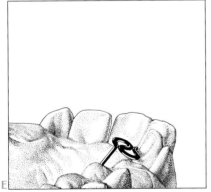

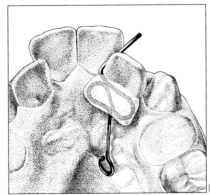

A
B
C
D
E
F

FIGURE 5-9
Divided labial arches, described by Booy[35] and fabricated of 0.8-mm spring hard stainless steel wire, have certain advantages over a continuous labial arch. Divided labial arches can be activated well, generate small, long-lasting forces, and provide adequate labial guidance when distalizing canines (A, B). However, they easily deform. If the patient wipes his or her mouth with a sleeve, a labial arch can hook in a sweater and bend away.[29] Pigtail springs of 0.6 mm are suitable for distalizing premolars and canines. A large coil provides extra length and great flexibility (C, D). Before the plate is placed, the extensions of the springs have to be shortened. They have to be embedded in the acrylic resin at the cervical portion on the mesial side of the crowns when the anterior teeth are retracted. Protrusion springs cannot be combined with a bite plane used to reduce the deep bite (E, F), because these springs produce a reaction force that tends to move the plate away from the palate. In addition, these springs make the plate so thick in the anterior region that the distance between the molars becomes more than 1.5 mm. These shortcomings are avoided when, instead of a protrusion spring, an elastic is extended from a button on the palatal side of the involved tooth to a hook on the continuous labial arch, as explained in chapter 3.

The height of the bite plane should be increased stepwise. The procedures involved and essential factors to consider have been described in chapter 3. While the canines are distalized, the deep bite can still be corrected. After that is accomplished, the bite plane serves only as vertical support for the mandibular anterior teeth when the posterior teeth occlude.

Occlusion on metal parts, and the hindrance of distal and buccal movement of premolars by the metal parts, should be avoided. The end of the clasp around the third molar rests at the tube but is not in contact with the buccal side of the molar. In addition, when the plate is removed the clasp is pushed away from the tooth, leading the end of the clasp to bend buccally over time.

The labial arches should not be in contact with the buccal surfaces of the premolars as long as these teeth have to move buccally. Furthermore, proper trimming and buildup of the margin of the plate are essential (Fig 5-9).

FIGURE 5-10

The correct positioning of a labial arch can be controlled through finger pressure (A). Where the wire makes contact and how much force is exerted locally can be checked with a piece of silk floss placed under the arch. A long, narrow, tapered acrylic resin bur should be used to trim the margin. For retrusion of the maxillary incisors, the orientation of the side of the acrylic resin bur should correspond to the palatal surface of the incisors (B). A labial arch can be folded back to move a first premolar or canine palatally (C). The end of a labial arch can be modified to intrude an incisor (D). Resin composite buildups can provide more retention and facilitate the extrusion of teeth.[48]

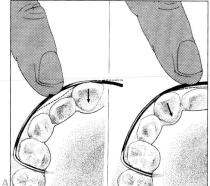
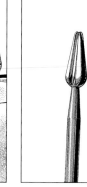
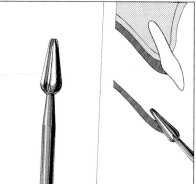
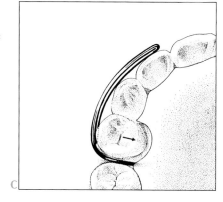
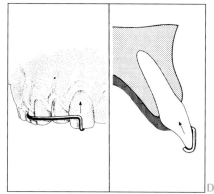

Effective use of a plate depends largely on the fixation of the plate. In that respect, not only a correct fit and anchorage are important. Occluding on metal parts is not only uncomfortable but also causes the plate to dislodge and increases the chance of breakage and deformation of metal parts.

Besides clasps, labial arches provide some retention, for which they have to be activated. Of course, for effective clasp function, the acrylic resin has to be in close contact with the palatal side of the teeth involved.

In retracting incisors, good fit of the acrylic resin at the canines and premolars provides extra retention. That applies particularly to the mesial side of the canines.

When labial arches have to work selectively, firm control over the points where they touch is essential (Fig 5-10, A). Strategic trimming of the margin of the plate is also key to success (Fig 5-10, B). When incisors are being retracted not only the acrylic resin palatal to the crown but also the acrylic resin located more cranially at the alveolar process should be removed. The roots should have the freedom to move palatally, and the overlying alveolar process should have the freedom to remodel.

According to the need, a labial arch can be modified, for example, to move a premolar palatally or to intrude an incisor (Fig 5-10, C and D). An incisor can be extruded by placement of a resin composite stop at the labial surface and placement of the labial bow on top of it. An incisor can be intruded in a comparable way; however, this will cause a reaction force that tends to move the plate away from the palate. Therefore, effective retention of the plate is required, particularly in the anterior region. Furthermore, a plate with a bite plane has the additional advantage that the movements of posterior teeth are not hindered by the occlusion.

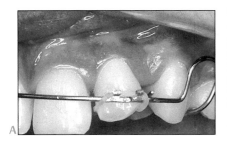
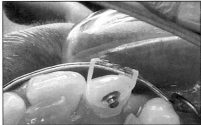

FIGURE 5-11

Simultaneous reduction of a deep bite and protrusion of a maxillary incisor can be carried out with a bite plane and an elastic on a continuous labial arch (A, B). Thereafter the appliance can be changed to divided labial arches.

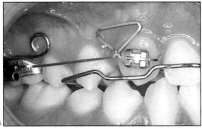
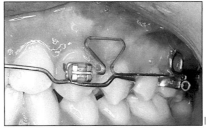
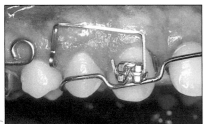
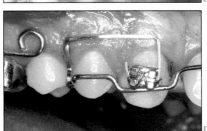

FIGURE 5-12

Canines can be uprighted with a bracket and a sectional wire (A). The labial arch should lie against the bracket when extrusion has to be prevented (B). A rectangular uprighting spring that is hooked under the labial arch also can be used. This construction results in a reciprocal force that is transmitted to the canine and prevents its extrusion when the labial wire is in contact with the bracket before the spring is attached (C). The spring should fit precisely in the bracket and be ligated tightly (D). With this construction, teeth also can be rotated.

As explained in chapter 3, some movements can be performed more effectively with elastics than with springs (Fig 5-11).

A specific problem regards the uprighting of distally tipped canines. Such a correction is less often required for premolars, because they tend to be uprighted by the occlusion. Furthermore, they usually require movement over a shorter distance and are not tipped as far distally as the canines. Particularly in malocclusions with a large overjet and excessive space in the dental arch initially, a canine has to be moved distally over a great distance and will tip accordingly. The deviating angulation can be corrected by the placement of a bracket on the canine crown and a rectangular wire extending from the bracket to the molar tube, with or without a loop, to increase the flexibility. With this device, the canine can also be moved further distally (Fig 5-12, A and B). An uprighting spring, with its end hooked under the labial arch, also can be utilized (Fig 5-12, C and D). This construction offers better control, particularly in the vertical direction, but requires some dexterity by the patient, who has to release the extension when removing the plate for cleaning, and reattach it later, without deforming the device. Experience has revealed that most patients learn to do that well. Undesirable labiopalatal movements can be prevented by the margin of the plate and by the labial arch, and mesial movements can be prevented by the end of the pigtail spring, embedded in acrylic resin.

After a plate is added to the headgear, the inner bow has to be lengthened to avoid interference with the labial arches. The inner bow has to be widened when constructions, as described, are used in the posterior region. Of course, at every appointment it must be confirmed that the headgear and other appliances do not hinder or counteract each other.

Good results can be obtained with the combination of a headgear and a removable maxillary plate, although the possibilities are limited (Figs 5-13 to 5-18).

FIGURE 5-13

A boy aged 10 years 7 months had a Class II division 1 malocclusion, competent lip seal, and a profile that was normal for his age. The disto-occlusion, measuring the width of half a premolar crown, was due not so much to a deviating maxillomandibular relationship as to an abnormal positioning of the teeth. The maxillary incisors were tipped labially, while the overjet was only 4 mm. Sufficient space was available in both dental arches (A, B). At the age of 10 years 9 months, a cervical headgear was placed, and 7 months later a maxillary plate was added. At the age of 11 years 3 months, the occlusion had improved so much that the headgear could be discontinued. The bite was raised with the plate, and subsequently the anterior teeth were retracted. At the age of 12 years 4 months, an acceptable result was obtained (C, D). The records collected 5 years later, at the age of 17 years 3 months (E, F), as well as the records 10 years after treatment, at the age of 22 years 2 months (G, H), showed a stable situation.

The essential improvements in this treatment were realized with the plate. The headgear was needed only for a short period of time, because the growth pattern was favorable for the correction of the disto-occlusion. There was sufficient space to retract the maxillary incisors, which ended up in a good inclination, because of the initial eversion. Because the maxillary incisors were not arranged irregularly and did not deviate vertically, a simple maxillary plate without extra devices sufficed to reach a good result.

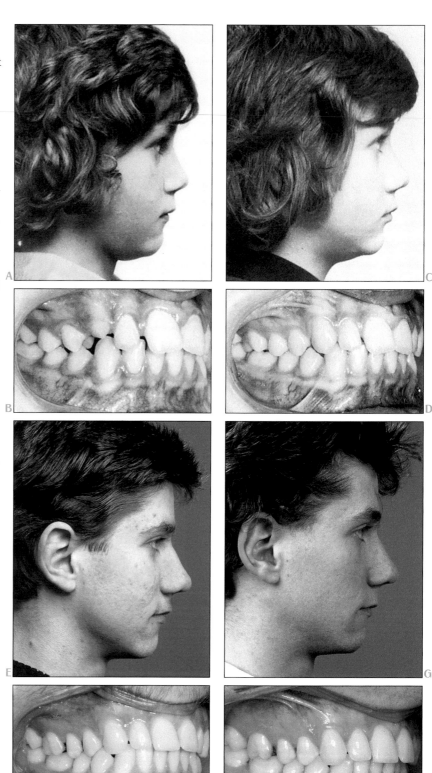

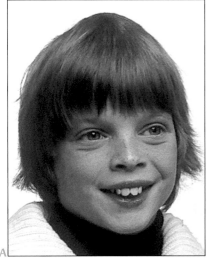

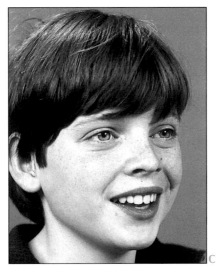

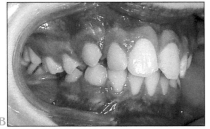

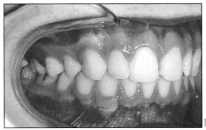

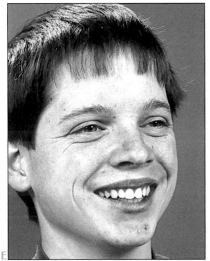

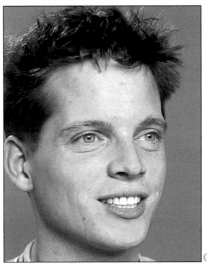

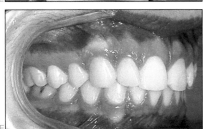

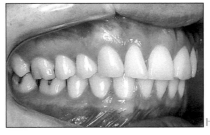

FIGURE 5-14

A boy aged 11 years 1 month had a Class II division 1 malocclusion with an overjet of 10 mm. There was sufficient space in both dental arches, which showed few irregularities. The primary maxillary second molars were still present (A, B). At the age of 11 years 3 months, a cervical headgear was placed. Quite some time later, at the age of 14 years 6 months, a maxillary plate was added. There was no need to add a plate earlier, because excessive space did not develop in the maxillary dental arch and the bite was not deep. With the plate, first the canines were distalized and subsequently the incisors were retracted and rotated. At the age of 15 years 4 months, the treatment was concluded and a pleasing result was obtained (C, D). In the following years, the intercuspation improved as the mandibular dental arch advanced slightly in relation to the maxillary dental arch. This change was apparent in the records collected 2 years later, at the age of 17 years 5 months (E, F), and 8 years later, at the age of 25 years 5 months.

An optimal result was obtained in this patient with only a cervical headgear and a maxillary plate. Initially, there was a distoocclusion measuring half a premolar crown width, some spacing was present in the maxillary dental arch, there were no abnormalities in the mandibular dental arch, and the maxillary incisors were not overerupted and not malaligned vertically. Furthermore, the appliances were worn as required, and facial growth was favorable.

FIGURE 5-15

A boy of 9 years 11 months had a Class II division 1 malocclusion and had prematurely lost the primary maxillary right canine. The maxillary incisors were not inverted but had drifted to the right side, and no space remained for the right canine. The overjet was 3 mm; the overbite was 2 mm (A, B). At the age of 10 years 5 months, a cervical headgear was placed to create more space in the maxillary dental arch. At the age of 11 years 0 months, a Crefcoeur plate was added; the separation was located at the site of the maxillary right canine. Later this canine was moved distally with an elastic attached from a button to the clasp around the molar. After sufficient space was gained at the age of 12 years 11 months, the Crefcoeur plate was replaced by a maxillary plate with divided labial arches to retract the incisors and improve the position of the canines. The treatment was concluded at the age of 13 years 6 months, but a solid occlusion of the premolars had not been reached on either side (C, D). Two years later, at the age of 15 years 8 months (E, F), and 5 years later, at the age of 18 years 8 months, no solid intercuspation of the premolars had been established on either side, although the interocclusal clearance had been reduced slightly (G, H).

As explained previously, a Crefcoeur plate is well suited for increasing space locally in the dental arch and for correcting midline deviations while reducing a deep bite at the same time.

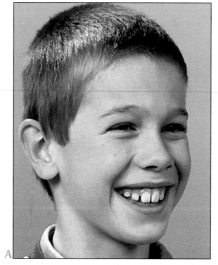

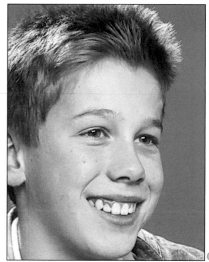

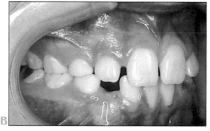

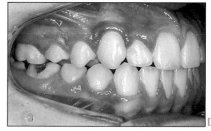

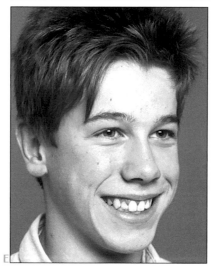

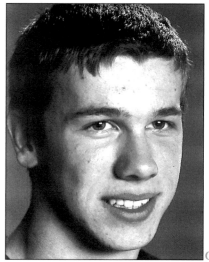

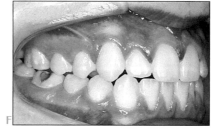

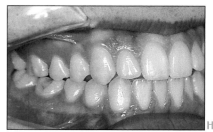

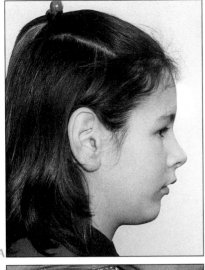

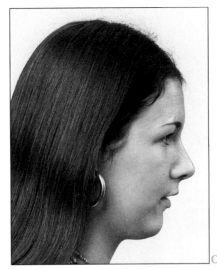

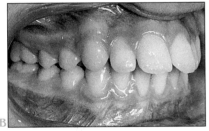

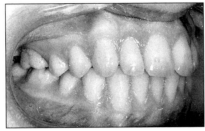

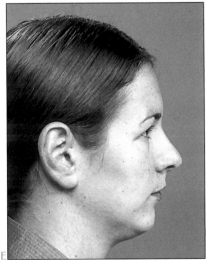

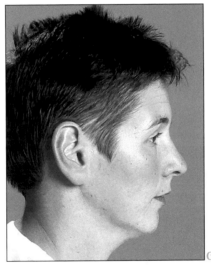

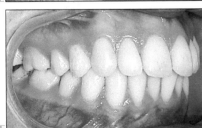

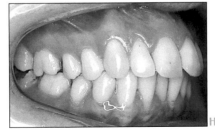

FIGURE 5-16

A girl who was 12 years 6 months of age had a Class II division 1 malocclusion with quite regular dental arches. The transition was completed, the premolars and canines were in disto-occlusion of half a premolar crown width, and the permanent first molars were in a complete disto-occlusion. The permanent second molars had emerged already (A, B). Regrettably, the treatment was postponed for 5 months, and then a cervical headgear was placed. Twelve months later, at the age of 14 years 1 month, a maxillary plate was added. The height of the bite plane was increased regularly, and the first premolars and canines were distalized with pigtail springs. The incisors were brought to the proper position with the labial arches. After the age of 15 years 6 months, the plate was kept in only during sleeping hours for retention purposes. The records collected at the end of the treatment, at the age of 16 years 8 months, showed a good result (C, D). Seven years later, at the age of 24 years 1 month, none of the realized improvements had been lost (E, F). The same was true 15 years after treatment, at the age of 34 years 1 month (G, H).

This treatment was started too late. The transition was completed, and the space that becomes available with the replacement of the primary molars by the premolars could not be utilized for the correction of the disto-occlusion. Nevertheless, a good result was obtained in this patient, because of the limited disto-occlusion (half a premolar crown width), the extra space available in the maxillary dental arch, and the eversion of the maxillary incisors.

FIGURE 5-17

A boy of 10 years 6 months had a Class II division 1 malocclusion with an overjet of 11 mm and an overbite of only 2 mm. The primary maxillary second molars were still present, and in both dental arches the available space was more than sufficient (A, B). At the age of 10 years 9 months, a cervical headgear was placed; 6 months later a maxillary plate was placed. The premolars and canines were distalized with pigtail springs. Thereafter, the incisors were retracted with divided labial arches. During the last 6 months of treatment, the plate was worn only during sleeping hours. The records collected at the age of 13 years 6 months showed that a good occlusion was reached in the posterior regions; however, the maxillary incisors were too upright. In addition, diastemata remained distal of the maxillary lateral incisors (C, D). In the following years, the maxillary incisors tipped more palatally and the diastemata closed, as was apparent in the records collected 2 years after treatment, at the age of 15 years 5 months (E, F), and 3 years after that, at the age of 18 years 7 months (G, H).

This patient is shown to demonstrate two important limitations of the approach presented in this chapter. With a plate, maxillary incisors cannot be torqued, and they cannot be intruded sufficiently. Both of these movements were required in this patient. If the mandible had experienced more growth in the anterior direction, the maxillary incisors would not have had to be retruded as far to reach sagittal contact and would not have attained such an upright position. However, when the lower lip covers the maxillary incisors excessively, a coverbite can develop.

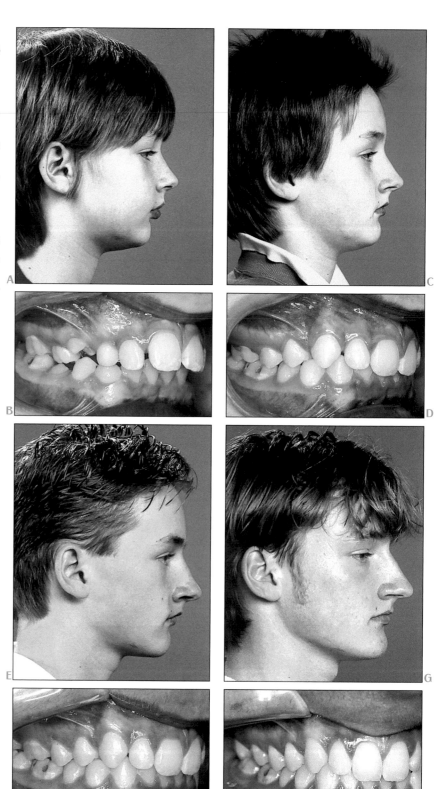

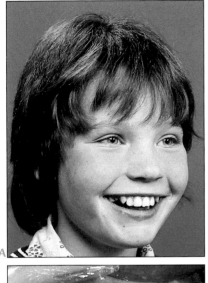

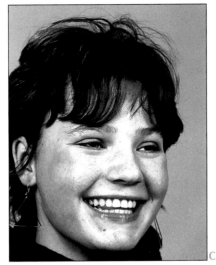

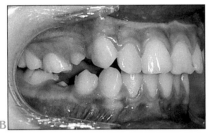

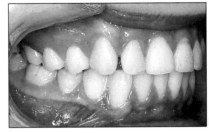

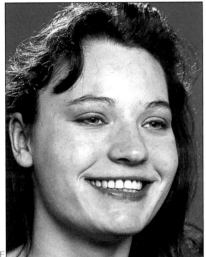

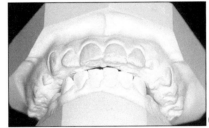

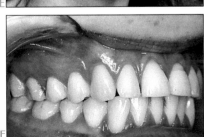

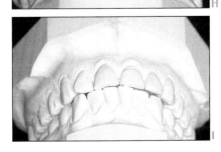

Figure 5-18

A girl aged 10 years 5 months had a broad face and a Class II division 1 malocclusion with a mild disto-occlusion. The primary maxillary second molars and the primary mandibular left second molar were still present. The overjet was 8 mm, the overbite was 3 mm, and in both dental arches sufficient space was present. However, a complete scissors bite existed on both sides (A, B, G). The inner bow of the cervical headgear was compressed to reduce the width of the maxillary dental arch. The disto-occlusion could be corrected without additional appliances, because of the anteriorly directed growth of the mandible. Six months after placement of the headgear, a removable maxillary plate with modified three-quarter clasps around the bands at the first molars, pigtail springs mesial of the first premolars and canines, and divided labial arches was placed. A bite plane was not required, because the overbite was small and the incisors were not in contact with each other. The clearance was sufficient, and the bite did not have to be raised. After the premolars and canines were distalized, the incisors were retracted. At the age of 14 years 1 month, the treatment was concluded. A good result with a solid intercuspation in the posterior regions was established. However, the maxillary right lateral incisor was still rotated (C, D, H). The records collected 5 years later, at the age of 19 years 3 months, showed that the result had been maintained. The diastema distal of the maxillary right lateral incisor had closed (E, F, I).

FIGURE 5-19

According to Bass,[11] a maxillary plate can be combined with a parietal headgear to intrude and torque maxillary incisors. The ends of the J-hooks are placed in the coils of the torquing springs, while the incisal edges are firmly embedded in the acrylic resin.

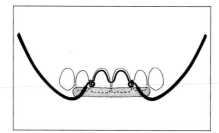
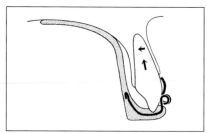

In malocclusions with a deep bite, a cervical headgear has distinct advantages over a parietal headgear. A cervical headgear can exert a mild extruding force on the permanent maxillary first molars, move the apices buccally, and control their mesiodistal angulation. Even with an open bite or non-occlusion in the anterior region, a cervical headgear is preferred. However, in patients with excess lower facial height, a parietal headgear has some advantages.

Bass[11] introduced a specially designed headgear and removable plate combination, aimed at intruding maxillary incisors and moving their apices palatally (Fig 5-19). In this design, the vertical support for the intrusive forces is provided by the acrylic resin that covers the incisal edges of the incisors.

With a headgear, molars can be rotated in their place, but they also can be moved distally to some extent. Most of the time, distal movement is hindered by the adjacent permanent second molar. When that molar is extracted, space for distal movement becomes available for the first molar. In patients with an asymmetric occlusion, the unilateral extraction of a permanent maxillary second molar can be a good solution. However, that only applies when the third molar is present.

When sufficient space is present in the maxillary dental arch, distal movement of the permanent first molars should be avoided. The modified three-quarter clasp offers insufficient resistance to such movement, but an additional straight piece of 0.9 mm-wire positioned against the distal surface is adequate.

For patients with Class II division 1 malocclusions and well-aligned dental arches, particularly young patients, treatment with an activator or similar appliance is preferred over a headgear.

Biologically based variations in reaction limit the predictability of results of orthodontic therapies. The estimated duration of the treatment is a good example of this phenomenon. The effects of the therapy also can deviate from the expectation. For example, a symmetric headgear may lead to an asymmetric outcome, and spontaneous widening of the maxillary dental arch does not occur in all instances. Sometimes premolars and/or canines do not have to be moved actively to the distal. Therefore, changes from the previous conditions should be carefully observed at every recall appointment.

Continuous wearing of the headgear and the use of excessive forces can result in large tooth movements and crowding of the permanent second and third molars. Furthermore, root resorption of permanent first molars has been observed.[112] Sometimes premolars and canines are tipped too far distally. In severe Class II division 1 malocclusions, the combination of a headgear with an activator might be the better solution.

Use of Activators and Other Functional Appliances

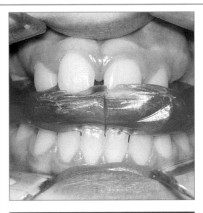

The activator was introduced in 1924 by a Norwegian, Viggo Andresen,[7] and has been further developed mainly in the German-speaking countries. For many years, the book *Funktionskieferorthopädie*, by Andresen, Häupl, and Petrik,[8] served as the standard work.

Many modifications of activators have been developed[84, 88], as have comparable appliances with a flexible rather than a rigid design.[21, 189] Furthermore, Fränkel[69, 70] has invented and advocated the function regulator.

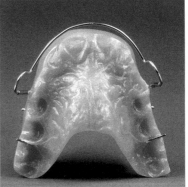

Activators and other functional appliances are used to correct malocclusions in young patients by influencing growth, eliminating functional disturbances, and correcting tooth positions. They are suited particularly to treating Class II division 1 malocclusions without further complications.

Activators and other functional appliances can correct disto-occlusions and deep bites, in addition to retruding or protruding mandibular and maxillary incisors, but cannot upright or torque teeth and are limited in improving rotations. Furthermore, these appliances do not provide sufficient control to complete treatments in which permanent teeth have been extracted.

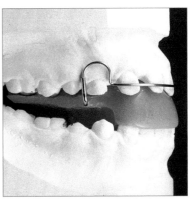

Activators and other functional appliances deliver the best results in patients who do not have a large lower anterior facial height and who exhibit anteriorly directed growth of the mandible. These appliances should not be used in patients with disturbed nasal passages or with limited intraoral space, because these patients are not able to keep the appliances in the mouth.

During the use of removable appliances, particularly those that are lying loose in the mouth, the motivation and cooperation of the patient are essential. Problems at the beginning of treatment should be anticipated.

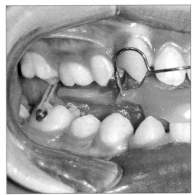

Many variations of the activator have been introduced, but the mode of operation is basically the same. The growth of the mandible is guided, particularly in the anterior and vertical directions, but the growth of the maxillary complex is also affected. About half of the improvements are realized by the movement of teeth.

6

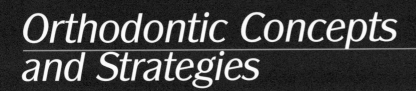

Orthodontic Concepts and Strategies

FIGURE 6-1

A Class II division 1 malocclusion that includes diastemata and eversion of the maxillary incisors and a normal mandibular dental arch can be treated well with an activator (A–D). Such treatment was carried out in this patient; the appliance is shown in Fig 6-2. The maxillary incisors were retracted with the labial arch. During the day, when the activator was not worn, the maxillary dental arch could adjust in width to the gradually more anteriorly positioned mandibular dental arch through interdigitation (rail mechanism). The obtained neutro-occlusion was secured by the solid intercuspation (E, F).

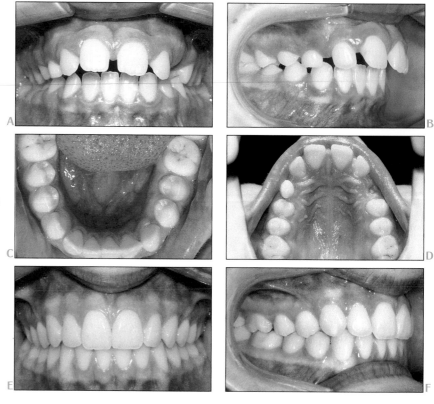

Treatment with activators should preferably start prior to the loss of the primary second molars, so the difference in mesiodistal crown dimensions between the primary molars and their successors can be utilized for the correction of the disto-occlusion. However, when treatment is started somewhat later, as in the patient shown in Fig 6-1, a satisfactory result can still be obtained when facial growth is favorable and has not been completed yet.

For the fabrication of an activator, a construction bite and a recent set of dental casts are necessary. Plaster bubbles on the occlusal surfaces of the casts should be removed.

The construction bite is made at the chair with the help of the set of dental casts (Figs 6-3 and 6-4). Because wax can make impressions of the gingiva, the areas where the wax has touched the mucosa should be cut away; otherwise, the construction bite will be stopped at the gingiva on the dental casts.

The activator has to be trimmed by the clinician and tried in the patient (Fig 6-2). The appliance delivered by the technician usually encroaches on undercuts, sometimes in the maxilla, but often in the mandible, leading to interferences that prevent the loose positioning in the mouth. These interferences should be trimmed away; the areas that restrict the eruption of the mandibular posterior teeth, namely the occlusal areas and lingual sides where the alveolar process has to remodel, should also be removed. When the acrylic resin is only in contact in the mandible with the occlusal surfaces of the incisors and the distal cusps of the most distally occluding molars, the curve of Spee can be leveled. The lingual wings of the activator should be sufficiently high to prevent the activator from being easily lost but should not have sharp facets that cause local irritations. The acrylic resin should be free of the lingual side of the mandibular anterior teeth.

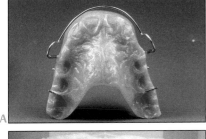

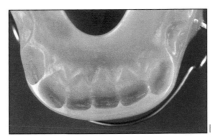

A

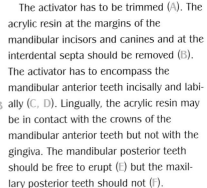

B

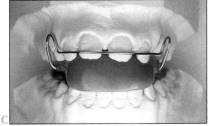

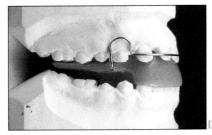

C

D

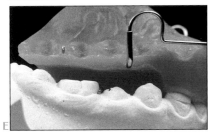

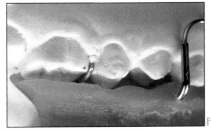

E

F

FIGURE 6-2

The activator has to be trimmed (A). The acrylic resin at the margins of the mandibular incisors and canines and at the interdental septa should be removed (B). The activator has to encompass the mandibular anterior teeth incisally and labially (C, D). Lingually, the acrylic resin may be in contact with the crowns of the mandibular anterior teeth but not with the gingiva. The mandibular posterior teeth should be free to erupt (E) but the maxillary posterior teeth should not (F).

In the maxilla, the acrylic resin is not trimmed palatal to the incisors, unless these teeth are retracted. In the posterior regions, the occlusal patterns are trimmed until only a plain acrylic resin surface remains on which the cusp tips touch, so that the posterior teeth are not hindered in their buccal movement.

The position of the support bars mesial to the permanent first molars should be checked at every appointment. These bars position the activator correctly, provide vertical support, and can also be used to block the mesial migration of the permanent first molars. The continuous labial arch should be in contact with the maxillary incisors and exert only a light pressure, while the U-loops should not touch the canines. The labial arch should be in contact with the incisal region of the maxillary incisors before the wire moves cervically, while the patient occludes with the activator in place. The acrylic resin should be trimmed from the alveolar region of an activator when incisors are retracted, to allow remodeling of the alveolar process. Unlike the mandibular posterior teeth, the maxillary posterior teeth should be blocked in their eruption by the plain occlusal surface. This approach has been advocated by Woodside,[239] on the assumption that use of an activator with a large interocclusal clearance to stimulate the mesially angulated eruption of the mandibular posterior teeth, and to block the perpendicular-to-the-occlusal-plane eruption of the maxillary posterior teeth, will result in a reduction of the distoocclusion. Others, who do not agree with this assumption, remove the acrylic resin from the occlusal surface of maxillary posterior teeth also but ensure that the support bars are located properly.

An activator has to be worn only during sleep; however, for the patient to get accustomed to the appliance, he or she should wear it some hours before going to bed. As soon as the patient awakens in the morning with the activator still in the mouth, he or she can discontinue wearing it before bedtime.

FIGURE 6-3

A construction bite should be made carefully (A, B). Two thirds of a red wax sheet is warmed by a flame, in a hot water container, or under a hot faucet (C, D). Subsequently, the soft wax is rolled without the inclusion of air (E, F). The wax roll is given a horseshoe shape and fitted on the recently obtained mandibular dental cast that encompasses the lingual sides of the alveolar processes to a sufficiently deep level. The wax roll is shaped further, given the proper width, and cut at the right length. Subsequently, the wax roll is placed again on the mandibular cast and pushed down until all teeth are covered to the occlusal half of their crown, so that the wax roll will fit well on the mandibular teeth (G, H). The patient should be informed in advance about the way a wax bite is made, and the procedure should be practiced while the patient holds a mirror.

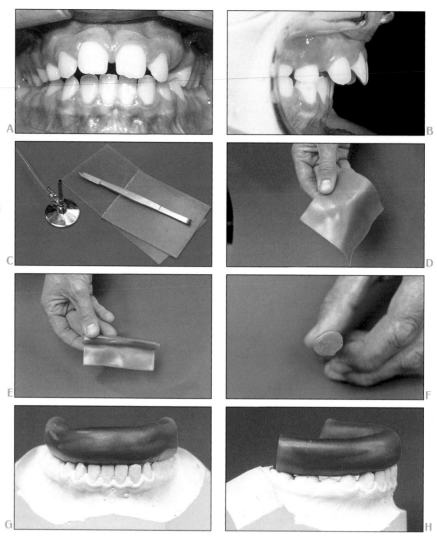

It is essential for the clinician to provide sufficient information and to demonstrates understanding of the feelings and discomfort of the patient as well as the concerns of the parents. The activator should be as convenient as possible, should not hurt, and should not cause sore spots. When the patient occludes, several teeth in both dental arches should make contact, to avoid overloading of individual teeth and to prevent movement of the activator.

Activators, as originally designed, are sturdy constructions with few metal parts, which do not deform readily; if they do deform, they can be easily returned to the correct shape. Few problems can arise between appointments, which can be 8 weeks or more apart and take little chair time. On these occasions, the patient should be asked if the appliance causes discomfort and is worn as required. The metal parts have to be examined and adapted, if needed. The mucosa must be inspected for sore spots and gingival lesions, particularly at the lingual aspect of the mandibular incisor region. Acrylic resin must be removed where teeth have to erupt and where the activator could interfere with spontaneous improvements.

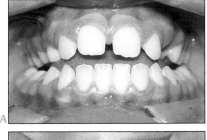

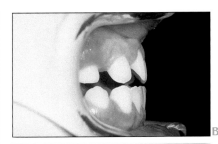

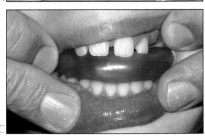

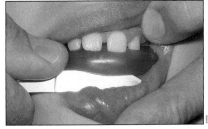

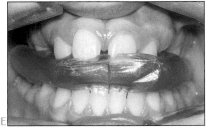

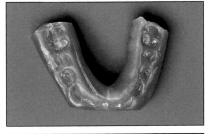

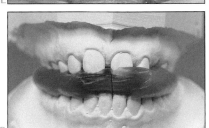

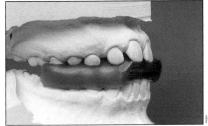

FIGURE 6-4

As a rule, a construction bite is made with the central incisors in an end-to-end position, with a distance of 3 to 4 mm between them (A, B). Under guidance, the patient occludes in the wax roll, positioned at the mandibular teeth (C), while the mandible is prevented from gliding posteriorly. Hence, starting in a more anterior position is recommended. Attention has to be paid to the aligning of the midlines of the two dental arches, which is facilitated by cutting wax away from the anterior region (D) and placing a vertical groove (E) that serves as guidance during further occlusion. After the construction bite has been removed and cooled (F), it is placed on the set of dental casts and moved around in the hand for inspection (G, H). As a rule, the midlines of the two dental arches should coincide in the construction bite. This was not done for the patient shown here, because the maxillary incisors had migrated to the right side.

In a favorable reaction to activator treatment, the maxillary posterior teeth will move away from the acrylic resin at the palatal sides. That is no problem, because the transverse position of these teeth is mainly determined by the intercuspation with the mandibular posterior teeth.

Some activators are designed with an expansion screw to widen the maxillary dental arch. However, there is no need for such a screw if the activator is worn only during sleeping hours, and the posterior teeth interdigitate well so that the "rail" mechanism can work during the day.

When a functional appliance is worn also during the day, the maxillary dental arch has to be widened actively, and a screw is appropriate. However, a standard activator is voluminous and interferes too much with speech, so that daytime wear is not feasible.

The author is not in favor of having patients wear functional appliances more than 12 hours a day, because normal physiologic processes that guide the development of the dentition, such as the rail mechanism, cannot occur.

FIGURE 6-5

The activator modified by Petrik[158] has support bars and sometimes one or more other wire constructions for tooth movement, for example, of a maxillary canine (A). Klammt[102] introduced an open activator consisting of two acrylic resin parts connected by a heavy wire (B). Bimler,[21] Stockfisch,[189] and others have designed flexible constructions that cover the mandibular incisors (C). Some of these appliances have clasps (D). Other designs contain a screw (E) or a Coffin spring (F).[107]

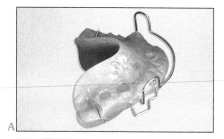
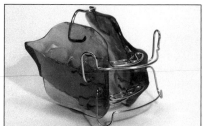
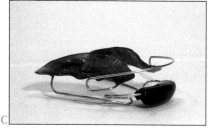
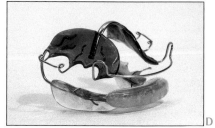
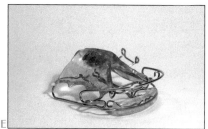
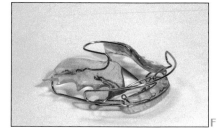
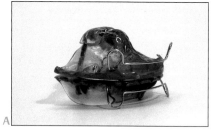
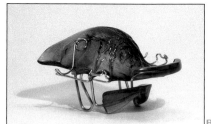

FIGURE 6-6

A stepwise advancement of the mandible in relation to the maxilla can be realized through the use of a screw placed between the two separated parts (A) or the use of heavy springs (B).[99, 235]

Indeed, the activator introduced by Andresen[8] is a rigid, firm appliance with a labial arch that incorporates U-loops at the maxillary anterior teeth. Petrik[158] reported that simple, stiff sections of wire mesial to the permanent first molars can stabilize the sagittal and vertical positions of the activator (support bars). In addition, he has introduced other stiff wire constructions that deliver forces, during occlusion, to specific teeth to promote their movement (Fig 6-5, A).[158]

To facilitate use of a functional appliance during the daytime, Balters developed a design that does not substantially disturb the speech. His bionator is free of acrylic resin palatal to the maxillary incisors.[9] The open acrtivator of Klammt is also free of acrylic resin lingual to the mandibular anterior teeth (Fig 6-5, B).[102]

While the patient occludes in the activator, teeth contact the acrylic resin. To the patient, this could feel like suddenly hitting a hard item, an unpleasant experience when only a single tooth is contacted instead of a group of teeth simultaneously. Subsequently developed, flexible functional appliance designs are more comfortable in that respect (Fig 6-5, C to F).

In addition to the appliances that force the mandible into an anterior position in one step, other designs for gradual advancement have been introduced (Fig 6-6).

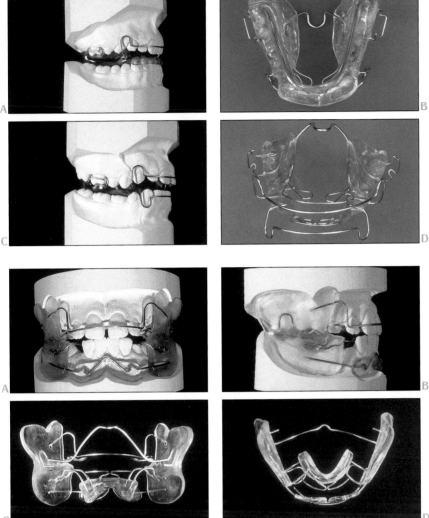

FIGURE 6-7

In open activators, the mandibular anterior teeth are usually vertically supported, and the clearance between the dental arches is substantial (A, B). When the anterior teeth have to be retracted in both jaws, two labial arches are needed (C). With springs at the lingual side of the incisors, the position of the incisors can be better controlled. With a heavy wire across the palate, the width of the appliance can be altered (D).

FIGURE 6-8

Fränkel's function regulator has buccal shields to keep the cheeks away from the posterior teeth and alveolar processes. In addition, this appliance has pads on the lingual side of the mandibular anterior region, which can be advanced (A, B). In the maxilla, the crossing wires only contact the occlusal surfaces, while in the mandible there is no contact between the appliance and the teeth (C, D).[70]

Open activators and other functional appliances with many metal parts are vulnerable and deform readily with careless use or when the patient rolls on top of the appliance during the night (Fig 6-7). Even for an experienced clinician, it is difficult and time consuming to correct such deformations.

Fränkel's function regulator is a vulnerable appliance, with its shields and pads to keep the musculature away from the teeth and alveolar processes and to bring the mandible gradually into a more anterior position (Fig 6-8). Fränkel required that his function regulators also be worn during the day.

An activator can also be utilized to prevent undesirable tooth migrations after premature loss of primary teeth (Fig 6-9).

Not all activator treatments are as uneventful as the case presented in Fig 6-10. That applies particularly to patients with open bites and with non-occlusions caused by tongue interpositioning that does not resolve. Nevertheless, if a solid intercuspation is not realized at the end of treatment, it still can come about years later (Figs 6-11 and 6-14). However, that does not happen often (Fig 6-15).

Individual teeth can be moved and rotated with auxiliaries such as buttons and elastics, as is sometimes indicated for permanent first molars (Fig 6-12). Crossbites also can be prevented or corrected in that way (Figs 6-13 and 6-14).

FIGURE 6-9

In a girl aged 9 years 9 months, with a Class II division 1 malocclusion and a disto-occlusion of half a premolar crown width, three primary molars were lost prematurely and the other primary molars were severely carious. The permanent mandibular right molar had moved mesially until the over-erupted primary maxillary second molar had blocked its migration. The arch length discrepancy in the mandible was –2 mm; in the maxilla, the discrepancy was +3 mm. The primary maxillary left canine and primary first molar and the three other remaining primary molars had to be extracted. Thereafter, the permanent first molars could migrate mesially and rotate. The mandibular incisors were tipped lingually, partly because of lip interpositioning (A–D). A few weeks after the extractions were carried out, an activator with a simple closed spring to distalize the permanent mandibular right first molar was placed. The other three permanent first molars were blocked in their mesial migration by the acrylic resin resting against their mesial surfaces. After 6 months, the lip interpositioning had disappeared, all premolars and permanent canines had emerged and erupted without space problems, a neutro-occlusion was reached, and the treatment was concluded. However, the premolars and canines were not in solid intercuspation, and 4 months later, when a slight disto-occlusion had reoccurred, the activator therapy was resumed (E–H).

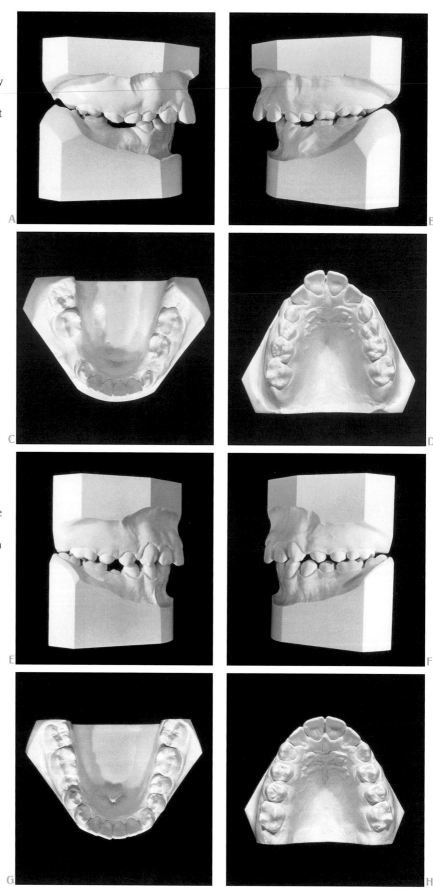

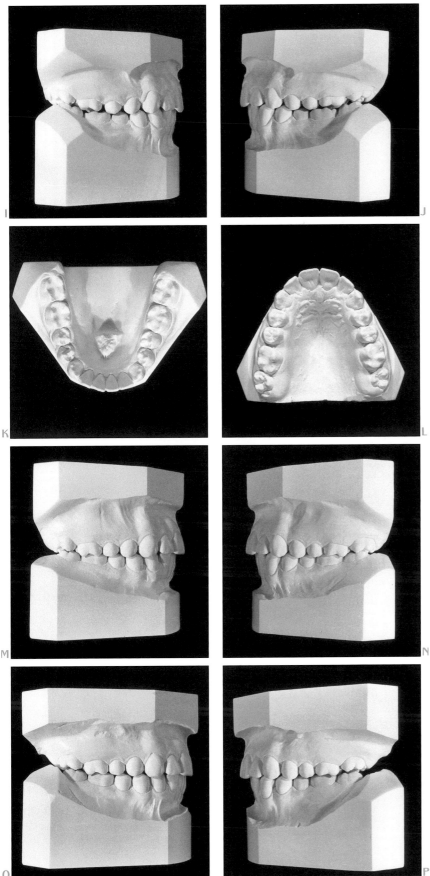

FIGURE 6-9 (CONTINUED)

After 3 months of additional activator treatment, a neutro-occlusion was established, but now with a solid intercuspation of the premolars and canines. Subsequently, some small tooth movements were generated by a positioner worn for 6 months. At the age of 11 years 7 months, the desired result was obtained (I–L). At the age of 14 years 2 months, the mandibular dental arch had attained a slightly more anterior position in relation to the maxillary dental arch than was found 2 years 7 months earlier (M, N). Three years later, at the age of 17 years 3 months, little had changed. The arrangement and occlusion of the dentition were still good (O, P).

Regardless of the way a disto-occlusion is corrected, there is no certainty regarding the permanence of the achieved neutro-occlusion when a solid intercuspation of premolars and canines is lacking; in most instances, part of the improvement will be lost. On the other hand, a solid intercuspation of the premolars and canines at the end of treatment will be maintained. Growth occurring after treatment, during which the mandible usually advances slightly, contributes to the stability of the improved occlusion.

FIGURE 6-10

A girl aged 10 years 0 months had a Class II division 1 malocclusion, without the usual associated facial appearance. She could breathe well through the nose and held her mouth closed at rest. The permanent first molars were in a disto-occlusion of one premolar width, the over-jet was 8 mm, and the overbite was 5 mm. The mandibular incisors contacted the palate. The dental arches were normal-ly shaped and had sufficient space for all teeth (maxillary arch length discrepancy: +5 mm; mandibular arch length discrepan-cy: +3 mm). The primary maxillary second molars had been lost shortly before. In the mandible, only the primary right second molar was still present (A, B). An activator was placed at the age of 10 years 3 months. Two years and 12 appointments later, at the age of 12 years 3 months, a fine result was obtained with a solid inter-cuspation in neutro-occlusion (C, D). The records collected 5 and 17 years later, at the ages of 17 years 11 months (E, F) and 29 years 11 months (G, H), confirmed the stability of the improvement.

This patient is an example of an ideal indication for treatment with an activator. She had a Class II division 1 malocclusion without additional complications such as crowding, rotations, or missing teeth. It was a typical Class II division 1 malocclu-sion, with all the secondary aspects expressed: a large overjet, a deep bite, an excessive curve of Spee, and a relatively narrow maxillary dental arch. With the acti-vator the primary factor, the disto-occlu-sion was corrected, but in the meantime all secondary aspects were managed. The activator was used only during sleep, and the recall appointments had been 2 months apart.

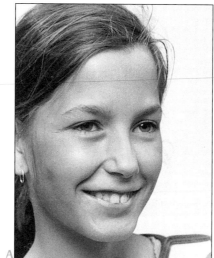

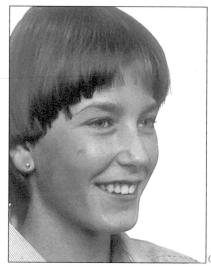

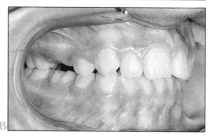

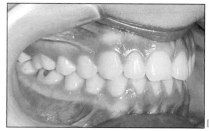

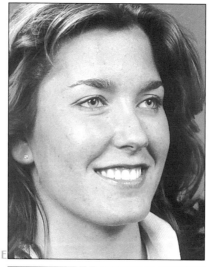

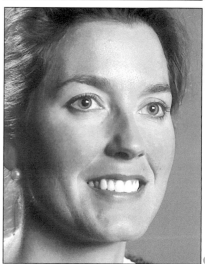

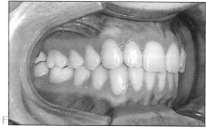

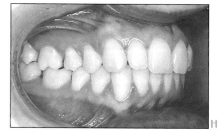

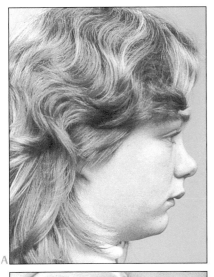

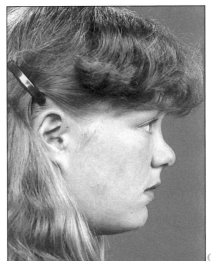

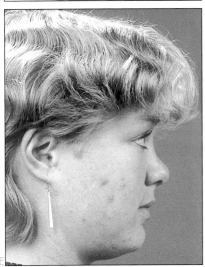

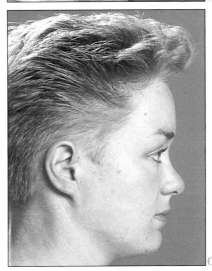

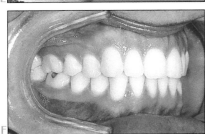

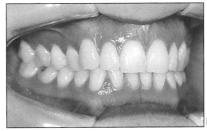

FIGURE 6-11

A girl of 11 years 5 months had a Class II division 1 malocclusion and a receding chin. The overjet was 11 mm and the overbite was only 2 mm, which involved a non-occlusion in the anterior region. The transition in the posterior regions was completed, and the canines and first molars were in a disto-occlusion measuring one premolar crown width. The mandibular dental arch had small diastemata (arch length discrepancy: +2 mm). In the maxilla more space was available (arch length discrepancy: +5 mm), including a central diastema and everted incisors (A, B). At the age of 11 years 9 months, an activator was placed. Two years later, the maxillary incisors had been retracted, the diastemata had been closed, and incisal contact was reached. However, in the posterior regions, there was a non-occlusion. Although the disto-occlusion was corrected, no solid intercuspation was established (C, D). Two years later, at the age of 16 years 1 month, there was a perfect occlusion with a solid intercuspation on both sides (E, F). At the age of 23 years 10 months, the dentition met the highest requirements, esthetically as well as functionally (G, H). The changes in the face that took place during as well as after completion of treatment were striking. The maxillomandibular relationships had improved markedly.

This patient is an example of the common phenomenon of displacement of an open bite or non-occlusion during treatment; in this patient, it migrated from the anterior to the posterior region. In addition, the patient is illustrative of the disappearance of open bites and non-occlusions during aging, which happens in about one third of patients.

FIGURE 6-12

A girl of 11 years 0 months had a Class II division 1 malocclusion with a disto-occlusion measuring three-quarters of a premolar crown width. She could breathe well through the nose and kept her mouth closed. The lower lip covered the rather upright maxillary central incisors for about one third of their crown height. The overjet was 6 mm; the overbite was 6 mm. The arch length discrepancy was +2 mm for the mandible and 0 mm for the maxilla. The permanent maxillary first molars were mesially rotated (A, B, G). At the age of 11 years 3 months, an activator was placed. Two months later, buttons were bonded at the distopalatal cusps of the permanent maxillary first molars; elastics were attached from these buttons to hooks fixed at the palatal sides of the activator in the first premolar regions. The acrylic resin prevented the mesiobuccal cusps of the maxillary first molars from migrating mesially. In that way, the rotations needed for a good occlusion of the permanent first molars could be carried out. After 2 years of activator treatment, a positioner was worn for an additional 6 months to improve some tooth positions. At the age of 13 years 9 months, a functional and esthetic result was obtained. The permanent maxillary first molars were correctly positioned and occluded well (C, D, H). At the age of 18 years 9 months, 5 years after treatment, the result was still satisfactory, although the maxillary incisors had attained a slightly more upright position. Indeed, the lower lip covered the maxillary central incisors for about half their crown height (E, F, I). The palatal tipping of the maxillary incisors could have been prevented if these teeth had been intruded, but that cannot be achieved with an activator.

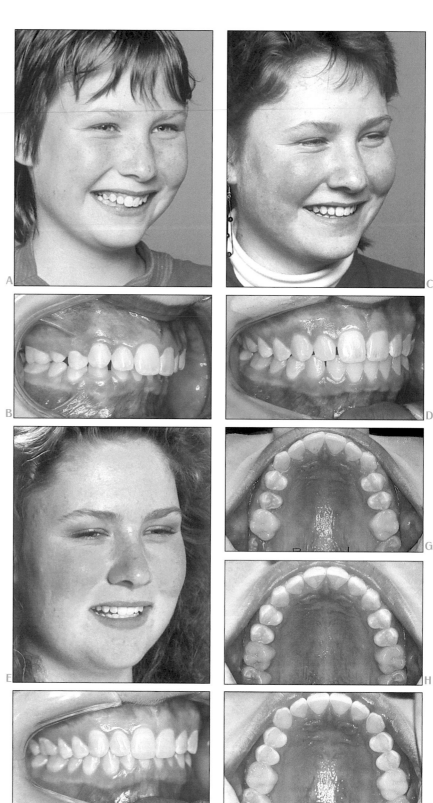

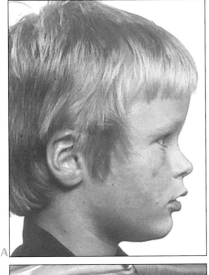

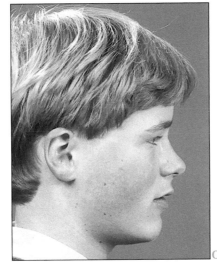

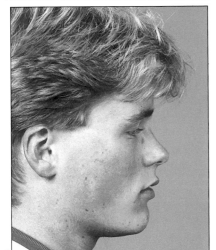

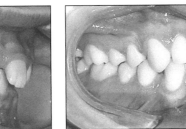

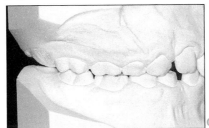

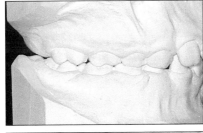

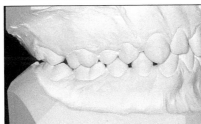

FIGURE **6-13**

A boy of 9 years 3 months had a Class II division 1 malocclusion with a disto-occlusion of a premolar crown width. Both the mandibular and maxillary incisors were everted, with diastemata between them. The mandibular arch length discrepancy was +6 mm; the maxillary arch length discrepancy was +4 mm. The maxillo-mandibular relationship was not deviating. The disto-occlusion was primarily of the dental kind (A, B). At the age of 9 years 4 months, an activator comprising two labial arches with U-loops was placed to retract the incisors in both arches. After 12 months, a neutro-occlusion was obtained and the use of the activator concluded (G). However, after another 12 months, the disto-occlusion had recurred, and a new activator was made (H). This activator was worn slightly more than 1 year, with a crossbite elastic for several months, to prevent the occurrence of a crossbite of the permanent right second molars. At the age of 15 years 5 months, an adequate result was obtained with a solid intercuspation of the posterior teeth (C, D, I). Further eruption of the maxillary canines in the following 2 years increased the sagittal securement of the neutro-occlusion, as was apparent in the records at 17 years 5 months of age (E, F).

Among other reasons, this patient is shown to demonstrate the partial loss of improvement in sagittal occlusion, which was due to the absence of a solid intercuspation. A solid intercuspation cannot be established when the flat, occlusally worn primary molars are still present. Conclusion of treatment at that stage results, as a rule, in a loss of about half the attained improvement in sagittal occlusion. A choice has to be made between continuing the activator therapy or refraining from treatment for some time, as was done in this patient.

FIGURE 6-14

A girl 10 years 8 months of age had a Class II division 1 malocclusion with a disto-occlusion of one premolar crown width and a non-occlusion in the anterior region. The incisors were tipped lingually in the mandible and labially in the maxilla. The overjet was 10 mm; the overbite was 1 mm. No vertical contact existed in the premolar region, where teeth were being replaced. The permanent right first molars were in crossbite. The arch length discrepancy in the mandible was 0 mm; in the maxilla, it was +2 mm (A, B). At the age of 10 years 10 months, an activator was placed. Two months later, an elastic was attached to buttons at the opposing permanent right first molars to correct the crossbite. Three months later, the same also was done on the left side to prevent a crossbite. At the age of 11 years 10 months, the permanent first molars were in good occlusion, and the incisors were in contact with each other. The labial arch had been used to retract the maxillary incisors. The mandibular incisors could protrude because the acrylic resin was maintained at the lingual side of the crowns and trimmed at the labial side, while the incisal edges rested at the acrylic resin plain surface. However, an open bite existed in the premolar region. It was decided to stop the activator treatment and wait for a while to see what would happen. The open bite in the premolar region disappeared, and the premolars and canines attained a good occlusion. At the age of 14 years 4 months (C, D) and also 5 and 10 years later, at the ages of 19 years (E, F) and 24 years (G, H), she had an esthetically pleasing dentition with a solid intercuspation of the posterior teeth. When the treatment is stopped for some time and no appliance is worn, periodic examination is recommended, for example, every 4 months, so that unpleasant surprises are avoided.

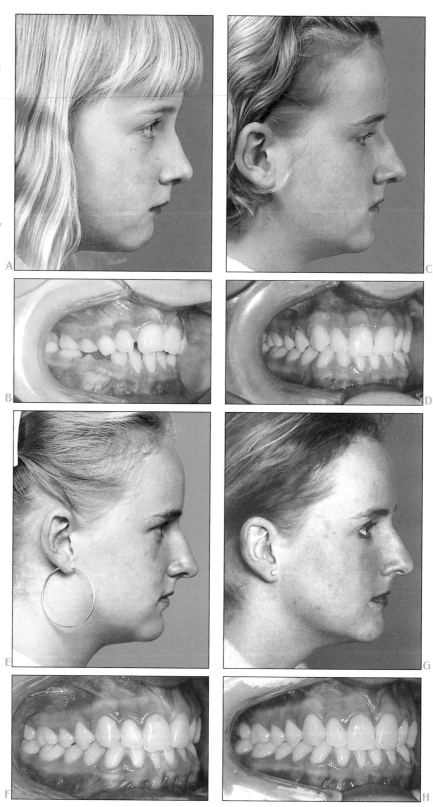

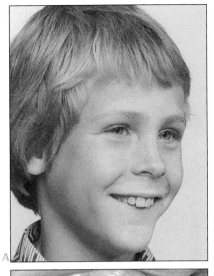

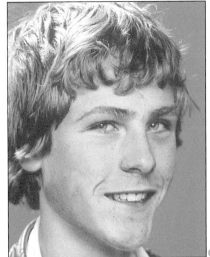

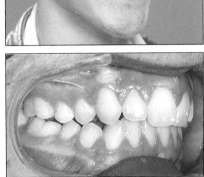

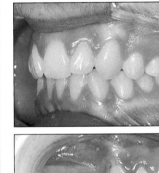

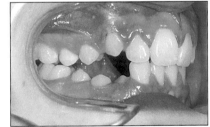

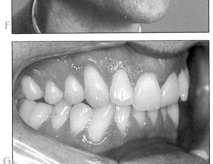

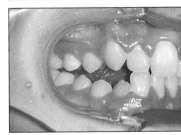

Figure 6-15

A boy aged 9 years 6 months had a large lower anterior facial height and a Class II division 1 malocclusion with a disto-occlusion of one premolar crown width. In the mandible, the primary canines were lost prematurely, and the permanent incisors were tipped lingually. The maxillary incisors were positioned normally. However, the overjet was 12 mm and the overbite was 1 mm. A non-occlusion was present not only in the anterior region but also in the primary right molar region. The arch length discrepancy in the mandible was −6 mm; in the maxilla, it was 0 mm (A, B). At the age of 9 years 9 months, an activator was placed. The sagittal occlusion improved and the mandibular incisors, not covered by acrylic resin on the labial side, moved anteriorly, providing space for the permanent canines. The support bars at their mesial sides prevented the permanent mandibular first molars from migrating mesially and thereby prevented a reduction in arch length. At the age of 11 years 9 months, after a treatment period of 22 months, treatment with the activator was concluded. A good molar occlusion and contact in the anterior region was established. However, there was still an open bite in the premolar regions, more on the right than on the left side, and a non-occlusion of the permanent right first molars. The open bite reduced in the following 12 months, as was shown in the records collected at 11 years 4 months (H) and 11 years 7 months of age (I). At 12 years 10 months of age, a satisfactory occlusion was reached on the left side but not on the right side (C, D, E). Fourteen years later, at the age of 26 years 10 months, a non-occlusion was still present on the right side (F, G).

FIGURE 6-16

In conjunction with activator treatment, crossbite elastics can be utilized to correct or prevent a crossbite (A). Elastics can also be hooked on the activator for tooth corrections (B).

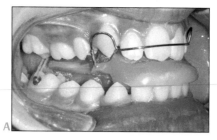
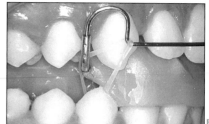

FIGURE 6-17

Fixed appliance treatment can be combined with the activator approach in a construction developed by Akkerman, the fixed appliance activator (A). The appliance is inserted in the headgear tubes of the permanent maxillary first molars (B).[229]

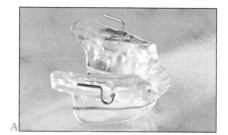
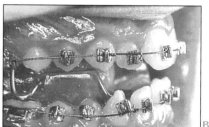

Activator treatment can also be supplemented with the use of elastics (Fig 6-16). In that way, teeth can be moved in various directions, especially mesially or distally. A good example of that approach is the mesial movement of the four permanent first molars in patients with agenesis of the second premolars, simultaneous with correction of the disto-occlusion and reduction of the overjet and overbite. Furthermore, the distal migration or lingual tipping of the teeth mesial to the missing premolars can be prevented.

An activator is particularly suited for the treatment of severe Class II division 1 malocclusions at an early age, especially when the lower lip is positioned palatal to the maxillary incisors and there is a great risk of tooth fracture. The early establishment of a normal lip position and a competent lip seal contributes to a favorable development of the dentition. As already explained, some of the achieved improvements are lost when the treatment is concluded before the premolars and canines have attained a solid intercuspation. When subsequent comprehensive orthodontic treatment is required for other reasons, a two-phase treatment is obviously the best approach. Indeed, many severe Class II division 1 malocclusions with additional complications are treated best by initial use of a facial orthopedic device, such as a headgear or an activator, and subsequent placement of fixed appliances to achieve the remaining corrections later.

Furthermore, an activator can be used as a retainer after fixed appliance treatment as well as in a modified form during that treatment (Fig 6-17).

Finally, the potentials of functional therapy and extraoral therapy can be combined in one system to increase the effect on facial growth and tooth movement, as will be explained in the next chapter.

Use of Headgear-Activator Combinations

By Herman van Beek and Frans P.G.M. van der Linden

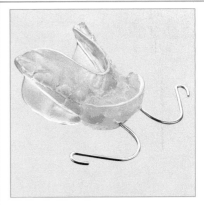

Since 1972, when Pfeiffer and Grobéty[159,160] proposed the idea of using a headgear and an activator at the same time, several approaches have been introduced in which both appliances are combined by placing extraoral force on the functional appliance.

Some constructions have tubes in the activator component, in which the inner bows of the parietal headgear can be inserted.[194] Many of these appliances have auxiliary devices, such as expansion screws, clasps, springs, buccal shields, and pads, to widen the maxillary dental arch, to hold the appliance in place, to move individual teeth, to keep the cheeks and the lips away from the teeth and alveolar processes, and to position the mandible in a more anterior position.[12]

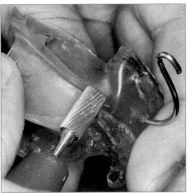

This chapter deals mainly with the Van Beek appliance.[203] The only one of its kind, his headgear-activator has no auxiliary components. The outer bows are embedded in the activator component, which has no parts that can be adjusted. Changes can be created only by trimming or building up the acrylic resin.

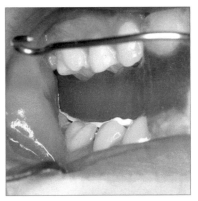

The appliance is well suited for the treatment of severe Class II division 1 malocclusions without additional complications in the dental arches. Prior to placement of the Van Beek appliance, irregular or palatally tipped maxillary incisors have to be corrected with a bite plate or partial fixed appliances. Subsequent to the use of the Van Beek appliance, a cervical headgear can be used to rotate permanent maxillary first molars, and a bite plate can be added. Finally, an ideal occlusion can be obtained in a relatively short period of time with fixed appliances.

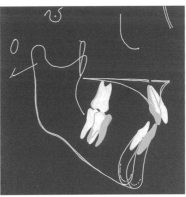

When extractions of permanent teeth are part of the treatment plan, the activator-headgear can be used as the first appliance to correct the sagittal and vertical deviations. However, without additional use of fixed appliances, an acceptable end result cannot be reached in extraction cases.

Orthodontic Concepts and Strategies

7

FIGURE 7-1

The Van Beek headgear-activator is low at the palate and has high wings lingually in the mandible (A). The short, wide headgear bows prevent irritation of the cheeks by the extensions of the parietal headgear (B).

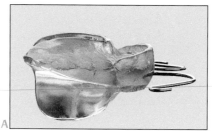
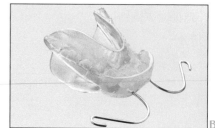

The Van Beek headgear-activator is a rigid appliance that does not break easily, and its heavy headgear bows do not deform (Fig 7-1). With good patient cooperation, the overjet reduces 1 mm per month, and appointments can be scheduled 3 months apart.

The technical aspects and handling of the appliance are explained, and the potential of the Van Beek appliance is illustrated with the records of treated patients.

The Van Beek headgear-activator works well for the correction of large overjets and deep bites in normally shaped dental arches. However, the treatment cannot be started when the position of the incisors interferes with the posturing of the mandibular dental arch in an overcorrected neutro-occlusion. Asthma and high fever present recurrent, but temporary, problems that are not contraindications to the use of the headgear-activator. Like all facial orthopedic appliances, it works best with favorable growth patterns. Deep bites are corrected by flattening of the curve of Spee, intrusion of the maxillary anterior teeth, or both. In a modified form, the headgear-activator also can be used in open bite patients, whether or not they have a large lower anterior facial height.

The main component of the Van Beek appliance is the activator, which forces the mandible into an anterior position through an avoidance reflex.[83,85] This reflex is evoked by the contact of the large wings with the mucosa in the mandibular premolar region when the patient does not position the mandible sufficiently to the anterior. The mandibular anterior teeth are kept free of the acrylic resin lingually but are covered incisally and labially over a distance of 2 mm. The maxillary incisor crowns are capped labially by the acrylic resin to prevent palatal tipping. The palatal cusps of the maxillary posterior teeth are capped by acrylic resin but not the buccal cusps. The palate is kept free, because the acrylic resin should not extend beyond the alveolar process. The headgear bows are embedded in the acrylic resin just below the contact points between the maxillary central and lateral incisors. The headgear bows should have a diameter of at least 1.3 mm and should not reach farther posteriorly than the maxillary canines. The bows should extend far enough laterally to prevent the elastics, which extend to the parietal headgear cap, from irritating the cheeks.

Screws, clasps, active wire components, shields, and pads are not needed. In addition, metal parts would complicate the strategic trimming of the acrylic resin. A central hole to facilitate breathing is not prepared, because the patient should be able to suck on the appliance, and an existing mouth-breathing habit should be stopped.

The acrylic resin has to be trimmed in such a way that, with the intended bodily palatal movement of the maxillary incisors, the maxillary posterior teeth become displaced buccally and distally (Figs 7-2 and 7-3). The distal movement of the posterior teeth will be smaller than the palatal movement of the incisors. That has to be the case, because in a severe Class II division 1 malocclusion with an overjet of 14 mm, the disto-occlusion at the permanent first molars only measures one premolar crown width, which corresponds to 7 mm. The tapered gothic maxillary dental arch has to change into a rounder, roman arch form (Fig 7-4).

The appliance is fabricated on a set of dental casts that should include the regions where the permanent second molars are located or will be located when they have emerged. The mandibular impression should be deep lingually, so that high wings can be made. The wax roll used for taking the construction bite should be firm and not too warm. The distance between the opposing incisal edges should be kept at about 10 mm but should be larger in open bites and non-occlusions. If possible, an end-to-end positioning of the incisors should be reached. To unload the temporomandibular joints when the construction bite is prepared, the patient's chin is pushed upward slightly. It is recommended that the procedure be practiced with the patient first, without the wax roll.

It is advantageous to fit the appliance in the wax stage, because it facilitates later acceptance of the device because undercuts are eliminated, and sore spots will occur less frequently. When the wax model is too high for insertion, some material has to be removed, not from the wings but from the superior side at the palate. Furthermore, in the wax stage it is possible to control whether the construction bite has been transverred correctly, and the headgear bows can still be repositioned.

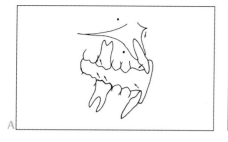
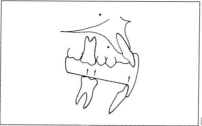

FIGURE 7-2

When the occlusal indentations are not removed from the mandibular posterior regions, the maxillary incisors will be exposed to an extruding and palatally tipping force, particularly when a large interocclusal clearance is present (A). This effect is dissolved after removal of the indentations (B).

Prior to placement, the appliance is shown to the patient and parents, and the mode of operation is explained. The discomfort and initial problems associated with habituation are discussed. The anticipated results with good and with poorer cooperation are illustrated.

When the appliance is tried in the mouth, it is placed on the mandibular arch first, and the patient is asked to occlude anteriorly. When the appliance has not previously been fitted in wax, some trimming may be needed at the superior side to allow insertion, and at other places to achieve perfect fit and relieve pain sensations.

The nasal passages are checked, and information about nasal drop medication is provided when indicated. It is important for the patient to practice swallowing with the appliance in place: first occluding, then sucking, and then continued occluding during the swallowing act. In particular, children with a deviating swallowing pattern have difficulty in practicing deglutition. However, the swallowing act, performed with active involvement of the chewing muscles, is essential to the effective application of the activator-headgear.

The force exerted by the parietal headgear should not be more than 150 g at each side. The extraoral traction keeps the appliance in place and blocks the eruption of the maxillary incisors. If the outer bows are bent upward, the incisors can be intruded.

Even with this small extraoral force and the standard recommended wear time of 12 hours a day, the anterior development of the maxilla is inhibited. However, the greatest contribution to the sagittal correction is provided by stimulation of the mandibular growth through the activator component. Forward rotation of the mandible by blocking of alveolar growth may also be applied as a mechanism, especially in patients with long faces. In addition, the appliance prevents the lower lip from being positioned palatal to the maxillary incisors and stimulates lip closure.

During the habituation period, the patient may have difficulty in sleeping, breathing through the nose, and swallowing. The appliance can be removed unconsciously during the night. Teeth can become painful, and sore spots can develop. A low construction bite causes more problems than does a high construction bite. A sore spot can be caused not only by a sharp edge but also by improper swallowing and incorrect biting in the activator. Besides local removal of acrylic resin, repeated instruction is important. Conscious and unconscious removal of the appliance is related to sore spots, restricted nasal passages, difficult swallowing, sensitive teeth, or irritation by the head cap. As far as possible, the causes are removed, and the head cap is fixed with hairpins if indicated. A paper antiallergic tape, loosely attached to the lips, is often effective.

The occlusal indentations of the mandibular posterior teeth are maintained until the patient is accustomed to the anterior positioning of the mandible. That is usually the case at the next appointment, 4 weeks later, and the indentations and the acrylic resin distal of the mandibular canines then can be removed. Thereafter, only the wings keep the mandibular jaw positioned anteriorly. If the indentations are removed before the patient becomes accustomed to this position, the wings will cause sore spots. The initial occlusal reference is essential for the patient's habituation and to master the desired positioning of the mandible. At the same session that indentations are removed, the acrylic resin at the superior side is trimmed for the distal and buccal movement of the maxillary posterior teeth (Fig 7-4 B).

The use of the headgear-activator varies according to facial height; the presence of a deep bite, non-occlusion, or open bite; and the need to expand the maxillary dental arch.

A deep bite can be reduced by leveling the curve of Spee; this is accomplished by maintaining contact in the mandible between the activator and the incisors anteriorly, and the occlusal surfaces of the permanent second molars posteriorly, and trimming away the acrylic resin between them to allow the other teeth to erupt further. In addition, this approach will prevent overeruption of the permanent molars and a posterior movement of the chin, for which the deep wings are so important. That also holds true in dentitions with a mild disto-occlusion. Eruption of the maxillary posterior teeth is prevented, because the mesial vector of their eruption path counteracts the correction of the disto-occlusion.

A deep bite can also be corrected by intrusion of the maxillary anterior teeth or by prevention of their eruption. Intrusion in the direction of the long axis of the teeth has the additional advantage of simultaneously reducing the overjet. This effect can be attained by bending the short headgear bows upward to the point just before the activator starts to incline.

Intrusion of the anterior teeth is most effective when the incisors are tipped labially and the acrylic resin contacting the occlusal surfaces of the mandibular posterior teeth is smooth and flat. When the indentations are not removed, they will transmit the forces evoked by the anterior positioning of the mandible as a posteriorly directed reaction force at the maxillary incisors, combined with a palatal tipping component. The anterior part of the activator will have the tendency to dislodge, particularly if a large interocclusal clearance is present, and the maxillary incisors will not intrude.

Another unfavorable side effect of maintaining the indentations is that they lead to mesially directed forces at the mandibular teeth, which can result in undesirable tipping (Fig 7-2).

How far the maxillary incisors have to be intruded depends on the size of the overjet and overbite and the desired height of the smile line.

The following guidelines apply for trimming the headgear-activator. The acrylic resin that completely covers the maxillary anterior teeth labially and lingually may not impinge on the cervical gingiva, and the interdental septa should not cause any disturbances. The mandibular anterior teeth should be in contact with the acrylic resin at the incisal edges and at the labial surfaces over a height of 2 mm. Their lingual surfaces should be free of the acrylic resin. The distal side of the mandibular canines should be well covered by the acrylic resin. A cylindrical acrylic resin bur, held perpendicular to the occlusal surfaces, is a practical tool for trimming the posterior regions. The trimming of the maxillary posterior regions is especially critical and should be performed with special care. The indentations have to be removed until only the cusp tips are in contact with the acrylic resin. The resulting plain surface should block the eruption of the maxillary posterior teeth (Fig 7-3). In addition, the acrylic resin in contact with the mesial sides of these teeth should be trimmed in such a way that, with the palatal movement of the maxillary incisors, a distally and buccally directed force is exerted on the posterior teeth. The maxillary anterior teeth are moved more or less bodily to the posterior by the extraoral traction transmitted through the activator, which has a firm grip at these teeth (Fig 7-4).

When the flat and smooth surfaces in contact with the maxillary posterior teeth are obliquely orientated to the midsagittal plane, the distally and buccally directed force will be exerted as required. For this fine trimming, a narrow, cylindrical acrylic resin bur with a smooth top is the preferred tool.

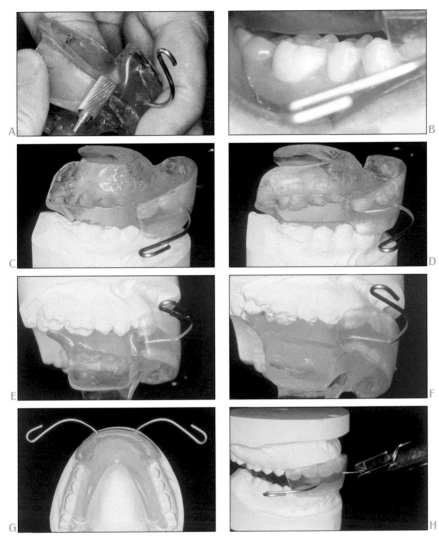

FIGURE 7-3

A cylindrical acrylic resin bur facilitates reaching a plain occlusal surface and straight lingual sides in the mandibular posterior regions (A). The acrylic resin should only be in contact with the distal cusps of the most distally occluding mandibular molar (B). When the permanent mandibular second molar is not present yet, the acrylic resin should extend to the area where this molar will emerge, to provide vertical support later. It is recommended that the appliance be fitted on the dental casts before trimming (C, E) and that the effect be regularly reexamined on the casts (D, F). In the maxilla, the acrylic resin extends over the most distally positioned molar but does not cover the distal half of the buccal surface of the canine. The headgear bows do not reach farther than the level of the maxillary canines, which are only partially covered by acrylic resin and are not covered at all on the distal side (G). The headgear bows are bent upward to obtain the intrusive effect (H).

Essential to the trimming procedure are the flatness and smoothness of the surfaces over which the teeth have to move. That applies to the surfaces in contact with the palatal cusps of the maxillary posterior teeth as well as the surfaces on their mesial side. The increase in maxillary dental arch width is also promoted by the occlusion, as the mandibular posterior teeth gradually attain a more mesial position in relation to the maxillary posterior teeth ("rail mechanism").

In patients with a large lower anterior facial height, an anterior open bite or non-occlusion, and a large overjet, every effort has to be made to prevent eruption of teeth. This aim can be realized for the maxillary teeth by the extraoral traction transmitted through the activator. For the mandibular posterior teeth, eruption is inhibited initially by occlusal contact with a high appliance and a large clearance. However, the eruption-inhibiting effect soon diminishes through growth of the mandible and adaptation of the masticatory muscles. Rebasing every 3 months, or preferably gluing gradually thicker rubber strips in the occlusal areas of the mandible, reactivates the bite block effect (Fig 7-8, E and F).

When the increase in height of the alveolar processes is stopped, mandibular growth will result in an anterior movement of the chin and a reduction in the overjet and open bite. The short headgear bows are not bent upward when intrusion is not intended. Long headgear bows should not be used because they tend to extrude the maxillary incisors and to create a "gummy" smile. Furthermore, long headgear bows will counteract the anterior rotational growth of the mandible through the canting of the occlusal plane.

Indeed, an additional reason to avoid eruption of mandibular molars in patients with a large lower anterior facial height is that an increase in the height of the alveolar process will lead to a posterior movement of the chin point. In these cases, it is better not to level the curve of Spee and only to remove the indentations and flatten the areas of the activator in contact with the mandibular posterior teeth, to prevent the patient from "hanging" with the mandible in the activator. The high wings will still provoke the avoidance reflex. Furthermore, if there is a deep bite in these patients, which is rarely the case, it should be corrected by intrusion of the maxillary incisors.

In most Class II division 1 malocclusions, the maxillary dental arch has to become wider. This is realized with the headgear-activator by shifting of the maxillary posterior teeth to a more anterolateral position in relation to the appliance. The extraoral traction, in combination with the mesiopalatally contacting oblique guiding surfaces, results in a distal and buccal movement of the posterior teeth (Fig 7-4). In a maxillary palatal crossbite, this movement is insufficient, so prior active expansion is required. On the other hand, in a maxillary buccal crossbite, the maxillary dental arch should not be expanded, and the capping of the cusps of the maxillary posterior teeth should be maintained (Fig 7-5). Occasionally, expansion of the mandibular dental arch is required (Fig 7-5, E and F). For partial scissors bites, the approach has to be modified (Fig 7-5, I to L).

In the normal course of events with a headgear-activator in a growing patient, the overjet will reduce 1 mm a month, independent of the age of the patient. This is the result of the intrusion and retraction of the maxillary incisors, blocking of the increase in alveolar height, and growth of the mandible. A decrease of less than 1 mm a month is a certain sign of insufficient cooperation, and this is indisputable. Only ankylosis of a maxillary incisor could explain the occurrence of too little progress.

Extraoral forces of more than 150 g will not provide faster or better results. Furthermore, greater forces involve the risk of devitalizing the maxillary incisors, particularly when intrusion is the goal. Wearing the appliance for more than 12 hours a day will lead to a faster result, but the effect is more dental than skeletal, and the treatment goal is not reached. The aim is not only an overcorrection of the disto-occlusion, the overjet, and the overbite, but also a reduction of the skeletal convexity of the face. In the choice for the best moment to start treatment, the risk of trauma to everted incisors is a key factor. If that is the reason for starting in the mixed dentition stage, the extraoral force has to be kept small when the permanent canines emerge; otherwise they will erupt buccally. When there is no lip interpositioning, it is better to wait until the maxillary canines have erupted and the mandibular second molars have emerged.

In patients with a vertical facial growth pattern, early intervention by stopping habits and active treatment are indicated. The vertical development may be progressive and lip incompetence can result. A competent lip seal is an essential condition to achieve a satisfying result, particularly in this type of treatment.

An important advantage of the headgear-activator is that this appliance offers control over the vertical position of the maxillary incisors. Overeruption in patients with lip interpositioning can be avoided, and maxillary incisors can even be intruded.

Consequently, the appliance is well suited for the treatment of Class II division 2 malocclusions. However, prior to placement of the headgear-activator, the palatally inclined maxillary incisors have to be tipped to a slightly exaggerated labial inclination, because the maxillary incisors will upright somewhat during retraction.

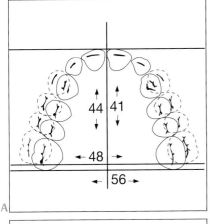

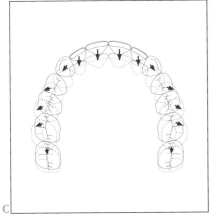

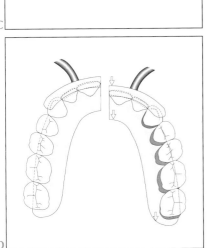

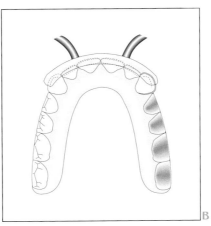

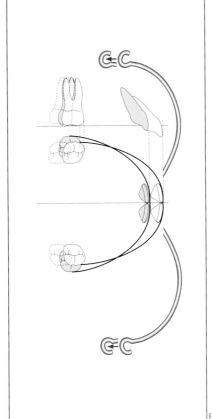

FIGURE 7-4

The changes in position of the maxillary teeth that have resulted from headgear-activator treatment are elucidated with a superimposition of occlusograms. The arch width increased progressively, more in the molar than the canine region, and the arch depth decreased (A). To attain these changes, the acrylic resin has to be trimmed in such a way that the maxillary posterior teeth are only touched by a flat surface occlusally and mesiopalatally (B: TRIMMED ON THE RIGHT SIDE BUT NOT ON THE LEFT SIDE). The maxillary incisors will move palatally, while the other teeth migrate distobuccally, except for the most distally occluding molars, which are displaced not buccally but only distally. Some acrylic resin can be removed from the labial surface of the lateral incisors so that they migrate less palatally than do the central incisors (C). With the movement of the maxillary teeth, the positions of the canines, premolars, and first molars change in relation to the appliance, because they attain relatively more anterior and lateral positions within the appliance (D: LEFT, BEFORE MOVEMENT; RIGHT, AFTER MOVEMENT). The central incisors upright slightly in their movement, and move more posteriorly than do the permanent first molars (E: DARK SHADING, AFTER MOVEMENT). The position where these molars should be, if the acrylic resin had not been trimmed from the posterior regions, is indicated by dotted lines.

When the molar occlusion is overcorrected and the incisors have reached an end-to-end position (in corrected open bites a slight overbite), the retention phase can start. For that purpose, the appliance is worn only during sleep, and the extraoral traction is abandoned. When the activator, without this traction, is not lost during the night, the headgear bows can be removed. During the retention phase, the distally tipped maxillary posterior teeth will upright because the mandible grows more anteriorly than does the maxilla. The crowns will move mesially, but the apices will not or will only slightly move (Fig 7-12). As a rule of thumb, the retention phase should last as long as the active treatment but longer in patients with a large anterior facial height, preferably until growth has ceased.

Additional treatment with fixed appliances should not be started before the molars and premolars have improved their angulation; otherwise the disto-occlusion can return. Following the fixed appliance therapy, retention is provided with a maxillary plate and a wire bonded lingually to the mandibular anterior teeth.

Like every treatment method, the headgear-activator therapy has unfavorable aspects and undesirable side effects. One of these is the occurrence of mandibular crowding. However, the development of crowding and the increase in existing crowding are general phenomena that occur during adolescence and early adulthood even without preceding orthodontic treatment.[133, 185] The tendency to develop crowding is great during and after headgear-activator treatment, particularly when the mandibular incisors have been inclined labially. With the reduction in the skeletal convexity and the decrease in the overjet, the lower lip will exert more pressure at the mandibular incisors. Furthermore, during the active treatment phase, normal occlusion is lacking, so undesirable migrations will occur more readily. If the acrylic resin is not removed in due time from the buccal side of the maxillary canines, the mandibular canines can migrate too far lingually.

Furthermore, if the patient sleeps with the head reclined, the mandible drops down and the mandibular teeth rest at the wings. The chance that this will happen is greater in mouth breathers, in patients with a small interocclusal clearance, or if the appliance has short wings. Crowding in the mandibular anterior region can develop when indentations are not removed or the acrylic resin coverage of the anterior teeth extends to the distal surface of the mandibular canines. This development can be counteracted by a retention wire placed lingual to the mandibular anterior teeth or by the use of a removable Essix retainer during the day.

Sometimes a lateral open bite develops if the extraoral force is too great, the headgear bows are too long, or the bows have not been bent upward. This also can occur in patients with upright maxillary incisors. Lateral open bites and non-occlusions do not disappear when the tongue interpositioning is maintained.

An anterior open bite or non-occlusion can develop as a result of too much intrusion but also through lip biting or lip sucking, and the anterior lower facial height can increase rapidly. These patients often have problems swallowing with the appliance in the mouth, and occasionally grinding facets can be seen at the wings. In these patients, relapse cannot be prevented (Fig 7-11).

With an otherwise favorable anterior rotational growth of the mandible, the maxillary incisors can intrude too much and become insufficiently visible during speaking and smiling. In these patients, long headgear bows are permitted, and the deep bite should be corrected by trimming away the acrylic resin occlusal to the mandibular premolars and molars. For these patients, a cervical headgear with a maxillary plate or a conventional activator is a good alternative. The development of or increase in a concave profile should be prevented.

Ninety percent of patients treated with a headgear-activator will reach a neutro-occlusion. One of 10 patients cannot cope with the appliance for one reason or another. However, other therapeutic approaches are often also unsuccessful in these patients. The long-term results are not always of the quality that was initially projected. Five years after treatment, only 50% of the headgear-activator patients have anterior guidance, and 25% have an overjet of up to 4 mm, but that is not obvious and is not experienced as disturbing. However, 25% have a visible overjet, although it is always smaller than the overjet that existed prior to treatment.[204] Relapse occurs in all facial types and is primarily caused by deviating functional aspects in the orofacial region. Open mouth posture and red lips are indicative of that condition. It is recommended that the chances of relapse be discussed with the patient and his or her parents prior to the start of treatment.

A number of aspects relevant to headgear-activator treatment are clarified by the records of patients treated with this appliance (Figs 7-6 to 7-11).

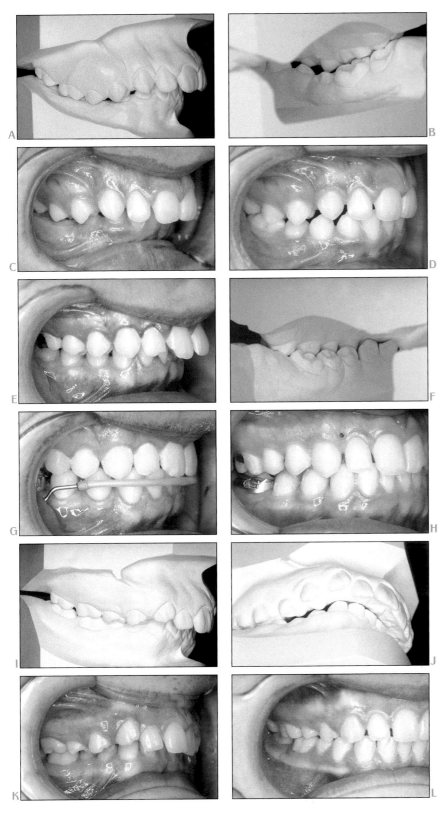

FIGURE 7-5

In crossbites, the occlusal surfaces in contact with the maxillary posterior teeth, which are buccally positioned, should not be removed. The correction of the crossbite will depend on the successful advancement of the mandibular dental arch in relation to the maxillary dental arch. If that advancement is too small, the crossbite will not resolve adequately. After an appropriate transverse relationship has been obtained, the indentations are trimmed. An extreme deep bite and an excessive eruption of the posterior teeth sometimes accompany a complete scissors bite (A–C). In this case, the complete scissors bite and the deep bite were corrected over a period of 18 months with a headgear-activator that was not trimmed in the maxillary posterior region. The molar occlusion was overcorrected, and the premolars and molars were tipped distally (D). Expansion of the mandibular dental arch can contribute to the correction of the scissors bite, particularly if mandibular teeth are missing. This approach was followed in a patient with a complete bilateral scissors bite with an extreme deep bite, in whom the permanent mandibular first molars had been extracted some years before (E, F). With a headgear-activator and a lip bumper of 0.045-inch stainless steel wire at the permanent second molars, a considerable improvement was obtained (G, H). In partial crossbites in which only the maxillary premolars are in non-occlusion, the acrylic resin on the permanent molars has to be trimmed and the coverage of the premolars must be maintained (I, J, K). Concomitant with the correction of the crossbite, other improvements can be realized, such as the correction of the distoocclusion, the intrusion of the maxillary incisors, and the flattening of the curve of Spee (L). To limit occlusal interferences, which move back the teeth involved in the correction of the crossbite, the headgearactivator has to be worn more than the standard 12-hour daily requirement.

FIGURE 7-6

A boy aged 11 years 10 months had a Class II division 1 malocclusion with a disto-occlusion of one premolar crown width and an overjet of 8 mm. There was sufficient space in the dental arches, which were otherwise normal. He had an open mouth posture, although the nasal passages were not impeded (A, B). At the age of 12 years 1 month, a Van Beek headgear-activator was placed. The overjet decreased 1 mm a month, and the maxillary dental arch gradually widened, while the occlusion in the posterior regions improved. At the age of 12 years 7 months, after 6 months of treatment, sagittal contact was reached in the anterior region, but solid intercuspation of the posterior teeth was not yet established. The decision was made to discontinue the extraoral traction, to remove the headgear bows, and to utilize the appliance only as an activator (C, D). During the retention period of 2 years 6 months, facial growth continued, and a solid intercuspation of the posterior teeth was established. The records collected at the age of 15 years 1 month revealed a successful treatment result (E, F), as did the records obtained at 20 years 2 months (G, H).

The initial malocclusion was well suited to treatment with a headgear-activator. The dental arches showed no malpositioning, except those related to the secondary aspects of the disto-occlusion, such as the large overjet and overbite, the deep curve of Spee, and the relatively narrow maxillary dental arch. No additional treatment with comprehensive appliances was needed. This patient can be considered a good example of successful treatment with a headgear-activator, resulting from a favorable initial situation, good patient cooperation, and favorable facial growth during and after treatment.

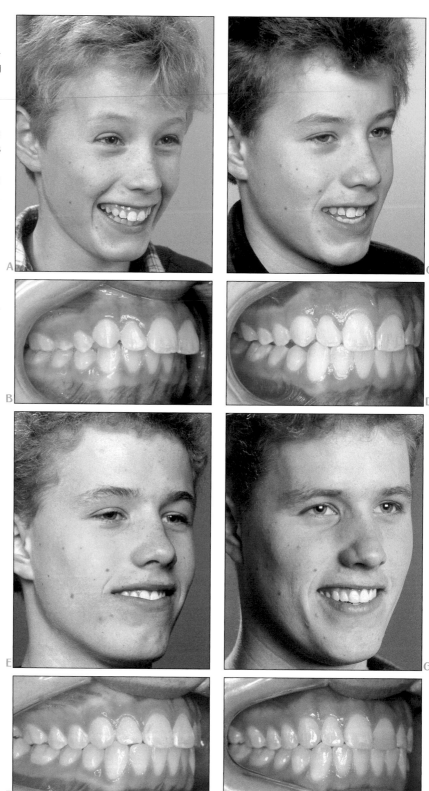

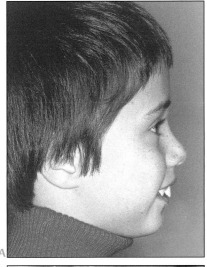

A

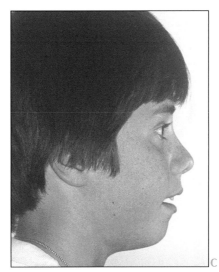

C

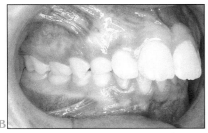

B

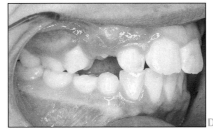

D

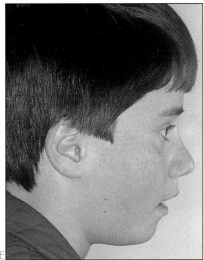

E

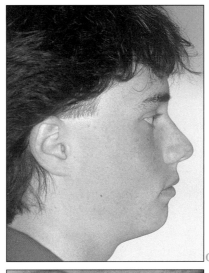

G

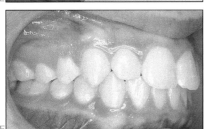

F

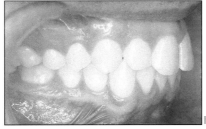

H

FIGURE 7-7

A boy who was 10 years 6 months of age had a Class II division 1 malocclusion with a disto-occlusion of one premolar crown width and an overjet of 9 mm. The mandibular incisors had overerupted and were in contact with the palate. The dentition dominated in the face, which still had much growth to experience. He could not keep his mouth closed, and the lower lip was located palatally to the maxillary incisors at rest (A, B). At the age of 11 years 6 months, after a headgear-activator treatment of 10 months, the situation had improved considerably. The maxillary right first premolar had emerged and tipped considerably distally (C, D; SEE ALSO FIG 7-12). One year later, at the age of 12 years 6 months, the goal of the active treatment was reached, the headgear bows were removed, and the patient was asked to wear the appliance for retention during sleep. Facial growth was not yet completed, and at rest the lips were not closed (E, F). The retention phase was lengthy and was not concluded until a competent lip seal was established. At the age of 19 years 6 months, 2 years after the retention was stopped, facial growth was almost completed, the soft tissues had increased and matured, and a competent lip seal was realized (G, H).

This patient is a good example of late growth of the facial skeleton and late maturation of soft tissues in boys. In girls, facial growth and maturation are completed earlier, in general by 15 years of age. In boys, this stage is not reached until 20 years of age or later. Hence, boys require a longer retention phase than girls, particularly when a competent lip seal has not yet been reached.

FIGURE 7-8

A girl who was 11 years 6 months of age had a Class II division 1 malocclusion with a sizeable anterior open bite, a large lower anterior facial height, and an open lip posture; however, the nasal passages were not obstructed (A, B). The treatment with a headgear-activator went well and lasted 2 years. At the age of 16 years 0 months, the retention was concluded, and a fine result was obtained. The open bite had disappeared, the posterior teeth occluded well, and the profile and vertical dimensions of the face were quite acceptable (C, D).

In patients with an open bite and a large lower anterior facial height, the eruption of the posterior teeth should be prevented to guide the growth of the mandibular condyles in anterior direction, resulting in an anterior movement of the chin. A headgear-activator with a large intraocclusal clearance and plain surfaces in contact with the posterior teeth usually offers adequate control over the development of the lower face. This control is improved substantially by the gluing of rubber strips to the occlusal surfaces in contact with on the mandibular posterior teeth and increasing the thickness of these strips every 3 months (E, F). Through this procedure, the space between the condyles and the articular fossae was enlarged (G). During the treatment of this patient, the lower facial height increased little (H).

Patients with a large lower anterior facial height and a large anterior open bite are difficult to treat, and it is by no means simple to reach a satisfying result. Even if the desired goal has been realized, much of what has been achieved can be lost when facial growth continues after retention is concluded. Therefore, to maintain the obtained improvement, retention has to be continued until facial growth is completed.

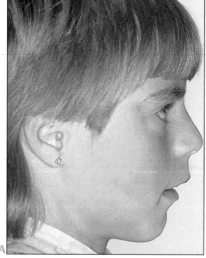
A

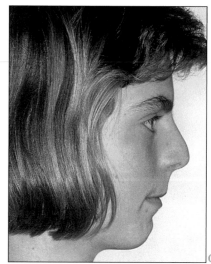
C

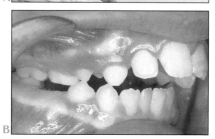
B

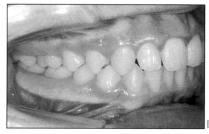
D

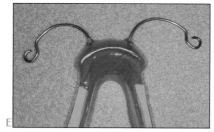
E

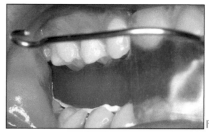
F

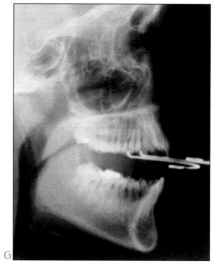
G

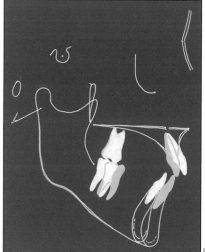
H

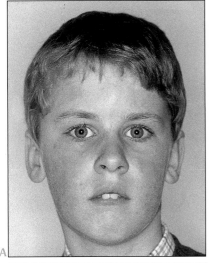

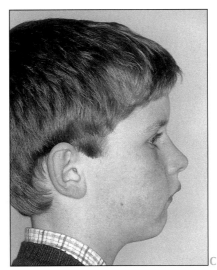

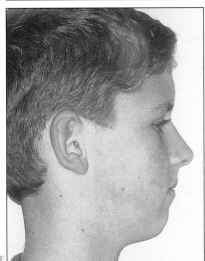

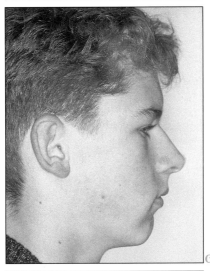

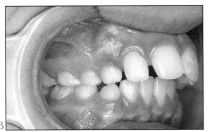

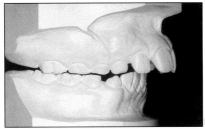

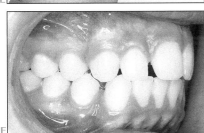

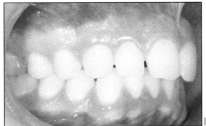

FIGURE 7-9

A boy aged 11 years 4 months had a Class II division 1 malocclusion with a disto-occlusion of one premolar crown width, an overjet of 10 mm, an anterior open bite, and a large lower anterior facial height. At rest, the lower lip was positioned palatal to the maxillary incisors (A–D). Rubber strips, as illustrated in Fig 7-8, were glued to the occlusal surfaces in contact with the mandibular teeth to control the vertical development of the lower face. At the age of 13 years 10 months, after 2 years 6 months of active treatment, a satisfying result was obtained. However, a competent lip seal was not reached, and facial growth was not completed (E, F). For retention, the headgear bows were removed, and the activator was worn during sleep to control the height of the lower face. At the age of 17 years 6 months, the retention was concluded. The lower facial height had increased only slightly. Facial growth was favorable, and an acceptable profile with a competent lip seal resulted (G, H).

The active treatment in this patient was lengthy because of the late and slow transition of the posterior teeth. The maxillary incisors had not been intruded. However, the diastemata between them were not closed, because the interdental acrylic resin relief in the maxillary anterior regions had not been removed. During the retention period, the diastemata disappeared in the mandible, and the overbite increased slightly. Later, the maxillary incisors moved more palatally and the diastemata closed there also.

FIGURE 7-10

A boy who was 12 years 4 months of age had a Class II division 1 malocclusion, a disto-occlusion measuring one premolar crown width, and a sagittal overbite of 10 mm. The maxillary incisors had overerupted, and the mandibular incisors were in contact with the palate (A, B, G). At the age of 12 years 6 months, a headgear-activator combination was placed; the appliance had extra-short headgear bows, bent far upward, to intrude the maxillary incisors. Patient cooperation was excellent, and after 18 months the maxillary anterior teeth were intruded more than was necessary. When the boy smiled, the maxillary incisors were not sufficiently visible (C). With fixed appliances, the positions of the teeth were improved further, while Class II elastics contributed to extrusion of the maxillary incisors to the desired level (D, E). At the age of 14 years 4 months, the fixed appliances, which had been used for 6 months, were removed. The vertical positioning of the maxillary incisors was correct, and the posterior teeth occluded well. The overjet and overbite were overcorrected (F, H).

Intrusion of the maxillary incisors leads to reduction of the overbite and overjet. In addition, the tendency of the lower lip to be positioned palatal to the maxillary incisors lessens. In patients with significantly overerupted maxillary incisors, the outer bows have to be bent upward directly after the appliance has been accepted, so that the intrusive force is applied as soon as possible. If fixed appliances with Class II elastics are used after the headgear-activator, overintrusion of the maxillary incisors in the first treatment phase is indicated.

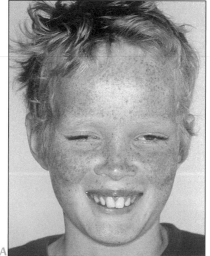

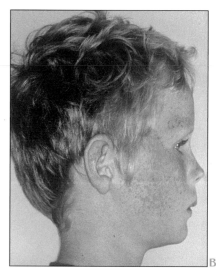

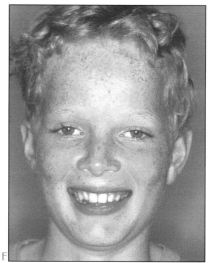

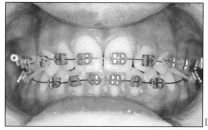

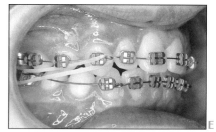

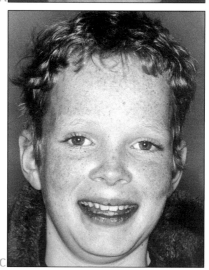

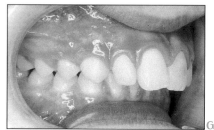

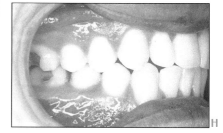

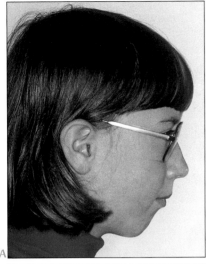

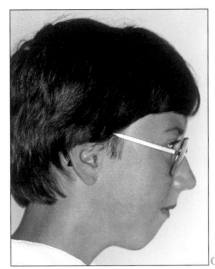

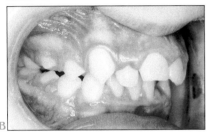

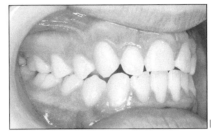

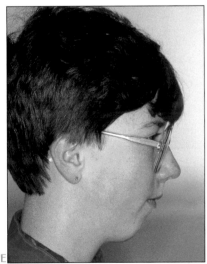

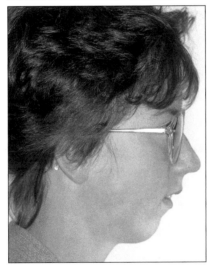

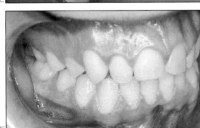

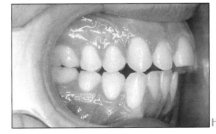

FIGURE 7-11

A girl who was 12 years 2 months of age had a Class II division 1 malocclusion, characterized by a disto-occlusion of three-quarter premolar crown width, malaligned maxillary anterior teeth, and a non-occlusion in the anterior region. In addition, she had a large lower anterior facial height, an open mouth position, and a lip-biting habit (A, B). First, a plate was used to align the maxillary anterior teeth. Subsequently, a headgear-activator was placed, with the addition of rubber strips at the occlusal surfaces in the mandibular posterior regions. With this approach, a neutro-occlusion was reached, but neither contact in the anterior region nor a competent lip seal was obtained. Furthermore, the lower anterior facial height had increased, as was indicated by the records collected after the active treatment was concluded at the age of 13 years 8 months (C, D). After the headgear bows were removed, the activator was worn during sleep for 3 years as a retention device. During that period, the occlusion improved, and the vertical proportions of the face stayed more or less the same. At the age of 16 years 8 months, the positions of the teeth and the occlusion were quite acceptable. However, no competent lip seal had been established (E, F). Seven years later, at the age of 23 years 8 months, much of the improvement obtained through treatment was lost. An anterior open bite with malaligned maxillary anterior teeth was present, and a transverse end-to-end occlusion was found in the posterior regions. Remarkably, the patient was satisfied with the result. The suggestion to improve the profile through surgical correction of the chin was not accepted (G, H). As explained previously, it is difficult to obtain a satisfactory result in patients with a large lower anterior facial height. Furthermore, the improvements realized by treatment can fade away in subsequent years, and the situation can worsen. This type of undesirable development should be expected in patients with deviating functional conditions.

FIGURE 7-12

The maxillary posterior teeth will become distally inclined during active treatment with a properly trimmed headgear-activator but will upright during the retention phase. These changes in angulation are illustrated with roentgenograms and tracings of the patient shown in Fig 7-8. Prior to the onset of treatment, the maxillary canine, premolars, and first molar were angulated mesially (A, B). At the end of the active treatment with the headgear-activator, their angulation had been changed through distal tipping (C, D). During the retention phase, the crowns of the maxillary posterior teeth moved anteriorly, and the angulation improved (E, F). These illustrations also demonstrate the potential of the headgear-activator to intrude maxillary incisors.

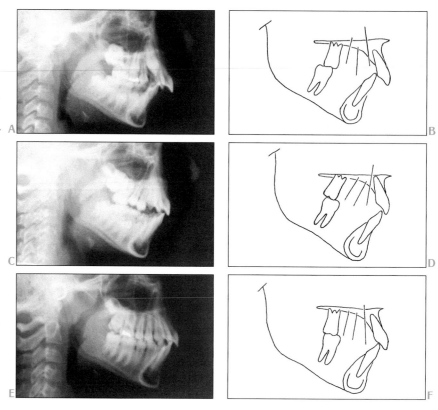

In headgear-activator treatment, the maxillary posterior teeth tip distally. That also happens with primary molars, which carry the unerupted premolars distally with them. The degree of distal tipping depends on the magnitude of the extraoral traction, the way the acrylic resin has been trimmed, and the number of hours the appliance is worn. When the occlusal surfaces are not trimmed, as recommended for crossbites, the maxillary posterior teeth will tip further distally than they will when the occlusal indentations are removed. When mandibular growth during treatment is extensive, the distal tipping will be lessened. During the retention phase, the previously distally tipped maxillary posterior teeth will be uprighted, as the mandible grows more anteriorly than the maxilla. The crowns will move mesially; the apices will exhibit little or no movement (Fig 7-12). In a retention phase without growth, no uprighting will occur. The same applies to patients in whom, during the retention phase, the mandible grows not anteriorly but caudally.

In conclusion, a Van Beek headgear-activator is a useful appliance for the correction of large overjets, deep bites, and open bites. Its mode of operation is based mainly on the inhibition of the vertical development of the alveolar processes in the posterior regions, which stimulates the anterior rotational growth of the mandible, and on the retrusion and intrusion of the maxillary anterior teeth.

Validity of Facial Orthopedics

In the preceding four chapters, various aspects of facial orthopedic therapy have been elucidated. However, the changes occurring after treatment have been discussed only occasionally.

Indeed, a number of studies have demonstrated that the direction of growth of the facial skeleton can be altered. The same applies to the amount of growth that takes place. However, it also has become clear that the effect is limited to a change of a few degrees in the direction of growth and to a change of 3 to 4 mm in the amount. The latter also applies to dental movement.[4, 56, 94, 127, 129, 151, 154, 199, 202] In addition, considerable variations in growth patterns and in reactions to facial orthopedic therapies have been found. Children can have a favorable or an unfavorable growth pattern for the correction of a Class II malocclusion. On average, the sagittal maxillomandibular relationship alters little or not at all in children, especially before the start of puberty. However, in some children, the maxillomandibular relationship improves spontaneously; in others, it worsens. A comparable variation is found in the reaction to facial orthopedic therapy. Most children respond favorably, some very favorably; however, some do not show any improvement, despite their dedicated wearing of the appliance.[201]

First the variation in maxillomandibular growth and its importance for orthodontic treatment are discussed. Subsequently, average growth patterns are presented, followed by the explanation of the limited value that can be attached to the extrapolation of data from these patterns to individual patients. The results of cervical headgear treatment are demonstrated in research findings that cover a long period of time. As a clinical example, a girl for whom records were collected 2 years before the start of treatment is shown. The short- and long-term effects of a parietal headgear treatment are also demonstrated through the records of a patient.

Special attention is given to the relatively short period of the total facial growth during which facial orthopedic therapy is applied. In this chapter, in which emphasis is placed on the long-term results, images of six patients who have been followed for many years are shown to elucidate various aspects involved. In that context, the return to the original growth pattern, and the possibility of preventing this, are discussed. Finally, the interaction between facial growth and the development of the dentition during treatment will be explained. The importance of a solid intercuspation to maintaining a good occlusion and to stabilizing the results will be emphasized.

Orthodontic Concepts and Strategies

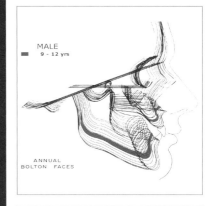

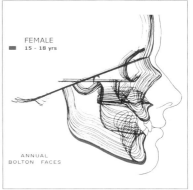

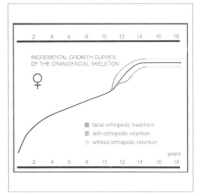

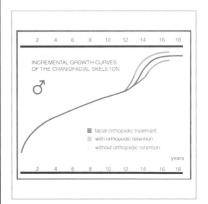

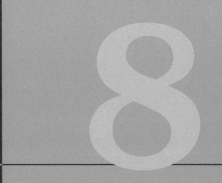

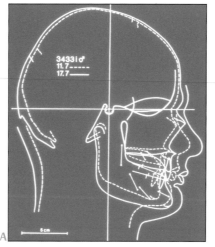
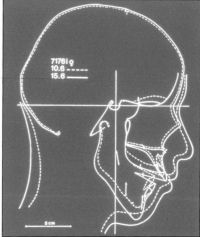
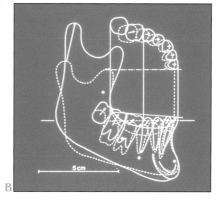
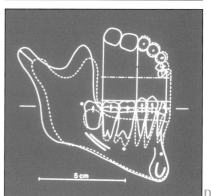

FIGURE 8-1

Tracings of cephalograms of two non–orthodontically treated persons in whom metal implants were placed. In A and C, the superimpositioning is at the anterior cranial base, and the movement is indicated with arrows. In B and D, the superimpositioning is at the implants.

The individual on the left side had a small lower facial height, a Class II division 2 malocclusion, and an excess of external soft tissues. With growth, the mandible rotated anteriorly and the symphysis moved forward, almost horizontally (A). The growth at the condyles was extensive and directed anteriorly, and the mandibular teeth migrated mesially (B).

The individual on the right side had a large lower anterior facial height, a Class II division 1 malocclusion with an open bite, and a relative shortage of external soft tissues. With growth, the mandible rotated posteriorly and moved caudally, and the chin moved downward perpendicularly (C). The growth at the condyles was directed posteriorly, and the mandibular teeth erupted perpendicular to the occlusal plane (D).[27]

One of the most valuable contributions to the knowledge of facial growth has been delivered by Björk,[24] who placed small metal implants in the craniofacial skeleton prior to taking standardized lateral cephalograms, long before implants were introduced in clinical dentistry. Prior to these studies, he had published the article, "The Face in Profile," which laid the basis for many cephalometric radiographic studies performed in the second half of the 20th century.[23]

The use of implants made it clear where growth occurred and at which surfaces bone was deposited and resorbed. This method also revealed a large variation in growth patterns. In addition, it became clear that the mode in which the craniofacial skeleton enlarges is not uniform.[25, 26, 28] In some individuals, growth at the sutures contributes most to the increase of the midface; in others the deposition of bone at surfaces is responsible for such growth. Figure 8-1, A and C, shows the cephalometric tracings of two individuals who differ markedly in skeletal morphology, facial configuration, and dentition. Their growth patterns and mode of growth also vary widely. The direction of growth at the condyle differs considerably between the two individuals, as does the pattern of deposition and resorption of bone at the mandibular border and at the posterior surface of the ramus. Furthermore, the movement of the teeth in the arches is different (Fig 8-1, B and D).

The first longitudinal studies of cephalometric radiographs provided information about average growth patterns. Broadbent[37, 39] introduced the "Bolton standards," which include the period from 3 to 18 years of age (Fig 8-2). Brodie[40] studied facial growth in children aged 3 months to 8 years of age and concluded that the facial pattern is determined at an early stage and remains constant.

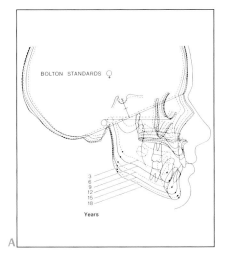

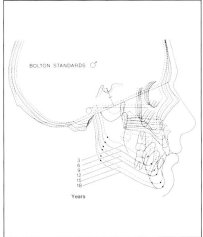

FIGURE 8-2

These illustrations, from Broadbent,[39] of the development of the craniofacial skeleton are based on the averages of 16 boys and 16 girls with corresponding, similar-looking facial configurations. Girls grow less than boys and have a smaller adolescent growth spurt than boys, and the adolescent growth takes place about 2 years earlier in girls than in boys. Furthermore, in contrast to boys, girls exhibit little or no growth after 15 years of age and attain a less straight profile. The data on which these illustrations are based were collected more than 60 years ago. At the present time, the adolescent growth spurt takes place 1 to 2 years earlier and the growth in girls is completed earlier.

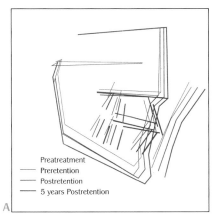

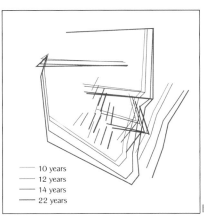

Preatreatment
Preretention
Postretention
5 years Postretention

10 years
12 years
14 years
22 years

FIGURE 8-3

Changes in 26 boys with a Class II division 1 malocclusion treated with a cervical headgear, usually with the addition of a maxillary plate (A), and 18 untreated individuals (B). The records were collected at the beginning of treatment, the beginning of retention, the completion of retention, and 5 years postretention. The records of the control group coincided in age.

There is a large variation in facial patterns in children at 3 months of age.[40]

However, this is already the case 6 months after conception, as was found in a cephalometric radiographic study on 30 fetuses.[128] From the many studies published in the last 60 years of the 20th century, it became clear that variation exists not only in initial facial patterns but also in the changes in facial configuration realized by further growth. Both variations are probably caused mainly by factors located outside the facial skeleton, of which functional components play a dominating role.[219]

The alterations in direction and amount of growth caused by facial orthopedic appliances are illustrated with data from a long-term study of cervical headgear therapy (Fig 8-3).[89] Children from the "Nijmegen Growth Study" served as control.[164] A significant difference was found between the two groups at the age that treatment was concluded. The same difference existed 5 years later and regarding a more posterior positioning of the lips, of the anterior sides of both arches, and of the permanent maxillary first molars in the original Class II division 1 group. This study further revealed that, in the cervical headgear group during treatment, the mandible mainly grew in the caudal direction with a substantial increase in ramus length. The latter confirmed the observations of Baumrind et al,[16] published in 1981. Of particular importance was the finding that, in the 2 years following treatment, the mandible grew mainly anteriorly and very little in the caudal direction. In the control group, such a dichotomy between vertical and sagittal growth was not observed. During treatment with a cervical headgear, the direction of facial growth was altered, but, with growth taking place in the years following, the previous facial configuration returned. The changes illustrated in Fig 8-3 and desribed above were also found in the female samples of 24 experimental and 17 control individuals. However, the changes and differences were less marked in girls than in boys.[89]

FIGURE 8-4

A girl aged 7 years 2 months had a severe Class II division 1 malocclusion, an anteriorly located midface, and a posteriorly positioned mandible. She had sucked her thumb intensively until 2 months previously (A, B). At the age of 9 years 8 months, 2 years 6 months later, the facial configuration had improved spontaneously, and a headgear was placed (C, D). Ten months later, fixed appliances were added. At the age of 12 years 2 months, after active treatment of 2 years 6 months, retention was started (E, F). This involved a retention plate in the maxilla and a canine bar in the mandible, which stayed in until the age of 15 years 6 months (G, H). In all respects, an excellent result was obtained. The facial photographs revealed the spontaneous pretreatment improvement of the facial configuration, to which the cessation of the sucking habit contributed (A, C). The facial changes during treatment were rather small. The midface became somewhat less prominent and the mandible was repositioned more anteriorly, but only slightly (C, E). However, the improvements in the profile in the 3 years following active therapy were striking (E, G). In the first 18 months of that period, a maxillary retention plate was used. It is not realistic to assume that this plate or the mandibular canine bar affected facial growth. This patient happened to have a very favorable facial growth pattern, which indeed was altered during treatment, but that resulted in a beautiful face mainly through growth that took place after treatment.

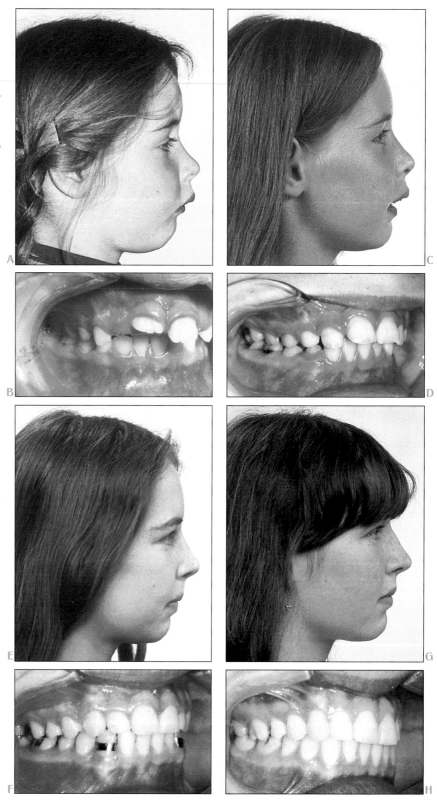

Figure 8-4 shows a girl with a favorable growth pattern who was treated with a cervical headgear and fixed appliances. It is clear that the beautiful face she developed was the result of a very favorable growth pattern.

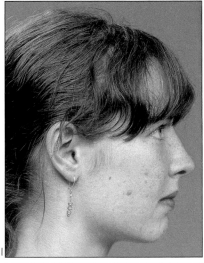

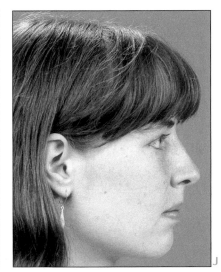

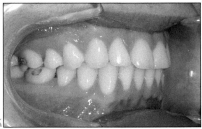

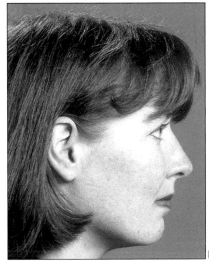

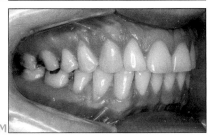

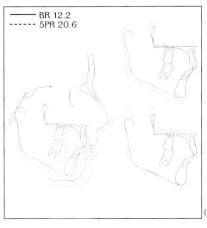

I

J

K

M

L

```
——— BT 9.7
------ BR 12.2
```

N

```
——— BR 12.2
------ 5PR 20.6
```

O

FIGURE 8-4 (CONTINUED)

The photographs obtained at the age of 20 years 6 months indicated that the profile and the dentition had undergone no or few changes in the preceding 5 years (I, K). Over the years, the face matured, as was apparent in the photographs taken at 25 years of age (J, M) and 30 years of age (L), which show an older but certainly no less beautiful face.

For many years, the author believed that the excellent development illustrated here was achieved mainly through the orthodontic treatment and its accompanying influence on facial growth. About 8 years ago, the author started to realize that this assumption was incorrect. Indeed, an ideal occlusion was realized by the treatment and facial growth was affected. However, the beautiful face she reached cannot be attributed to the treatment. Of course, without treatment, the disto-occlusion and large overjet and overbite would not have been improved or would have improved only slightly. The malocclusion would have been maintained, but would have been camouflaged largely by the favorable facial growth. The superimposition of the tracings revealed that, because of the use of the cervical headgear, the anterior part of the maxilla did not move anteriorly during the active treatment phase, and the mandible moved only slightly anteriorly but mainly caudally (N). The reverse happened in the years thereafter (O). These records were collected at the beginning of treatment (BT), the beginning of retention (BR), and 5 years postretention (5PR). These changes conform to the ones shown in Fig 8-3, B, in which the effects of a cervical headgear during and after treatment are illustrated.

FIGURE 8-5

A girl aged 9 years 9 months had a Class II division 1 malocclusion with a disto-occlusion the equivalent of half a premolar crown width, an anterior non-occlusion, and extensive crowding in both dental arches (A, C). All four first premolars were extracted, and a parietal headgear and fixed appliances were used. A parietal headgear was applied purposely because she had a large lower anterior facial height. The active treatment lasted 1 year 4 months, followed by a 6-month retention phase with a positioner. At the age of 12 years 2 months, when the use of the positioner was concluded, an ideal occlusion and harmonious face were reached (B). However, 1 year later, the contact in the anterior region was lost, although the incisors still overlapped each other. Fifteen years later, at the age of 27 years 11 months, the lower face had become markedly longer, and an anterior non-occlusion was still present (D, E). The superimpositions of the tracings showed that the total facial height and the lower anterior facial height barely increased during treatment. The growth of the maxilla was inhibited, and the chin had moved anteriorly (F). The vertical development after treatment was considerable. The permanent maxillary first molars erupted significantly, the condyles experienced extensive vertical growth, and the lower facial height increased substantially (G). These records were collected at the beginning of treatment (BT), at the completion of retention (RC), and 10 years postretention (10PR). Obviously, the direction and amount of facial growth were influenced effectively by the treatment. Thereafter, the former growth pattern was reestablished because growth was not completed yet. After the age of 12 years 2 months, the nose became considerably larger, and the jaws grew further anteriorly, but the increase in lower anterior facial height was most striking.

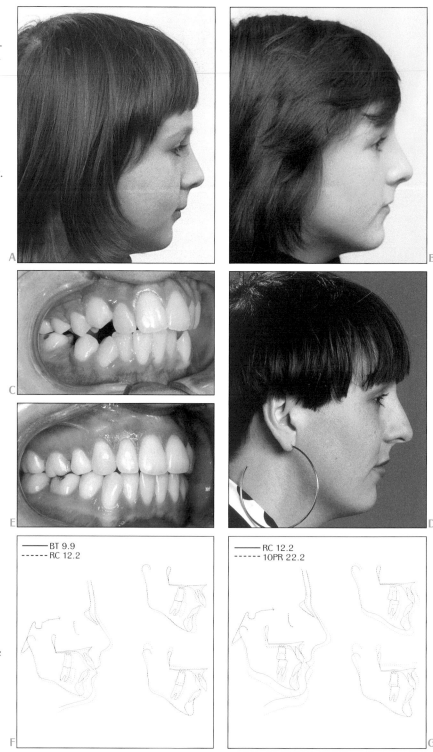

Figure 8-5 presents a girl with a large lower anterior facial height, in whom a parietal headgear had restricted the caudal development but marked vertical development occurred after treatment.

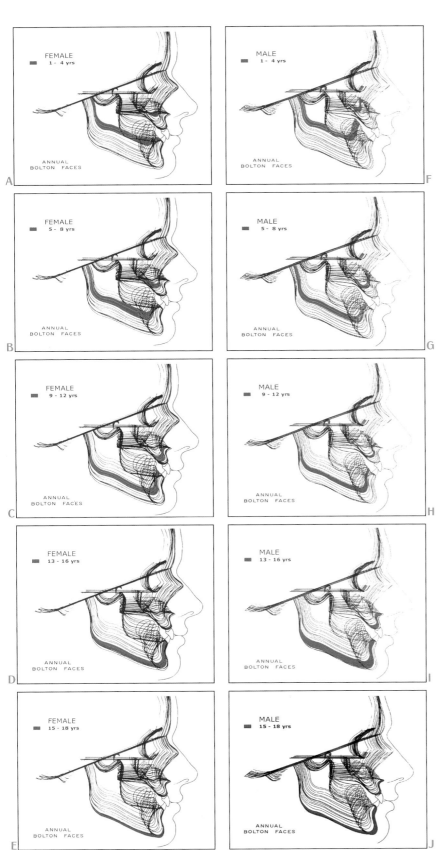

FIGURE 8-6

The Bolton standards presented in Fig 8-2 are reproduced with coloring of areas representing 3-year periods of maxillo-mandibular growth. This is done to indicate the amount of growth and the differences at various age periods between girls (LEFT) and boys (RIGHT). Many treatments are carried out between 9 and 12 years of age, during which girls experience the adolescent growth spurt (C, H). However, it is still questionable if the majority of girls truly undergo such a growth spurt in the face.[30] Indeed, most boys experience a facial growth spurt, which occurs at a later age (I). Of importance also is the amount of growth remaining after treatment, which is much greater in boys than in girls.

Review of these illustrations makes it clear that facial orthopedic therapy affects only a small part of the total facial growth over time. Considerable growth takes place before treatment and often thereafter. It is not realistic to assume a permanent effect of facial orthopedic therapy when growth continues. Furthermore, the Bolton standards are based on 16 selected, similar-looking individuals with ideal occlusion and well balanced faces of each gender[18]; periods of rapid growth, and particularly the adolescent growth spurt, vary in the age at which they take place. Like the start of puberty, the onset of the adolescent growth spurt has a normal range of variation of ± 2 years around the mean. This variation leads to the smoothing of peaks in growth curves based on more than one individual. Average growth curves portray a smaller and longer-lasting growth spurt than is experienced individually.[134] Furthermore, the standards are based on yearly observations, also leading to the recording of smaller and longer-lasting growth spurts than occur in reality in the individuals observed.[208]

Figure 8-6 illustrates the average amount of growth occurring in 3-year periods, clarifying that the quantity of growth influenced by treatment is relatively small.

FIGURE 8-7

The treatment of this girl, who had a Class II division 1 malocclusion, a disto-occlusion measuring half a premolar crown width, and an overjet of 8 mm, started at the age of 10 years 1 month (A, C). An activator was used to correct the disto-occlusion and retract the maxillary incisors. The limited tooth movements still needed were realized with a positioner, and the goal of therapy was reached at the age of 11 years 7 months (B). Not only an esthetically pleasing dentition and perfect occlusion but also a competent lip seal and a better facial appearance were obtained. Twenty years later, at the age of 31 years 7 months, the face had become larger and the profile was straighter. The arrangement of the teeth and the occlusion were good (D, E). The superimposed tracings of the cephalograms made at the start and at the conclusion of treatment demonstrated the changes in the skeletal structures and profile during treatment. The anterior development of the maxilla had been limited, while the mandible grew in the caudal direction (F). Much growth took place in the years following. The chin became displaced far anteriorly, but the anterior part of the maxilla also moved in that direction, although to a lesser degree. These changes resulted in the anterior movement of the lower face and the straightening of the profile (G). These records were collected at the beginning of treatment (BT), at the completion of retention (RC), and 10 years postretention (1OPR). The large amount of growth that occurred after the age of 11 years 7 months was striking. The growth occurred in the first years after treatment and was completed at 15 years of age.

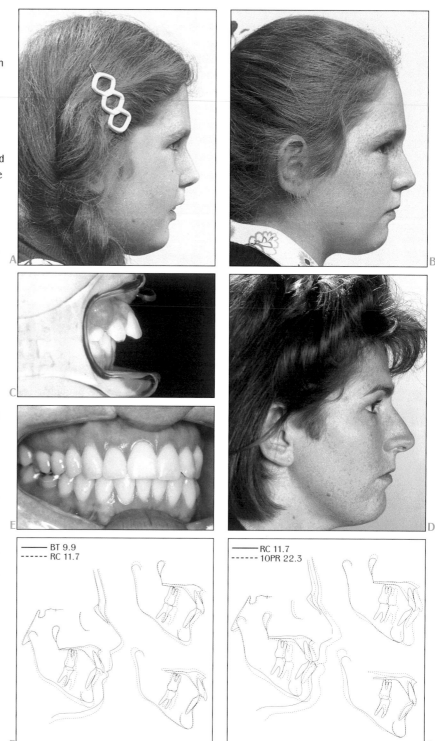

To demonstrate the changes over the long term, profile photographs and superimpositions of tracings of cephalometric radiographs of six patients are shown in Figs 8-7 to 8-12, the first three of whom are girls. When girls are treated at an early age, considerable growth can take place afterward. However, facial growth is completed in most girls at about 15 years of age or earlier. When treatment is carried out at a later age and concluded when growth is finished, few changes will occur subsequently, and the result obtained is largely permanent.

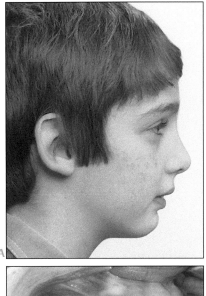

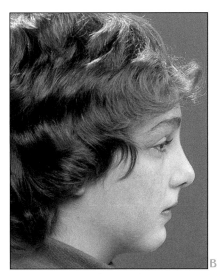

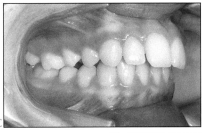

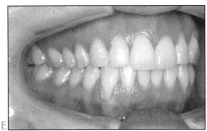

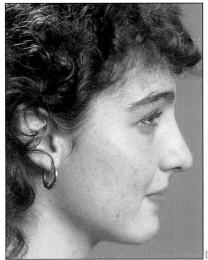

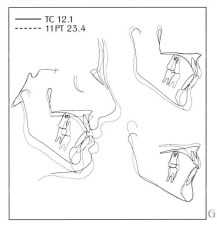

A

B

C

D

E

F

BT 10.0
TC 12.1

TC 12.1
11PT 23.4

G

FIGURE 8-8

This girl, 10 years 0 months of age, had a Class II division 1 malocclusion with a disto-occlusion of one premolar crown width and a receding chin. All permanent teeth, except the third molars, were already present in the mouth. The upper lip was short, and she exhibited a 2-mm gingival zone when smiling. (A, C). She was treated with a parietal headgear, a maxillary plate, and fixed appliances at the maxillary incisors. At the age of 12 years 1 month, after 24 months of treatment, a good result was obtained (B). In the years following, the dentition showed only minor changes; however, facial growth was substantial. At the age of 23 years 4 months, more than 11 years after the conclusion of treatment, the patient had a nice profile and an esthetically pleasing and well-functioning dentition (D, E). The superimpositions showed that, during treatment, the anterior development of the maxilla had been inhibited and the permanent maxillary first molars had not erupted further. The height of the face and particularly the lower face did not increase or increased only slightly (F). The extensive growth after treatment occurred mainly between 12 and 14 years of age. During that period, the height of the face and the length of the mandible increased markedly (G). These records were collected at the beginning of treatment (BT), at the completion of treatment (TC), and 11 years posttreatment (11PT). The difference in development during and after treatment was remarkable. With the parietal headgear, the growth of the face in the caudal direction was inhibited, and the occlusion improved as the mandible became more anteriorly positioned in relation to the maxilla. After the conclusion of the treatment, the mandible grew further anteriorly, but the height of the face increased excessively, particularly in the midfacial region.

The situation is different in boys (Figs 8-10 to 8-12). Their adolescent growth spurt is greater, takes place about 2 years later, and lasts longer than that in girls.[150, 192] Regarding the second transitional period in the development of the dentition, the difference between boys and girls is smaller, and the primary molars and canines are replaced about 6 months later in boys than in girls.[213] When a treatment is started at the end of the second transitional period, in general, girls are already going through puberty, but boys are not.

Figure 8-9

A girl of 10 years 8 months had a Class II division 1 malocclusion with a receding chin, a short upper lip, and a "gummy" smile (A, C). After the disto-occlusion was corrected with an activator over a period of 9 months, the treatment was stopped. Eighteen months later, the disto-occlusion had returned somewhat, and a parietal headgear, attached to a Bass plate to intrude the maxillary incisors, was placed (SEE FIG 5-19). After 12 months, a neutro-occlusion was reached, and the maxillary incisors were intruded sufficiently. To improve the position of some teeth as well as for retention purposes, a positioner was used intensively for 1 month and subsequently during sleeping hours for 5 months. A well-arranged dentition and an acceptable facial appearance resulted, as was apparent in the records collected at the age of 15 years 1 month (B). Fifteen years after the treatment was concluded, at the age of 30 years, little had changed (D, E).

The superimposed tracings of the cephalograms, taken before and after treatment, demonstrated that the vertical development of the face occurred mainly in the midface, resulting in a descent of the mandibular border, and that the maxillary incisors were intruded. The chin had moved anteriorly, but the anterior part of the maxilla had advanced only slightly (F). The superimpositions demonstrating the changes that occurred after treatment revealed that, after the age of 14 years 10 months, little facial growth took place, and the facial configuration changed only slightly. The nose became somewhat larger, and the chin and mandible attained slightly more anterior positions (G). These records were collected at the beginning of treatment (BT), at the completion of retention (RC), and 10 years postretention (1OPR).

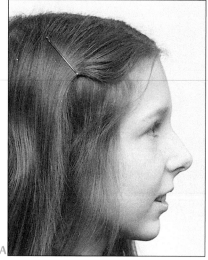
A

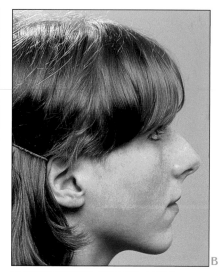
B

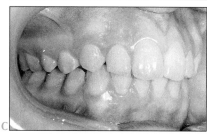
C

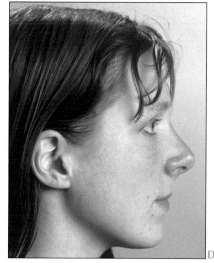
D

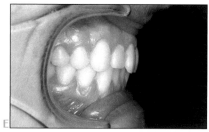
E

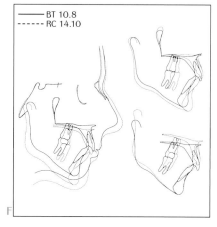

———— BT 10.8
- - - - - RC 14.10

F

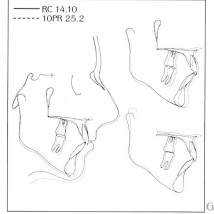

———— RC 14.10
- - - - - 1OPR 25.2

G

In boys, facial growth also can be guided. Treatment before puberty is preferred for psychological reasons and also has the advantage that the development of the dentition can be guided. However, as a consequence, the treatment will not benefit from the adolescent growth spurt in the face, and often substantial growth will occur after active treatment has been concluded.[161]

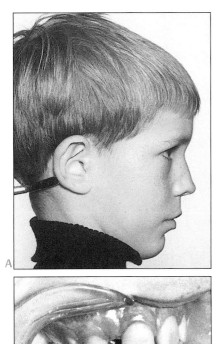

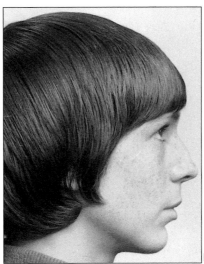

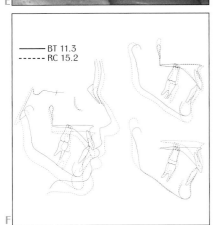

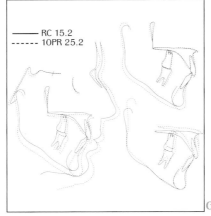

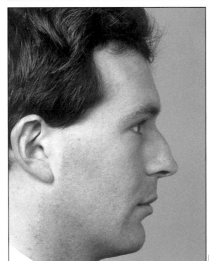

A

B

C

D

E

F

G

BT 11.3
RC 15.2

RC 15.2
1OPR 25.2

FIGURE 8-10

A boy aged 8 years 2 months had a moderate Class II division 1 malocclusion with crowding in both dental arches, which had resulted in premature loss of primary anterior teeth (A, C). To correct the asymmetric arrangement of the incisors and improve their positions, the remaining primary canines were extracted successively. At the age of 11 years 2 months, a lingual arch was placed to increase the space in the mandibular dental arch. For the same purpose, but also to correct the disto-occlusion, a cervical headgear was placed in the maxilla. Later, a maxillary plate was added. After active treatment for 2 years 3 months, all appliances were removed and a positioner was placed; it was used for 1 year 8 months. The photographs made at the age of 15 years and 2 months showed a harmonious profile for that age (B). At 25 years 1 month of age, the face had matured, but the dentition showed little difference from the situation 10 years earlier (D, E). The superimpositions showed the changes in the facial skeleton that occurred during treatment, including the retention period. Facial height had increased substantially, while the mandible had moved more to the anterior than had the maxilla (F). In the years following, the face grew more anteriorly than caudally, resulting in a more anterior positioning of the mandible and the chin. The maxilla also attained a slightly more anterior position (G). These records were collected at the beginning of treatment (BT), at the completion of retention (RC), and 10 years postretention (1OPR). The records of this patient demonstrate clearly the large amount of growth that can take place in boys after 15 years of age, resulting in a harmonious face and straight profile.

It also holds true for boys that, after facial orthopedic treatment, the former growth pattern returns.[131] The chance of this happening is greater in boys than in girls, because boys exhibit more growth after treatment. When facial growth is within the range of normality, this aspect is of little importance. However, problems can arise in patients with a large lower anterior facial height, which is often accompanied by an anterior open bite. The same applies to patients with a small lower anterior facial height, which is often accompanied by a deep bite.

FIGURE 8-11

A boy who was 11 years 7 months of age had a Class II division 1 malocclusion with an anterior open bite. He had a long, narrow face, a small nose, a large lower anterior facial height, and a steeply inclined mandibular border. He could not breathe well through the nose, and he had an open mouth posture (A, C). In view of his large facial height and lip incompetence, the disto-occlusion was corrected with a parietal headgear. Later, a maxillary plate was added to distalize the premolars and canines and to retract the incisors. The active treatment lasted 1 year 5 months. The disto-occlusion was corrected, and the incisors were retracted but without reaching contact with the mandibular anterior teeth (B). The active treatment was not followed by retention, which was an error in judgment and a clinical mistake. In patients with an incompetent lip seal and a restricted nasal passageway that necessitates mouth breathing, it must be anticipated that the maxillary incisors will move labially again. In this patient, the six maxillary anterior teeth and the first premolars should have been splinted together by a bonded, thin dead-soft braided wire. The neutro-occlusion in the posterior region was maintained, but the open bite and eversion of the maxillary incisors had returned. Furthermore, facial height had increased excessively (D, E).

The superimposed tracings showed that, during treatment, the height of the midface increased slightly and that of the lower face barely changed. The eruption of the maxillary first molars had been arrested (F). In the years following, the face exhibited excessive vertical development. The maxillary molars extruded, and the length of the ramus and the height of the midface increased markedly; however, most striking was the increase in lower anterior facial height (G). These records were collected at the beginning of treatment (BT), at the completion of treatment (TC), and 8.5 years posttreatment (8.5PT).

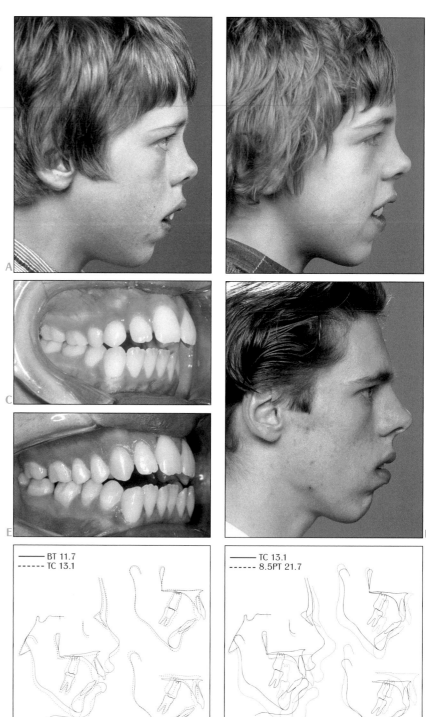

When data from growth studies carried out years ago are interpreted, the secular trend in growth has to be taken into account. That term refers to the gradual shifting of the start of puberty and the adolescent growth spurt to an earlier age.[191] In addition, the population of the western world is becoming gradually taller, with Dutch people at the lead.[73] However, the Netherlands is also the country in which more growth data have been collected in the last 60 years than in any other country in the world.[54, 74, 169, 231]

Furthermore, growth curves are based mostly on averages; as a consequence, peaks are smoothed and growth spurts are estimated as lasting longer than they actually do (Fig 8-6).

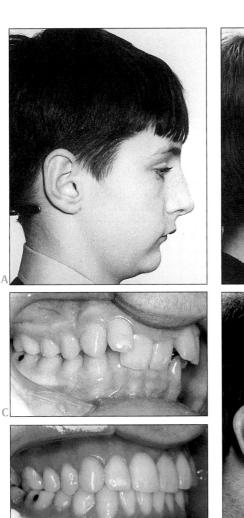

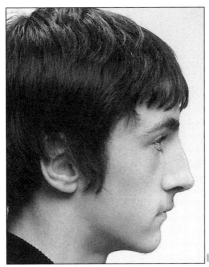

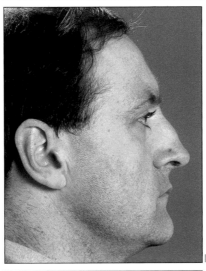

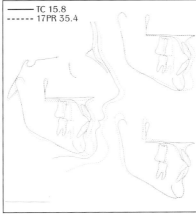

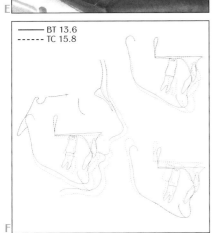

FIGURE 8-12

A boy aged 13 years 6 months with a Class II division 2 malocclusion had a posteriorly located mandible and a short upper lip. The lower lip covered the maxillary central incisors completely and was positioned palatally of the lateral incisors (A, B). To correct the disto-occlusion and increase the lower anterior facial height, a cervical headgear was placed. In the mandible, a lingual arch was used. The treatment lasted a total of 2 years 1 month and was completed with fixed appliances. At 15 years 8 months of age, a good result was obtained and the maxillary incisors were not covered excessively by the lower lip (C). In the mandible, a canine bar was placed for retention; it was removed after 2 years 6 months. The maxillary retention plate was worn day and night for 6 months and then used only during sleep for 1 year. At 35 years 4 months of age, 17 years after retention was ended, the dentition had changed little (D, E). The superimposed tracings showed that, during treatment, the mandible exhibited extensive growth in the anterior and caudal directions, while the maxilla did not move anteriorly (F). Following the active treatment, the growth of the mandible was accompanied by an anterior rotation, leading to a reduction of the lower anterior facial height (G). These records were collected at the beginning of treatment (BT), at the completion of treatment (TC), and 17 years postretention (17PR). Boys still can exhibit considerable facial growth after 15 years of age, which can be favorable or unfavorable. In this patient, a retention plate with a bite plane should have been worn during the night until facial growth was completed, which seldom occurs in boys before around 20 years of age.

Adolescent growth spurts do not occur at the same time in the various regions of the body. First the extremities undergo the growth spurt, then the trunk, followed by a more rapid broadening of the shoulder region. Furthermore, the extremities can be subdivided in that respect: first the foot, then the lower leg, and finally the upper leg experiences the growth spurt. The period of accelerated growth for a single anatomic structure is rather short, and that probably also applies to the mandible, as one of the last structures in the body that undergoes acceleration of growth.

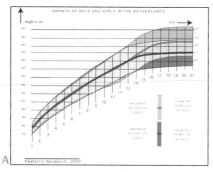
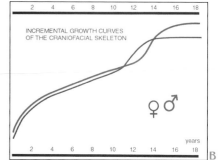

FIGURE 8-13

Recently collected data on the increase in stature in the Dutch population demonstrate the difference between boys and girls (A). The facial growth spurt starts much earlier and ends much sooner in girls than in boys (B).

FIGURE 8-14

It is assumed that facial orthopedic therapy will increase or decrease the rate of growth of specific skeletal structures, resulting in a higher or lower course of the growth curve (green). After treatment, decreased or increased compensatory growth takes place (yellow), and a return to the original growth curve occurs (A, B). When the active treatment is followed by a facial orthopedic retention period (orange), lasting until growth is completed, the effect of the treatment will be probably maintained to a large extent (C, D). The same applies when the facial orthopedic treatment is carried out at the end of the growth phase (E, F). This "catch-up" phenomenon has been observed in longitudinal growth studies in humans and animals. A child who experiences a long-lasting illness or is severely underfed will not grow. When the health and living conditions have returned to normal, accelerated growth will compensate for the deficiency until the child is caught up. However, when poor conditions continue until the epiphyseal disks are closed, the potential stature will not be reached.[192]

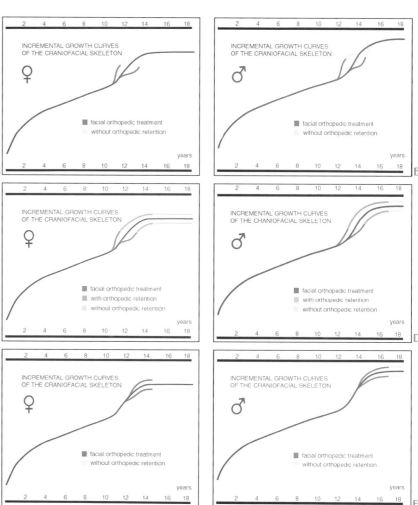

The difference in the course of growth between boys and girls becomes clearly evident in the most recently collected Dutch data (Fig 8-13, A). The hypothesized average values for facial growth are presented in Fig 8-13, B, in a comparable way. These values have been used to express the assumed effect of facial orthopedic therapy during treatment and thereafter (Fig 8-14).

The end result of facial orthopedic therapy depends on the amount of growth that occurs after treatment and on the application of facial orthopedic retention.[52, 98, 153, 237] Although in general no permanent effect remains of facial orthopedic therapy, that does not mean that such a treatment does not have advantages.

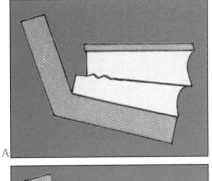

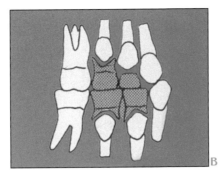

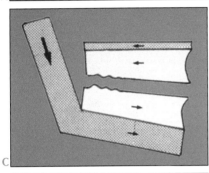

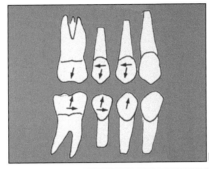

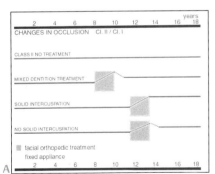

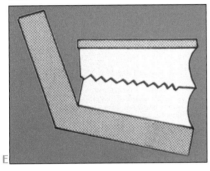

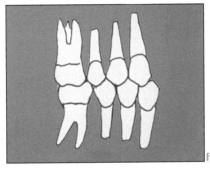

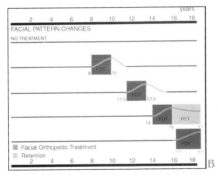

FIGURE 8-15

A solid intercuspation does not exist in the mixed dentition in either normal occlusions or Class II division 1 malocclusions. The occlusal surfaces of the primary molars become flat through attrition, and permanent first molars do not interdigitate rigidly (B). In an effective facial orthopedic therapy, the length of the ramus increases, the mandible attains a more anterior relationship to the maxilla, and the sagittal occlusion improves (C). Through the increase in lower facial height, the erupting posterior teeth can be guided over a larger distance, facilitating their guidance to the correct mesiodistal positions. Emerging premolars are easier to redirect when advantage is taken of the extra space that becomes available in the dental arches when their predecessors are shed (D). When the premolars and canines occlude with a solid intercuspation after treatment, the realized improvement in occlusion of the posterior teeth will be maintained (E, F). Subsequent changes in the sagittal relationship between the two jaws will not affect the occlusion, because a partial or complete return to the original facial pattern will be accompanied by a compensating migration of the teeth within the arches.

FIGURE 8-16

Changes in the occlusion of the posterior teeth will only be maintained if a solid intercuspation exists. That is not the case in patients with occlusally flat primary molars or open bites and non-occlusions in the posterior regions (A). Changes in the facial configuration are not preserved when growth continues after treatment has been concluded (B).

Indeed, essential advantages are the temporary improvement of the sagittal maxillomandibular relationship and the increase in lower facial height through which it becomes easier to reach a neutro-occlusion in a biologic way (Fig 8-15). When Class II division 1 treatments are concluded with a solid intercuspation, the neutro-occlusion will be maintained (Fig 8-16). However, that does not apply to Class III malocclusions, because continued mandibular anterior growth can lead to mesio-occlusion again.

In growth occurring after treatment, the mandible moves more anteriorly than does the maxilla, which contributes to the stability of a corrected disto-occlusion. Dental arches with a solid intercuspation will shift within the growing jaws as one unit. The associated tooth movements are quite extensive even after all permanent teeth, except the third molars, have attained full occlusion, and that applies particularly to boys (Fig 8-17, A).

FIGURE 8-17

A solid intercuspation maintains both the sagittal and the transverse occlusions in the posterior regions. In a growing face, the teeth migrate within the arches under the guidance of the occlusion. When a solid intercuspation exists at the end of treatment (A: BLACK, BEFORE TREATMENT; RED, AFTER TREATMENT) the migration of the opposing posterior teeth will be coordinated (B: GREEN, AFTER GROWTH IS COMPLETED). However, when no solid intercuspation is obtained, the migration of the opposing teeth will not be coordinated, and with continuing growth of the face improvements in the occlusion are often partially lost. The mandibular and maxillary posterior teeth will migrate independently of each other in the growing face (C, D).

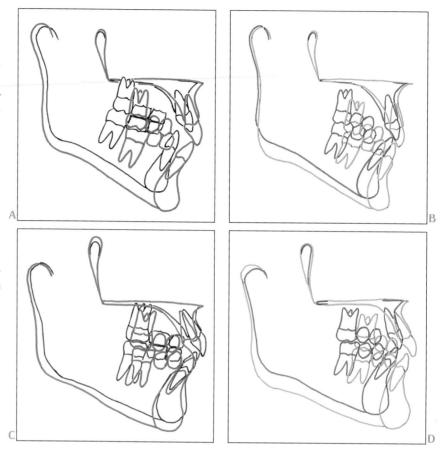

However, if a solid interdigitation does not exist, the movements of the opposing teeth will not be coordinated as the mandibular teeth shift independently of the maxillary teeth in the growing face. Correction of disto-occlusion or mesio-occlusion will be partially lost (Fig 8-17, B).

Proffit[166] has recommended that patients with a large anterior facial height wear a parietal headgear or a high bite block in the posterior regions as a retention device during sleep until facial growth is concluded. However, this is more theory than practice. Boys are not inclined to follow this protocol and to remain faithful to it until the end of growth, somewhere around 20 years of age. More cooperation is encountered for the continued use of a face mask with anterior traction to the maxilla to prevent the recurrence of a reversed anterior overbite and the return of an unpleasant facial and lip appearance. The suggestion that orthognathic surgery can be avoided with this approach is helpful in gaining compliance. However, orthognathic surgery is also an option for patients with a large facial height when this condition is experienced as a facial disfigurement by the patient and those in his or her social environment.

Prospective randomized clinical trials have demonstrated that, with facial orthopedic therapy at an early age, the facial pattern is improved and subsequent treatment with fixed appliances will be of shorter duration than is the case when no facial orthopedic treatment has preceded.[59, 77, 100, 201, 236] However, a few years after conclusion of the second treatment phase, no differences can be observed between the patients who have undergone a two-phase treatment and those who have undergone only a one-phase treatment with fixed appliances.[201]

In conclusion, it irrelevant in which way a solid intercuspation has been reached. Permanent maxillary first molars can be distalized, for example, with a pendulum appliance, or with an effective facial orthopedic appliance, such as a Herbst appliance, and the end result seems not to differ.

However, without question, although facial orthopedics may not have a permanent effect, it facilitates the attainment of a good occlusion and, when used at an early age, provides several other benefits: Functional conditions can be improved early, lip closure is stimulated, and the risk for fractures of maxillary incisors is reduced.

Use of Partial Fixed Appliances

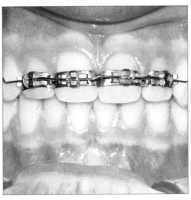

Complete fixed appliances are not always needed to reach a satisfactory result in the correction of malocclusions.[215] That holds particularly true for Class II division 1 malocclusions, for which much improvement can be achieved with headgears, activators, and combinations of both, as explained in preceding chapters. In addition, quite an improvement can be reached with a removable plate; this also applies to Class I malocclusions. However, when three-dimensional control of the maxillary anterior teeth is needed, only fixed appliances at the incisors and permanent first molars can lead to a satisfying result. Rotations, vertical deviations, mesiodistal angulations, and labiolingual inclinations can be corrected with a resilient wire in the brackets attached to the incisors.

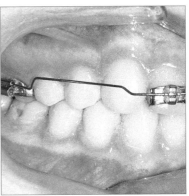

Undesirable alterations in the dentition occurring at a later age, such as tertiary crowding in the mandibular anterior region, can be treated efficiently with partial fixed appliances. The same holds true for the correction of relapse after orthodontic treatment, especially of the mandibular incisors. Alignment of these teeth can be carried out in a relatively short period of time with a resilient wire placed through the brackets at four or six anterior teeth and tubes at the molars, particularly if the space needed has been generated by interproximal stripping.

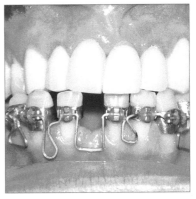

When the malocclusion is limited to the congenital absence of maxillary lateral incisors, partial fixed appliances can occasionally suffice to provide the required positioning of the teeth to allow substitution of the lateral incisors with a fixed partial denture or by means of an implant. That also applies when a mandibular incisor has to be extracted.

Indeed, partial fixed appliances are a useful means to correct malalignments in the mandibular and maxillary anterior regions, particularly when additional esthetic improvement is provided with resin composite.

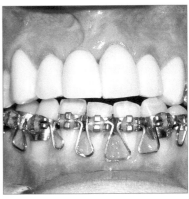

In this chapter, various aspects essential to treatment with partial fixed appliances are discussed, and the results that can be obtained are illustrated. Some of the patients shown were treated prior to the introduction of resin composites in dentistry. They are included to demonstrate the long-term results of partial fixed appliances.

Orthodontic Concepts and Strategies

9

FIGURE 9-1

In an esthetically optimal arrangement of the maxillary anterior teeth, the incisal edges are horizontally aligned so that the edges of the lateral incisors are located 0.5 mm more cervically than are the edges of the central incisors and the cusp tips of the canines (A). The cervical borders of the central incisors and canines are at the same level; those of the lateral incisors are slightly more occlusal (B). Grinding or extension with resin composite can compensate for deviations in crown heights (C). The clinical crown height can be increased by gingivectomy (D).

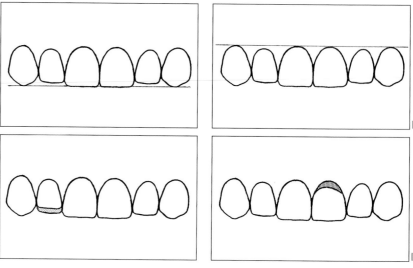

FIGURE 9-2

Esthetically well-arranged maxillary anterior teeth add to the facial animation when these teeth are fully shown during laughing without exposure of a zone of gingiva and, in addition, when the incisal line runs parallel to the curvature of the lower lip (A).[178] Differences in heights of the cervical borders of the central incisors can be visually disturbing (B). That also holds true, although to a lesser extent, for too large a difference in height between the lateral and central incisors (C). A straight incisal line reduces the liveliness (D).

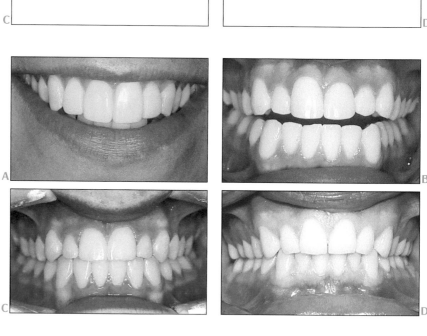

The use of fixed appliances was simplified and facilitated with the introduction of bonding, because bands on anterior teeth are not needed anymore. Currently, brackets have a preprogrammed design, different for every tooth, so that straight archwires without loops or torque can provoke the required movements. In addition, various highly resilient, preformed archwires that deliver small, long-lasting, well-controlled forces are available.

For the patient and the surrounding social environment, the position of the maxillary anterior teeth is the most important criterion for evaluating the success of orthodontic treatment. Prior to the introduction of resin composites in dentistry, the position of the teeth in fixed appliance treatment was difficult to evaluate, because bands obscured the observation, and proper positioning at the end of treatment was more difficult to obtain. Bands covered the crowns over a large area and interfered with the establishment of approximal contacts. It was difficult to determine if adjacent anatomic contact points were properly located.

Since it became possible to bond attachments to the enamel, not only can the position of the teeth be judged better, but also the teeth can be brought in contact with each other in ideal positions, for which specific criteria apply regarding the height of the incisal edges and the height of the cervical margins of anterior teeth.

In addition to orthodontic treatment, the removal of enamel at incisal edges and approximal surfaces, supplemented with esthetic dentistry and gingivectomy, can be carried out to reach an ideally esthetic anterior region (Figs 9-1 and 9-2).[170, 214]

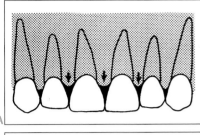
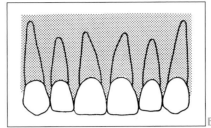
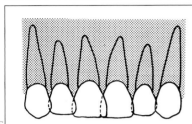
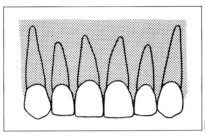
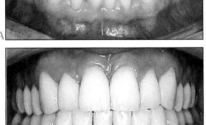
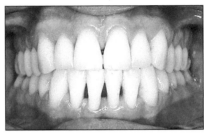

FIGURE 9-3

The papillae between maxillary incisors retract with aging when the contact between adjacent surfaces does not reach half of the crown heights (A). The contact area should not be farther away from the alveolar bony crest than 5.0 mm.[193] A contact that is located too far occlusally can be caused by an excessive mesial angulation of the maxillary incisors and by the shape of the teeth (B). Wide, triangular crowns can be changed in form by approximal grinding, so that the contact areas can extend more cervically (C, D).

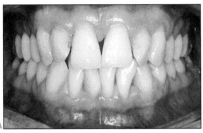
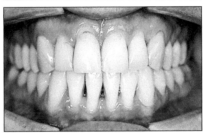

FIGURE 9-4

Black triangles can develop during the orthodontic correction of crowding of maxillary incisors with triangular crowns, particularly in adults (A). In this patient, approximal grinding could not be carried out to the required extent because the crowns would have become too narrow (B). The cervical regions of the crowns were built up with resin composite to fill the remaining open spaces (C). Ten years later, the papillae were still present (D).

For a pleasant appearance, not only the position of the anterior teeth, but also how much they are shown in speaking and smiling, is important. In addition, the presence or absence of interincisal papillae plays a large role. Whether papillae will be present at the end of treatment or will retract later depends largely on the shape of the crowns and on the angulation of the teeth, for which specific criteria also apply (Figs 9-3 and 9-4).[105, 141, 242]

It is difficult to pass judgment on the position of the maxillary anterior teeth when the patient is lying or sitting in the dental chair. The patient should be asked to rise, so that the clinician can look at the patient at an equal height and observe him or her from different angles. When the best-looking side is compared with the other side, it becomes clear where improvements are indicated.[243]

Adult patients are more demanding and critical than are children, particularly regarding the position of the maxillary incisors. With aging, the maxillary incisors become less visible as the upper lip increases in length and becomes less mobile. However, the mandibular anterior teeth are shown more, which may necessitate treatment at a later age. Such a request quite often arises from patients who have had relapse or who have developed tertiary crowding of the mandibular anterior teeth. After these deviations are treated, the result should be stabilized with a bonded lingual retainer.

Figure 9-5

When brackets with built-in angulation, torque, and compensating thickness in the base are used, the bracket slots have to be placed parallel to the incisal edges and positioned 0.5 mm more superior in relation to the incisal edges at the central incisors than at the lateral incisors (A). In the mesiodistal direction, the bracket should be positioned at the center of the crown (B). In normally shaped crowns, the lower side of the bracket base should be parallel to the incisal edge (C). The bracket slots of the maxillary incisors are not oriented perpendicular to the long axes, but deviate slightly, by 2 degrees for the central incisors and 5 degrees for the lateral incisors (D).

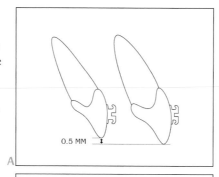
A

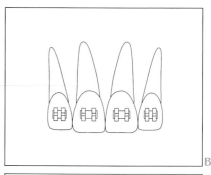
B

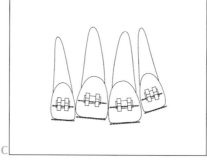
C

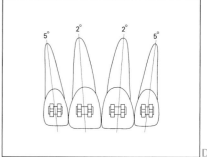
D

Figure 9-6

A flexible horseshoe-shaped archwire, which must be adapted to the form of the dental arch, is bent up behind the molar tubes to prevent the forward movement of the incisors. The archwire can be fastened in the bracket slots with soft 0.010-inch stainless steel ligatures or elastic rings (A). For rotational movement, only the bracket wing that lies close to the archwire is used initially, as is shown here for the left lateral incisor (B). At a later visit, when some movement has occurred, the archwire can be tied fully into the bracket (C). Teeth such as the left central incisor can be rotated further with a rotation wedge (D).

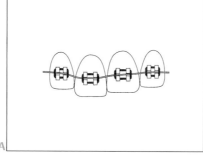
A

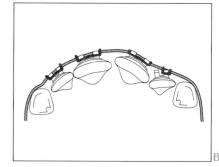
B

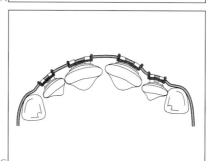
C

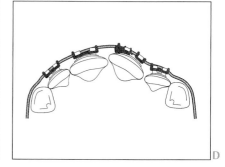
D

Partial fixed appliances are well suited to align maxillary anterior teeth. The brackets available now are designed to act with straight wires to lead the teeth automatically to the proper positions. Specific rules related to the ideal arrangement of teeth apply to the location of the brackets (Fig 9-5). Furthermore, the line between the maxillary central incisors should be parallel to the midsagittal plane of the face. When that is the case, a slight deviation of this line in relation to the midsagittal plane of the face will not be noticed.[97]

The commercially available preformed arches vary considerably in material composition, shape, cross-section, dimension, and properties. They have in common that they can generate small, long-lasting forces, when applied properly. Proper usage is clarified with drawings (Figs 9-6 to 9-10).

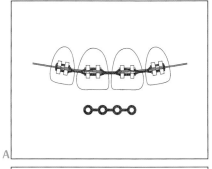

A

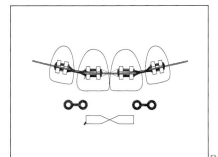

B

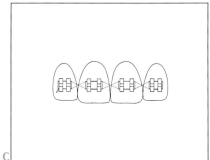

C

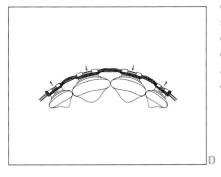

D

FIGURE 9-7

An "elastic chain" is used to pull the teeth together along the archwire (A). When contact between the adjacent teeth is established, the correction is maintained by tying a soft 0.008-inch stainless steel ligature around the brackets (B). Once all spaces have been closed, the teeth are held together with a 0.008-inch ligature laced across the four teeth (C). When an elastic chain is used across a curved arch segment, flattening of that curve has to be expected. To prevent undesirable flattening of the maxillary anterior teeth, the use of an elastic chain should be discontinued once all the spaces are closed (D).

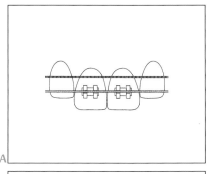

A

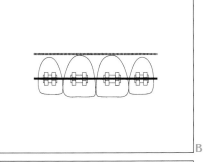

B

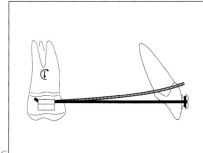

C

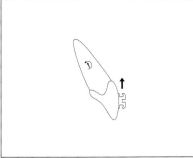

D

FIGURE 9-8

Maxillary incisors can be intruded with a braided archwire (the broken lines represent its passive position) (A). For simultaneous intrusion of the four maxillary incisors, it is also possible to use a stainless steel solid archwire (B). The reaction force at the molars has the effect of extruding and tipping them distally. If the force is so large that the molars do tip, then the archwire no longer has an intrusive effect at the incisors (C). Because the intrusive force at the incisors is directed vertically and is applied to the teeth anterior to their center of resistance, a couple is developed, which tends to rotate the incisors in the sagittal plane. The incisal edges will move labially, while the apices move palatally (D).

Unerupted maxillary canines can become impacted with the use of a partial fixed appliance, as the roots of the maxillary lateral incisors can move the canines to other positions. In addition, the roots of the lateral incisors can resorb.[19] During early treatment with fixed appliances, indicated to correct severe rotations of maxillary incisors, attention should be paid to these aspects. However, early correction of severe rotations, before the cementoenamel junction has reached the alveolar crest, has the advantage that the supra-alveolar periodontal fibers are formed in the corrected positions.[110] Rotations and other irregularities in tooth position can be corrected with partial fixed appliances only when sufficient space is available and the occlusion does not hinder the improvements. Indeed, these restrictions apply to the use of all types of appliances.

Use of Partial Fixed Appliances

Figure 9-9

Maxillary incisors can be retracted with 0.022 × 0.028-inch brackets and a 0.019 × 0.026-inch archwire with stops mesial to the molar tubes and sections of open coil spring (0.010- to 0.030-inch). These coil springs are compressed with soft 0.010-inch stainless steel ligatures and activated at subsequent visits (A). The distally directed force can also be produced by elastic chains (B). The reaction force exerted at the buccal side of the first molars tends to tip the molars mesially and rotate them mesiopalatally. To counteract the tipping and rotation, the part of the archwire distal to the molar stops should be bent in the cranial and palatal directions (C). If the archwire is allowed to rest against the buccal surfaces of the canines, these teeth can be moved palatally (D).

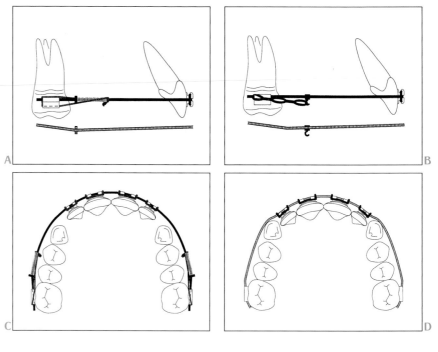

Figure 9-10

When maxillary incisors are steeply inclined, an archwire without torque will exert a palatally directed force at the apex (lingual root torque), and a labially directed force at the crown (labial crown torque). If the archwire is tied back, the root apices will move palatally (A). Lingual root torque will have also an extrusive effect on the incisors and an intrusive and buccally tipping effect on the anchorage molars (B). A cervical headgear with a Kahn spur can prevent extrusion and even cause intrusion of the incisors as well as enhance the torque because the force is applied anterior to the center of resistance (C). The creation of a central diastema and mesial tipping of the incisors can be prevented by the placement of a firmly twisted, soft 0.012-inch stainless steel ligature between and cervical to the brackets of the central incisors (D).

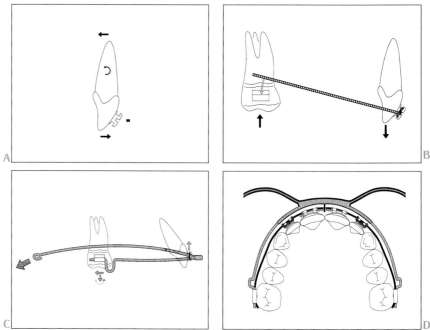

The vertical positions of the maxillary incisors are important not only for the appearance during speech and smiling but also for the stability of the treatment result. If the lower lip covers too much of the maxillary incisors after treatment, these teeth can be tipped to an upright position. To avoid overeruption of the maxillary incisors during treatment, or to intrude them, a cervical headgear with a Kahn spur can be utilized; this can also be used to extrude incisors (Figs 9-10 and 9-12). Furthermore, a parietal headgear with J-hooks can be applied to intrude the maxillary incisors (Fig 9-13).

When the maxillary incisors are intruded with partial fixed appliances only, use of too great a force has to be avoided to prevent the reaction force from causing distal tipping of the molars.

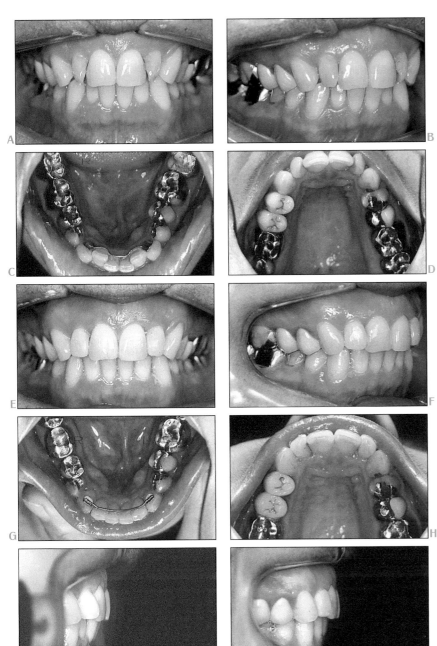

FIGURE 9-11

A woman aged 46 years 9 months had a Class I malocclusion and a good intercuspation in the posterior regions but crowding in the maxillary and mandibular anterior regions. To prevent a worsening of the irregularity of the mandibular anterior teeth, a cast chromium-cobalt bar had been fixed to all six teeth. The maxillary lateral incisors were in rotated positions. The overjet and overbite were normal (A–D, I). The chromium-cobalt bar was removed. The mandibular incisors were reduced in width, and enamel was also removed from the mesial sides of the canines. To these teeth and to the second premolars, 0.018 × 0.026-inch edgewise brackets were bonded, and a 0.015-inch dead-soft braided wire was inserted. To increase the flexibility of the arch, teardrop loops were bent mesial of the canines. After 6 months, the desired corrections were realized, and an adapted preformed retention bar was bonded lingually to the mandibular canines. One week later, the rotated position of the maxillary lateral incisors was camouflaged by grinding and buildup with resin composite. The combined treatment led to a satisfying result (E–H, J). Although the mesial sides of the maxillary lateral incisors were located too far mesially and labially, the effect was not unpleasant. The solid intercuspation of the premolars made it possible not to incorporate the molars in the partial fixed appliances.

On this page and the following pages, clinical examples of treatment with partial fixed appliances are shown (Figs 9-11 to 9-19).

Certainly, when a good occlusion is present in the posterior regions, limiting the appliances to the anterior teeth is an obvious solution. The forces should be kept small, particularly when teeth are being intruded. The force applied at incisors should be no more than 30 to 50 g. In adults, extra-light forces should be used, to prevent root resorption and loss of bone at the alveolar crest. The space needed to correct irregularities often can be obtained by reducing the tooth width through interproximal stripping.

FIGURE 9-12

A boy aged 8 years 6 months had a Class II division 1 malocclusion with a disto-occlusion of one premolar crown width and overerupted maxillary incisors. The primary canines and molars were still present, and in both dental arches sufficient space was available. He showed a broad gingival zone when laughing (A, B). First, an activator was made, which he did not wear regularly. The treatment was stopped for some time and resumed with a cervical headgear at the age of 9 years 11 months. In the meantime his attitude improved, and he used the headgear the prescribed 14 hours a day. Four months later, a removable maxillary plate was placed to correct the deep bite and move the first premolars and canines distally. At the age of 11 years 8 months, bands with 0.022 × 0.028-inch edgewise brackets were placed on the maxillary incisors, and a 0.019 × 0.026-inch archwire was inserted; loops between the central and lateral incisors were included to facilitate the correction of rotations and vertical irregularities and to retract the incisors with control over their inclination (C). Two months later, the cervical headgear was replaced by a headgear with a Kahn spur to intrude and torque the incisors (D). At the age of 12 years 3 months, all appliances were removed (E). To increase the stability, the supra-alveolar fibers around the maxillary incisors were sectioned, and the approximal surfaces of the mandibular teeth were flattened by stripping (see Fig 9-20). No retainer was used. Two years later, little had changed. The intrusion achieved with the Kahn spur was not lost, and when the patient laughed the gingiva was not visible (F, G). Ten years after treatment, the result was still satisfying (H, I).

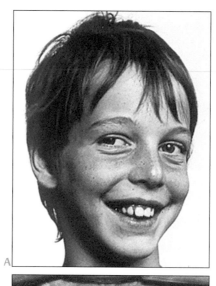
A

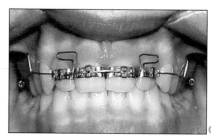
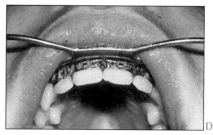
C

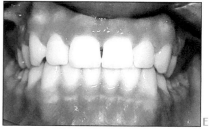
D

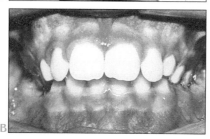
B

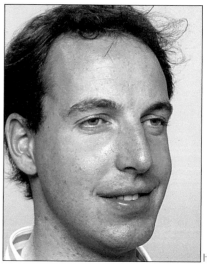
E

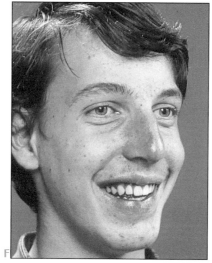
F

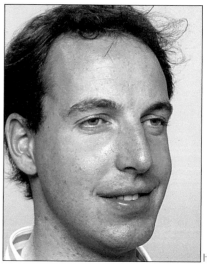
H

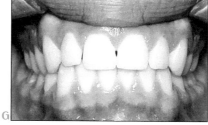
G

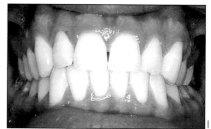
I

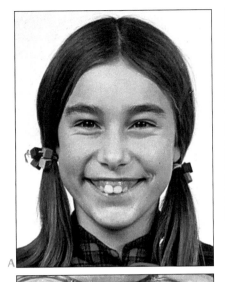

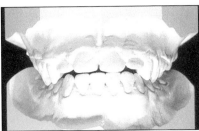

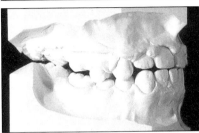

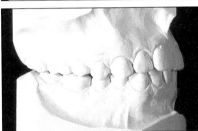

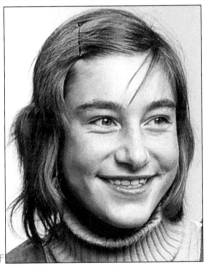

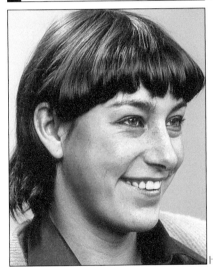

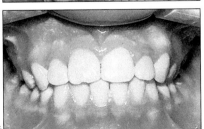

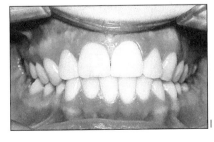

A

B

C

D

E

F

G

H

I

FIGURE 9-13

A girl who was 11 years 6 months of age had a Class II division 1 malocclusion measuring one premolar crown width and a large overjet. When laughing, she exposed a broad gingival zone; the lower lip was positioned palatal to the maxillary incisors (A, B). The treatment was started with a cervical headgear, which was worn as directed. Six months later, bands with 0.022 × 0.028-inch edgewise brackets were placed on the maxillary incisors and a 0.019 × 0.026-inch archwire with torque was inserted. A retracting force was generated with tied back coil springs resting against stops. After the diastemata in the posterior regions were closed, stops were soldered on the archwire, which rested against the molar tubes. The archwire had a slight intruding force and was fixed in the tubes with steel ligatures; the four incisors were anchored together with a figure-eight ligature. J-hooks were soldered at the archwire between the central and lateral incisors to allow attachment of a parietal headgear to reinforce the intrusion. Indeed, the maxillary incisors were overintruded and torqued. At the age of 12 years 3 months, when the treatment was concluded, the malocclusion was overcorrected and the maxillary incisors were positioned too far cranially (C, D). Retention was not applied. Two years later, the maxillary incisors were at the desired height level (E–G). Ten years after treatment, at the age of 22 years 2 months, the dentition and the smile line had a satisfactory appearance (H, I).

In this patient and the patient shown in Fig 9-12, control over the vertical position and inclination of the maxillary incisors was essential. The techniques applied to maintain that control many years ago are rarely used today. Nevertheless, the records of both patients are included to demonstrate the long-term effects of intrusion.

FIGURE 9-14

A girl 8 years 9 months of age had a Class II division 1 malocclusion that was camouflaged by an anterior forced bite over the maxillary right lateral incisor, behind which she could not bite in occlusion (A, B). After extraction of the primary maxillary right canine, the reverse overbite and forced bite could be corrected with a wooden tongue blade (C, D). At the age of 10 years 2 months, when the primary second molars were still present, a cervical headgear was placed to correct the disto-occlusion and to create more space in the maxillary dental arch (E, F). The arch length increased considerably, providing sufficient space for the permanent canines. A maxillary removable plate was added to correct the deep bite and to move teeth. At the age of 13 years 0 months, bands with brackets were placed on the maxillary incisors, mainly for intrusion. With the free sections of the edgewise archwire, the canines were moved palatally (G, H). At the age of 13 years 6 months, a satisfying result was obtained, and all appliances were removed (I, J). Retention was not applied. Twenty years later, at the age of 33 years 0 months, few of the improvements attained through the treatment had been lost (K, L). This patient, shown previously for other purposes in Fig 4-18, illustrates what can be achieved with simple means. However, a good treatment strategy and the use at the right time of various means, including partial fixed appliances, are essential to success.

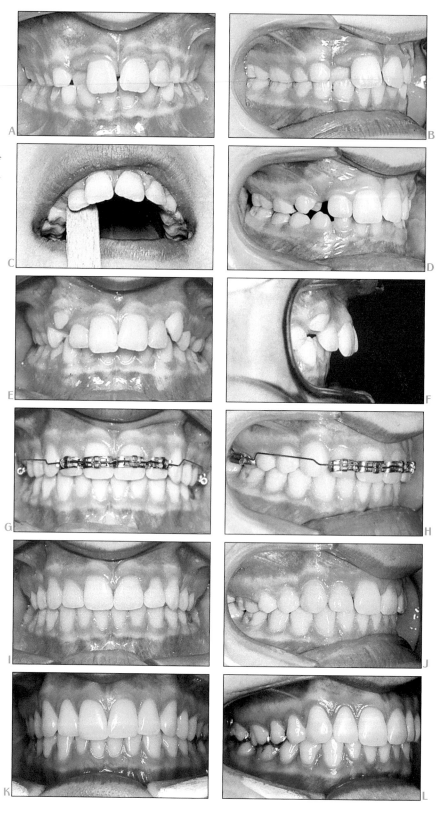

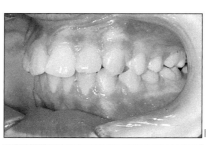

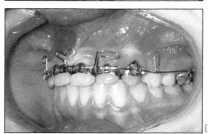

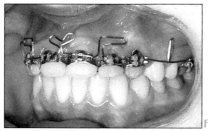

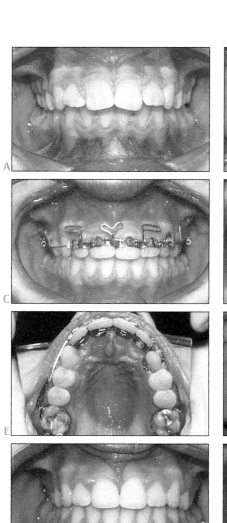

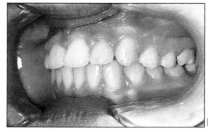

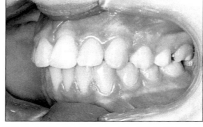

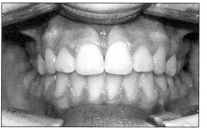

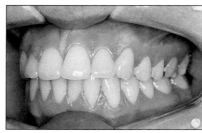

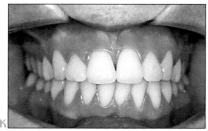

FIGURE 9-15

A girl aged 11 years 9 months had a Class II division 1 malocclusion with crowding in the maxillary anterior region and a mandibular dental arch without irregularities (A, B). The treatment was started with a cervical headgear to correct the disto-occlusion and to gain space in the maxillary dental arch. Eight months later, a plate was placed in the maxilla to reduce the deep bite and to distalize the first premolars and canines. Seven months later, at the age of 13 years 0 months, bands with 0.022 × 0.028-inch brackets were placed at the maxillary incisors, and a 0.016 × 0.016-inch archwire with several loops was inserted to move these teeth to the correct positions. The loops in the posterior regions closed the diastemata there and retracted the incisors. Later, a band with a bracket was placed on the left canine to rotate and properly position that tooth (C–F). At the age of 14 years 1 month, when all appliances were removed, a satisfying result was found (G, H). Retention was not applied. One year later, the situation had not changed noticeably (I, J). The same applied 15 years later, at the age of 29 years 6 months (K, L).

The last photographs are included to demonstrate that, in the long term, the central papilla will not fill the space cervical to the contact point if that is located incisal to the midpoint of the height of the crowns (this was also the case in the patient shown in Fig 9-12). Furthermore, in this patient, the central incisors were angulated too far in the mesial direction; they should have been uprighted more. However, the central papilla would not have retracted if the shape of the central incisor crowns was modified by mesial grinding, so the contact area could have been raised to half the height of the crowns.

FIGURE 9-16

A girl aged 10 years 10 months had a Class II division 1 malocclusion with disto-occlusion of one premolar crown width and sufficient space in both dental arches. The mandibular left central incisor was slightly rotated (A, B, E). The treatment was started with an activator and continued with a cervical headgear. A maxillary plate was added to raise the bite, to distalize the premolars, and to improve the position of the anterior teeth. After the plate was used for 8 months, it was obvious that partial fixed appliances were needed for the final detailing. Edgewise 0.018 × 0.026-inch brackets were bonded to the maxillary incisors and a 0.0175-inch braided wire was inserted, to be replaced later by a 0.016 × 0.016-inch archwire. The required improvements were realized in 6 months' time. After 3 years 3 months of treatment, a good result was obtained (C, D, F). A retention plate was worn in the maxilla day and night for 6 months; for the following 1 year, it was worn only during sleep. Two years later, the mandibular left central incisor was positioned lingually (G). Eight years later, at the age of 25 years 7 months, the malalignment in the mandibular anterior region had increased to the extent that the patient wished to have it corrected (H). After the mandibular anterior teeth were stripped, 0.018 × 0.026-inch brackets were bonded to them, and tubes were placed at the first molars. First a 0.015-inch braided wire was inserted, to be replaced by a 0.014 × 0.014-inch archwire later. After 5 months, the appliances were removed, and a 0.015-inch braided wire was bonded to the lingual side of the six mandibular anterior teeth (I–L).

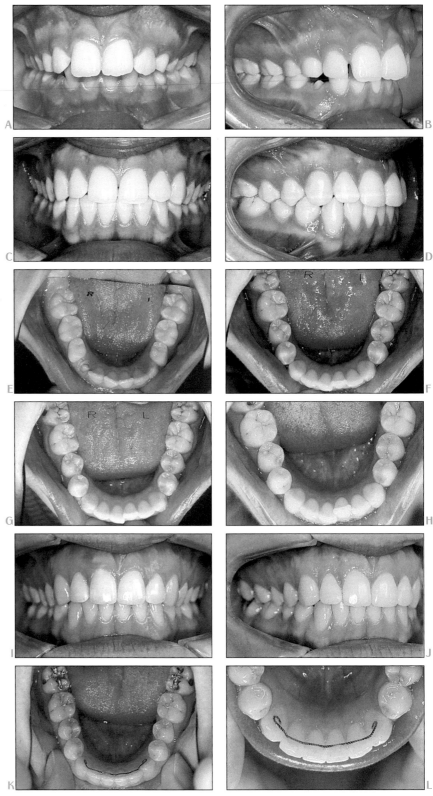

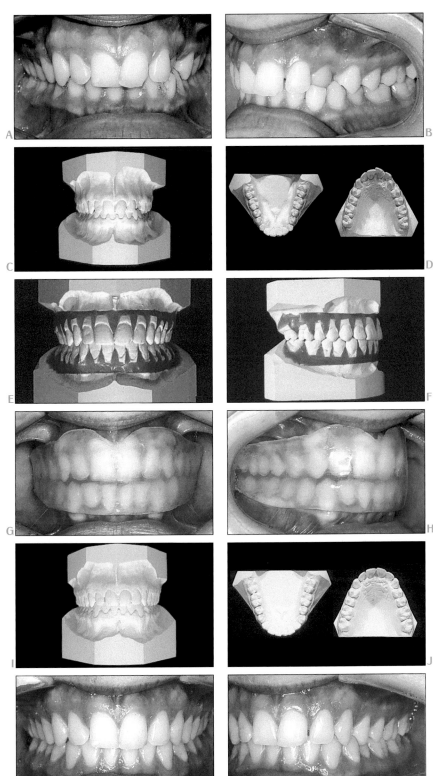

FIGURE 9-17

A boy of 17 years 10 months had a Class I malocclusion. The recently emerged maxillary left permanent canine was positioned palatally, and there was some overlapping of the maxillary incisors. The mandibular dental arch was well shaped, although the primary canines were still present. It was obvious that their successors would encounter space problems (A–D). After extraction of the mandibular primary canines, a plate was placed to move the permanent maxillary left canine buccally. The bite plane palatal to the maxillary incisors was sufficiently high to displace the canine without interference by the occlusion. In addition, the bite plane served to correct the deep bite. The position of the maxillary anterior teeth was improved with divided labial arches. Two months after the extraction of the primary canines, 0.018 × 0.026-inch brackets and tubes were placed at the mandibular teeth. A 0.075-inch braided wire was inserted, to be replaced 1 month later by a 0.016 × 0.016-inch archwire with push coils at the sites where the permanent canines had emerged in the meantime. After sufficient space had been gained and the canines had erupted further, brackets were placed on them, and they were moved to the correct positions. However, some irregularities still existed in the maxillary dental arch. It was decided to realize the required corrections with a positioner instead of fixed appliances; a diagnostic setup was made with the teeth in ideal positions (E, F). For the first 2 months, the positioner was worn for 4 hours during the day and while the patient was sleeping; for the subsequent 4 months, he wore it only at night (G, H). The final result was excellent, as was shown on the dental casts made at 18 years 9 months of age (I, J). Ten years later, the situation was still stable (K, L).

FIGURE 9-18

In a girl of 16 years 0 months of age, with a Class I malocclusion, the permanent maxillary lateral incisors were congenitally missing. The central incisors were tipped distally and were far apart. The canines were in contact with the first premolars but mesiopalatally rotated. The mandibular dental arch was normal; only the mesial side of the left central incisor was located too far labially. The posterior teeth occluded correctly. The maxillary central incisors were in habitual occlusion in contact with the mandibular incisors, and the overjet and overbite were small (A, B). The treatment was limited to the maxillary dental arch, where the central incisors had to be moved mesially and adjusted in angulation and the canines had to be rotated. To that end, these teeth were banded and provided with 0.022 × 0.028-inch Lewis brackets with rotation arms and anti-tip spurs; the first molars were provided with tubes. A swinging arch of 0.018 × 0.025-inch was inserted; stops were soldered on the segments that passed through the brackets of the incisors. The segments had to be shifted for activation. With this construction, reactivation and fixation could be accomplished, without removing the archwire, simply by opening the closing loop in the middle and closing the opening loops at the sides (C–F). The required changes were realized in 6 months' time (G, H). A retention plate with two artificial lateral incisors was used for retention; this was replaced by a spoon plate that served until the patient was 22 years 0 months of age (I, J). Subsequently, resin-bonded fixed partial dentures were placed.

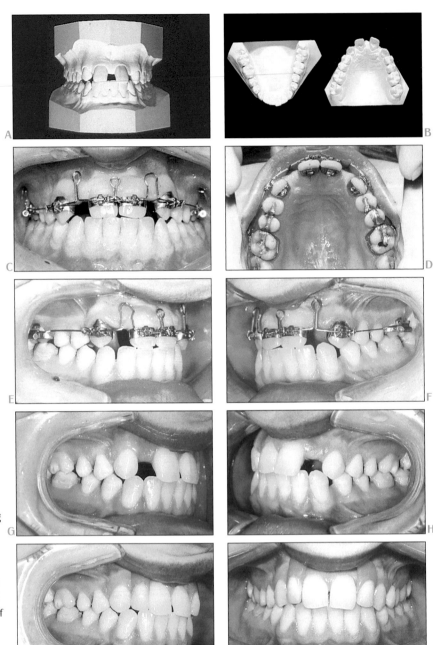

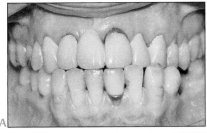

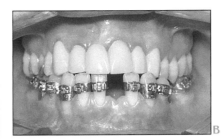

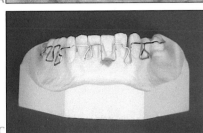

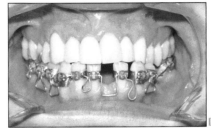

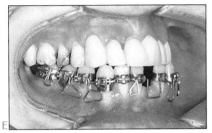

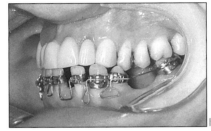

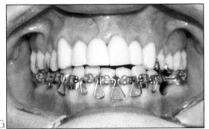

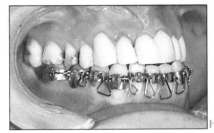

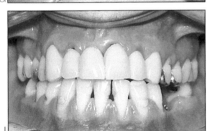

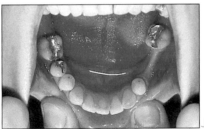

FIGURE 9-19

A woman aged 24 years 6 months had lost her maxillary right central incisor and fractured her mandibular left central incisor in an accident 4 years previously. A fixed partial denture was placed to substitute for the maxillary central incisor, and the mandibular central incisor was treated endodontically and restored with a crown. However, its root became resorbed laterally, and the tooth could not be saved. The mandibular incisors occluded too far anteriorly. On the right side, the incisors and canines occluded in an end-to-end position; on the left side, the lateral incisors, canines, and premolars were positioned in a reverse overbite (A). The mandibular left central incisor had to be extracted. The resulting diastema was to be closed orthodontically, with the additional aim of establishing normal occlusal contact in the anterior region and for the left premolars (B). The mandibular teeth were banded with 0.022 × 0.028-inch edgewise attachments. A 0.016 × 0.016-inch multipurpose archwire was inserted to close the diastema, control the angulation of the adjacent teeth, and narrow the dental arch (C–F). A removable maxillary plate with hooks in the acrylic resin for maxillomandibular elastics was used to support the lingual movement of the mandibular teeth (G, H). After a treatment time of 12 months, the goal was almost reached, and the remaining small diastemata were closed instantaneously with the retention plate (I, J). This patient has been included to illustrate that, with maxillomandibular elastics hooked to a well-anchored maxillary plate, fixed appliance movements in the mandibular arch can be controlled.

FIGURE 9-20

Contacts between mandibular incisors are often pointed and offer little stability (A). Reduction of the mesiodistal crown dimensions can provide flat contacting surfaces, which offer stability according to the roman arch concept (B).[156, 188]

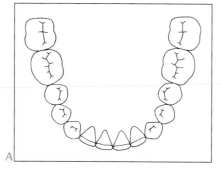
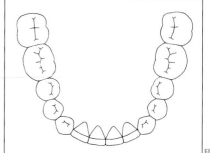
A B

FIGURE 9-21

Manual stripping can be performed with interproximal diamond strips. If they are moved 10 times up and down over a short distance, on average 0.1 mm of enamel is removed. It is practical to work first from the left side to the right side (A). Subsequently, the opposing surfaces are stripped (B). If the strip is folded over (doubled), adjacent sides can be reduced with the same strokes. The strip can be folded one more time to arrive at a three-layer thickness (C). The surfaces are smoothed and the corners are rounded with a narrow, fine-grained diamond strip.

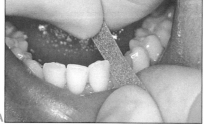
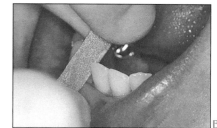
A B

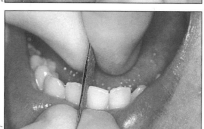
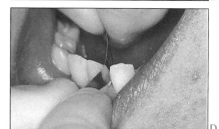
C D

As already mentioned several times, reduction of the mesiodistal crown dimensions by interproximal stripping can be of great help in correcting malalignment of anterior teeth (Fig 9-20). In the mandibular anterior region, 0.3 mm of enamel can be removed from each approximal surface. Including the mesial surfaces of the canines, a total of 3.0 mm can be gained in the mandibular anterior region. Stripping has to be performed carefully. Stripping by hand offers more control than does use of a rotating instrument (Fig 9-21).

As a rule, stripping at the start of treatment will not result in approximal surfaces that fit well against each other at the end of treatment. To reach that goal, the shape of the approximal surfaces has to be adjusted in the last phase of treatment; stripping should be followed by polishing with thin, fine-grained strips. Subsequently, the patient should rinse with a fluoride solution twice a day for 2 weeks.[242]

Finally, when fixed appliance components are combined with removable plates, the potential for controlled tooth movements with plates can be expanded, as will be explained in the next chapter.

Use of Removable Appliance–Fixed Appliance Combinations

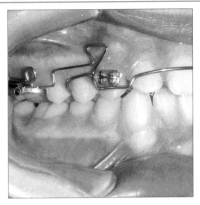

As clarified in chapter 3, full control over the magnitude and direction of forces can be established through the use of elastics hooked at brackets or buttons. This approach can be utilized not only with plates but also with activators, headgears, headgear-activators, and facial masks.

The course of the elastic determines the direction of the force; the length and thickness of the elastic control the magnitude of the force. An additional advantage of the use of elastics is that they keep the plate in place.

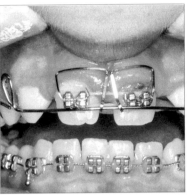

Parallel movement of teeth cannot be realized with a removable plate, even with the addition of elastics, without the use of auxiliary components. That also largely applies to uprighting, torquing, intruding, extruding, and rotating movements. However, most of these movements can be accomplished by the placement of brackets with extensions on appropriate teeth.

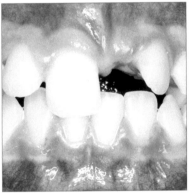

With the addition of this type of auxiliary component to a plate, the need for the use of complete fixed appliances can be reduced. Complicated treatments can be facilitated by performing specific movements with a combination of a plate and a small fixed construction, before the complete fixed appliance is used. That applies particularly to the uprighting of canines and the improvement of the angulation of maxillary lateral incisors that are going to replace missing central incisors. An advantage of this approach is that reaction forces not only can be counteracted but also can be utilized to effect other movements at the same time. Furthermore, teeth can be rotated by extensions placed in the brackets.

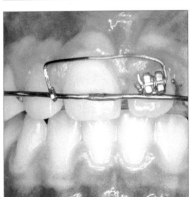

The concept of utilizing combinations of removable and fixed appliances is not complicated and does not require extensive explanation prior to the illustration of various procedures. Many clinical examples are shown to demonstrate how, with an effective design, complicated tooth movements can be carried out in a relatively simple way (Figs 10-1 to 10-46).

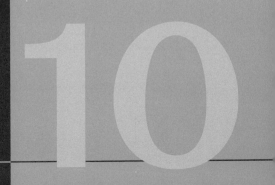

Orthodontic Concepts and Strategies

10

FIGURE 10-1

A protrusion spring at a maxillary incisor causes a reaction force that tends to move the plate away from that tooth. With an optimal use of clasps, the plate rarely will be fully adapted and will jump to the palate when the patient occludes on the far occlusally extending acrylic resin that covers the spring (A, B). When an elastic is used instead, the plate does not have to be as thick in that region, can be adapted well, and can also serve as a bite plane to reduce the overbite (C, D).

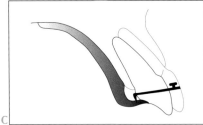
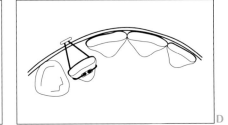
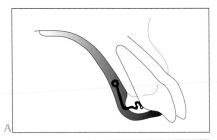
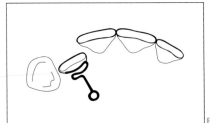

FIGURE 10-2

An incisor can be moved labially with an elastic extending from a button at its palatal surface to a hook at the labial arch (A, B). The plate will not have the tendency to dislodge from the palate, as is the case with a protrusion spring.

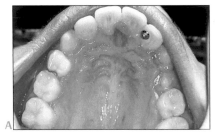
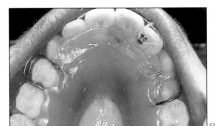

FIGURE 10-3

An incisor can be moved palatally through an elastic extending from its labial surface, on which a resin composite buildup is placed, to a hook in the plate. The margin of the plate should be fully in contact with the other anterior teeth (A, B). Clasps should provide sufficient retention. With resin composite buildups placed under three-quarter clasps, optimal fixation can be obtained, and the disadvantages associated with clasps located at the cervical margin are avoided (C, D).

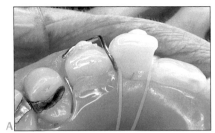
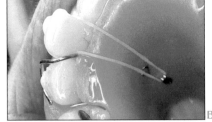
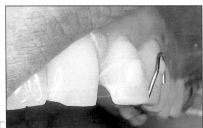
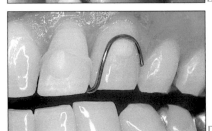

FIGURE 10-4

Incisors can be retracted with an elastic extending across the labial surfaces (A). Most of the time, mesial migration of the posterior teeth has to be prevented, as with the twisted steel ligatures in this case (B).

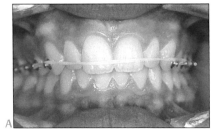
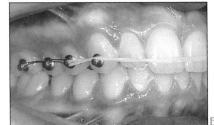

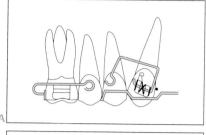
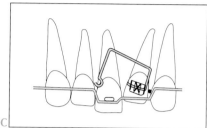
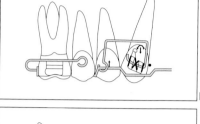
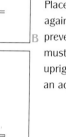

A

B

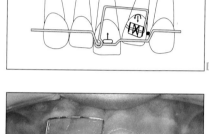

C

D

FIGURE 10-5

A tooth can be uprighted and extruded with a cervically angled edgewise wire section, ligated firmly into a bracket, with its end hooked under the labial arch. Placement of the continuous labial arch against the incisal side of the bracket can prevent extrusion (A, B). When the tooth must be extruded, the reaction force of the uprighting spring can be utilized to intrude an adjacent tooth (C, D).

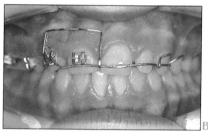
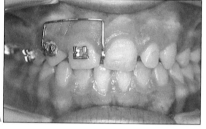

A

B

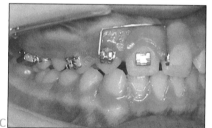
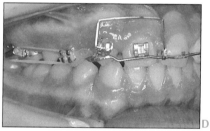

C

D

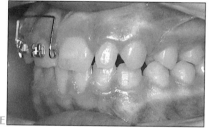
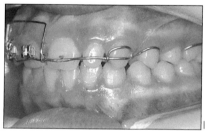

E

F

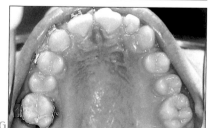
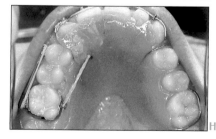

G

H

FIGURE 10-6

The uprighting of certain teeth with wire sections in brackets and the movement of other teeth with elastics can be carried out simultaneously. After the passive section is ligated into the bracket, it has to be activated to upright and extrude the canine. The reaction force working through the continuous labial arch at the bracket of the right central incisor, and at the resin composite buildup at the left lateral incisor, intrudes both central incisors. An elastic is placed between the end of the tube at the permanent right first molar and the bracket at the first premolar to close the space; no clasps are used on that side (A–D). On the left side, the plate is held in place by the returning part of the labial arch at the canine and two clasps in the posterior region. The hook welded at the labial arch allows placement of an elastic from the hook to the bracket at the right central incisor to move that tooth mesially (E, F). A button is not placed at the palatal side of the right first premolar, because only the buccal side of this tooth has to move distally. To move the first molar mesially, a hook is embedded in the acrylic resin to allow an elastic to run to the palatal side of that molar.

FIGURE 10-7

A buccally erupting maxillary second molar can be guided into occlusion with a crossbite elastic (A, B). The same applies to posterior teeth occluding in crossbite, provided that the elastic is worn 24 hours a day.

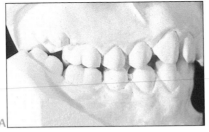
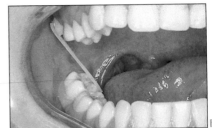

FIGURE 10-8

A canine can be moved distally with an elastic (A). A small piece of edgewise wire bent up at both sides of the molar tube serves as a hook (B). However, if an elastic is used alone, the canine will tip and rotate.

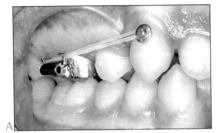
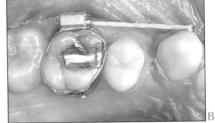

FIGURE 10-9

Teeth can be rotated with an elastic placed around the crown (A, B). This rotation will occur more smoothly when there is a diastema between the two teeth.

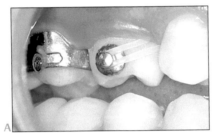
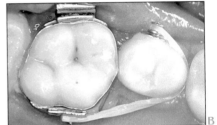

FIGURE 10-10

When an incisor is moved with an elastic attached to a button, adequate space should be available (B). After the needed movement is realized, the button should be removed and the acrylic resin margin should be built up to contact the tooth (A).

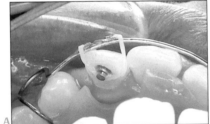
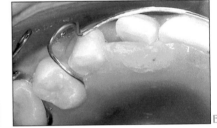

FIGURE 10-11

The primary canines have been extracted to provide the space for correction of the irregularities of the incisors and the reverse overbite of the left lateral incisor (A, B). The plate has a sufficiently high posterior bite plane to avoid occlusal interference in the movement of the left lateral incisor (C, D). Once the reverse overbite is corrected, the posterior bite plane should be trimmed away.

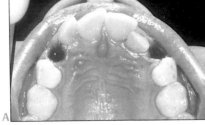
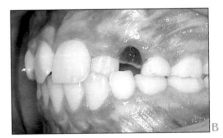
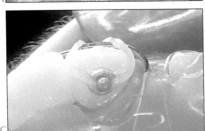
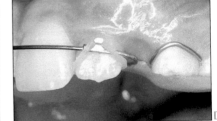

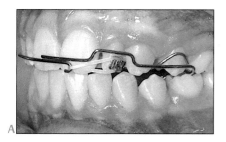

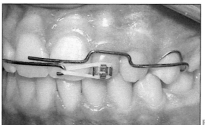

FIGURE 10-12

A hook is bent at the end of the right labial arch to place an elastic for rotation and mesial movement of the left lateral incisor (A). A satisfactory result is reached after 2 months (B).

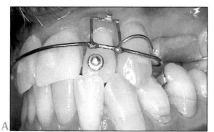

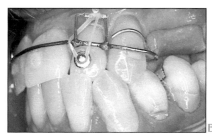

FIGURE 10-13

During intrusion with an elastic, the labial arch and the acrylic resin margin can provide guidance. The plate should be anchored firmly to counteract the reaction force; in this case, fixation is accomplished with resin composite buildups at the adjacent teeth.

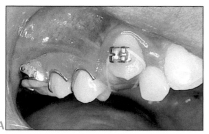

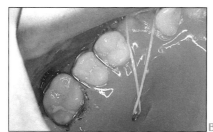

FIGURE 10-14

First, the right canine is moved distally and palatally with an elastic extending around the crown, on top of the bracket, to the hook in the plate (A, B). Thereafter, an extension is ligated into the bracket to rotate, upright, and extrude the canine (C). On the left side, the canine is uprighted and distalized with two vertical extensions. The palatal extension of 0.016 × 0.016-inch stainless steel wire is bent and directly bonded to the crown surface (D).

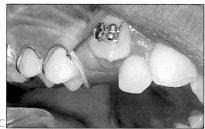

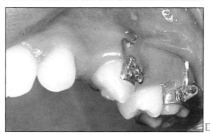

FIGURE 10-15

The maxillary right second premolar is extruded and moved buccally by an elastic extending through a guiding fork to the hook embedded in the acrylic resin (A, B). The patient should not occlude on the guiding fork.

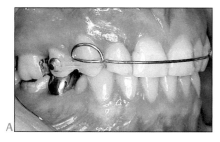

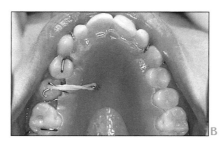

FIGURE 10-16

Through the use of palatally placed elastics extending from buttons to hooks in the plate, and buccally placed elastics extending from buttons to the returning parts of the labial arch at the canines, diastemata can be closed without the rotation of teeth (A, B).

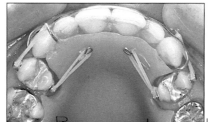

FIGURE 10-17

A compromise treatment with elastics can be used close a diastema between a maxillary right canine and central incisor in a simple and rapid way (A, B). A continuous labial arch with U-loops guides the movement of the teeth and retrudes the right central incisor (C, D). The elastic is placed at the cervically bonded buttons and extends not, as shown here, across the labial side (E) but around the palatal side (F). The elastic wraps around the crowns to rotate the teeth when they move together (G, H). Composite buildups are placed at the palatal sides of the crowns to keep the elastic correctly positioned. Such an elastic has the tendency to slide in the incisal or cervical direction and can lead to periodontal damage (I, J). Also, in this type of treatment, the labial bow and the margin of the plate should provide guidance for the movement of the teeth (D, K, L).

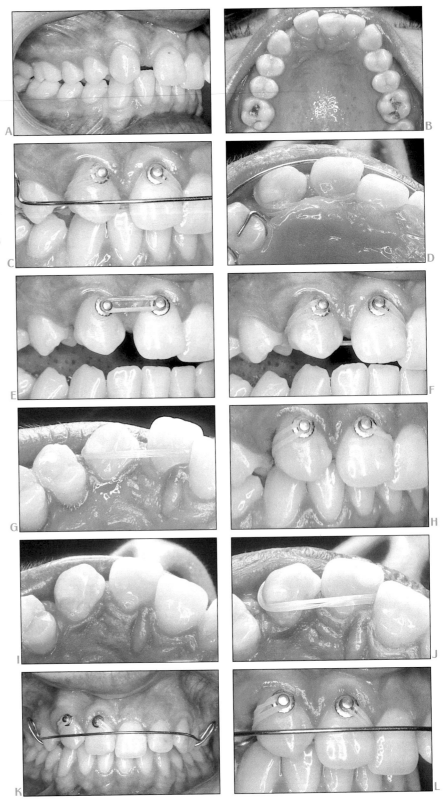

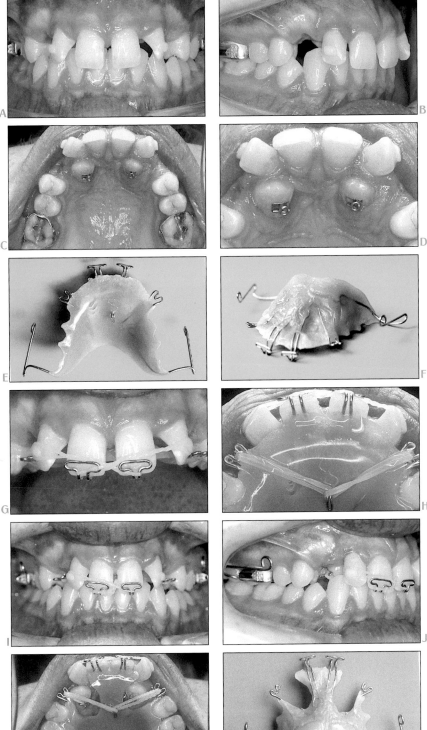

FIGURE 10-18

In a girl with palatally positioned maxillary canines, the movement of the canines and the required movement of the four incisors was carried out initially with a plate and elastics simultaneously. Resin composite hooks were placed on the lateral incisors (A, B), and cleats were placed on the canines to attach elastics for a controlled pulling force (C, D). The plate had modified claw clasps for the central incisors, to allow mesial movement of these teeth, and a hook at the middle of the palate (E, F). The elastics in front extended from the claw clasp at the central incisor on one side to the resin composite hook on the lateral incisor on the other side (G). On the palatal side, the elastics extended from the cleats on the canines, through guiding forks, to the hook in the plate (H, I). By the time the diastemata between the incisors were closed and the lateral incisors rotated, the canines had moved to the extent that the acrylic resin in that area had to be removed. The mesial fixation of the guiding forks was eliminated, and the remaining part was adjusted (J–L).

FIGURE 10-19

Molars sometimes have to be rotated. When mesial migration is allowed, such a rotation can be carried out with an elastic attached to a hook in the plate (A, B).

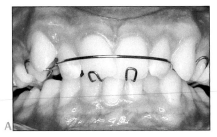
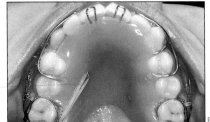

FIGURE 10-20

Acrylic resin has to be trimmed away from the mesial side of the molars. Generally, preformed molar bands have a palatal hook on which elastics can be placed. The clasps should be free of the crown mesiobuccally (A, B).

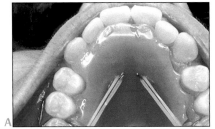
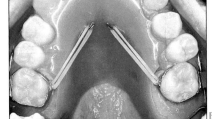

FIGURE 10-21

More than one tooth can be displaced with one elastic. At the same time, a canine can be moved palatally and a molar rotated (A). When the first premolar has to migrate buccally, the elastic can cross the palatal side of that tooth (B).

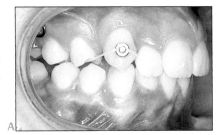
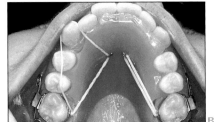

FIGURE 10-22

When molar bands are not needed, a button can be bonded alone; however, clasps should be used at the premolars (A, B). When bands are placed on the first molars, modified three-quarter clasps, positioned on top of the tubes, are preferred.

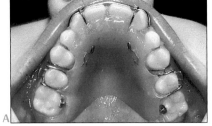
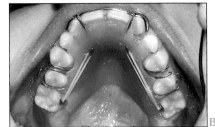

FIGURE 10-23

A button can be used as the point of application for a 0.7-mm stainless steel wire spring. A button is placed on the mesiobuccal cusp of a maxillary third molar to hook on the half-round end of the spring that runs distal to the second molar (A, B). With this construction, the third molar is distalized and uprighted (C, D). Such a design requires the patient to have the dexterity to release and replace the spring. Indeed, that applies to most of the systems shown.

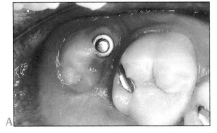
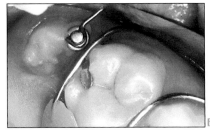
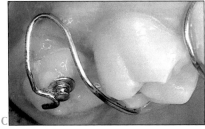
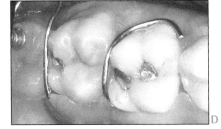

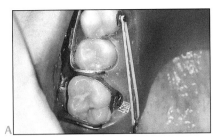
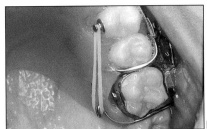

FIGURE 10-24

Instead of a pigtail spring, an elastic can be used to distalize and rotate a first premolar, especially when it erupts after the plate has been in use for some time (A, B).

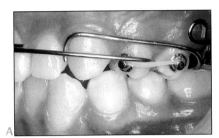
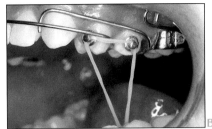

FIGURE 10-25

Crossbite elastics can be used to move premolars palatally, particularly if the opposing tooth has to be uprighted, as in this case (A, B).

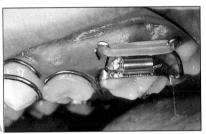
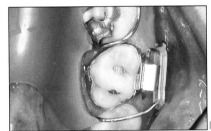

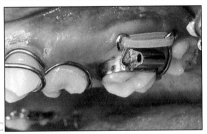
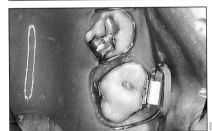

FIGURE 10-26

When the maxillary second molar is not fully erupted yet, the first molar can be distalized. To realize that movement, a close-fitting edgewise wire section with a hook at the mesiocervical side is placed in the molar tube, and the plate is provided with a stiff piece of wire with a hook at the end, some distance distal to that molar. An elastic is placed between the two hooks (A, B). After 2 months, the first molar has been distalized. At the intervening appointment it was confirmed that the metal parts, the acrylic resin margin, and the occlusion would not interfere with the movement (C, D).

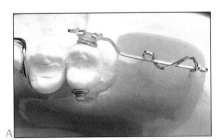
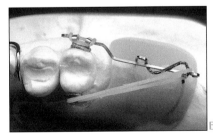

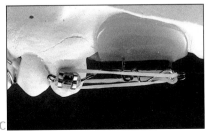
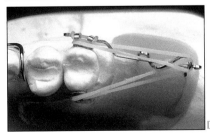

FIGURE 10-27

To move a maxillary second premolar bodily in the distal direction, a rigid edgewise wire section, placed in the bracket at that tooth, is fitted in a guidance construction (A). One elastic is placed around the end of the wire section and attached to a button at the palatal side of the premolar (B), and one elastic is extended buccally from the bracket to the end of the wire section (C). In that way, a force system that can distalize the premolar in a controlled manner over a large distance is developed (D).

Figure 10-28

A combination of a plate and fixed appliances can also be used in combination with extraoral traction. In a girl with a Class III malocclusion, a face mask was applied to move the maxillary complex anteriorly (A, B). The main purpose of the plate was to encompass the maxillary teeth rigidly, so that the force exerted by the elastics at the permanent first molars affected the maxilla as a whole (C, D, K). The elastics were placed on hooks attached to extensions welded to the palatal sides of the bands and on vertical wire extensions placed in the buccal tubes (E, F). The elastics extended to the bar in front of the mask (C, D, G, H). The retained primary mandibular second molars were ankylosed. If that is the case, these teeth may be used as solid anchorage units, like implants, to cope with undesirable reaction forces. In this patient, the ankylosed second primary molars were used as anchorage units to move the permanent first molars distally; on the right side, a push coil on a straight section of edgewise wire was used, and, on the left side, a sectional arch with a bent-in expansion system was used (I, J, L). In that way, the mesio-occlusion of the permanent first molars was partially corrected. In a later phase of treatment, the additional space gained, as well as the space that became available with the replacement of the primary second molars by their successors, was utilized for the retraction of the mandibular anterior teeth.

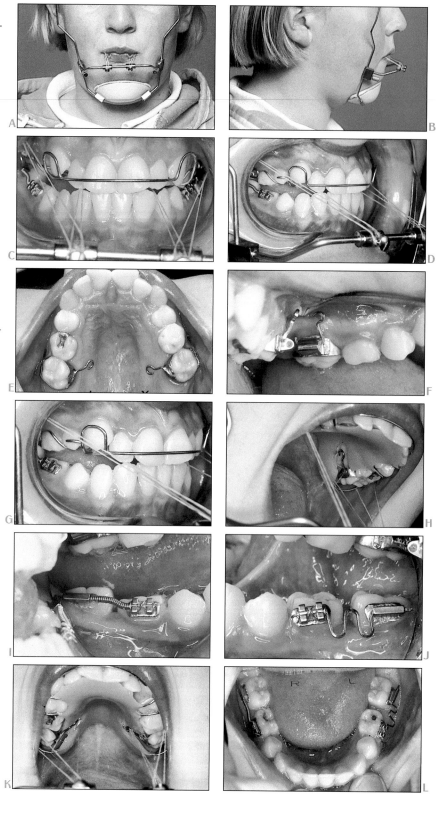

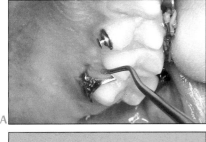

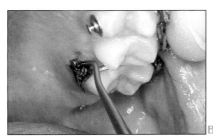

A
B

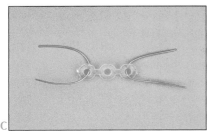

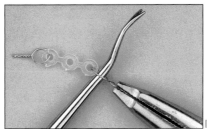

C
D

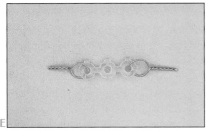

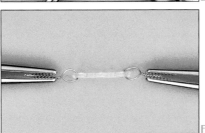

E
F

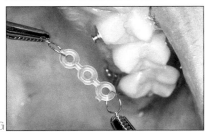

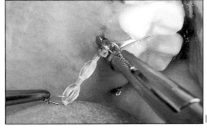

G
H

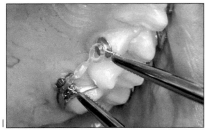

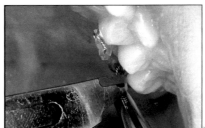

I
J

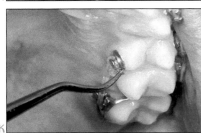

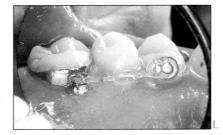

K
L

FIGURE 10-29

With the use of a plate, as well as with the use of complete fixed appliances, diastemata in the maxillary posterior region sometimes have to be closed. When, in addition, the first molar has to be rotated mesiobuccally and the first premolar distopalatally, a reciprocal design can be applied. Elastic chains fixed at buttons or hooks on the palatal sides of these teeth are well suited for that purpose. They are ligated with 0.012-inch soft stainless steel ligature wire, so that they will not come loose. When the hook on the molar band has been squeezed to avoid irritation, it can be lifted up with a small excavator (A,B). The ligature wire is shaped to a loop around the shaft of a ligature director by means of ligature-tying pliers (C–E). Subsequently, the tails are placed in two mosquito pliers (F). First the loop is placed around the hook at the molar band, and the tail is turned until the loop is closed (G, H). Then the other loop is tied to the button on the first premolar (I). Subsequently, the tails are shortened (J), and the ends are turned around with the ligature director (K, L). The tightening of the loops should be stopped in time to prevent the wire from cutting through the chain. This risk is avoided when first a knot is made in the ligature wire after it has been put through the end of the chain; the loop is then formed on this knot. When a cleat is bonded to the premolar, the elastic chain can be hooked directly to the cleat.

FIGURE 10-30

Elastics can also be used to move teeth in combination with an activator. When maxillary molars are being distalized, a notch in the posterior side of the activator can serve as a hook (A, B).

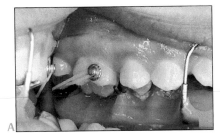
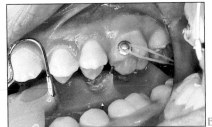

FIGURE 10-31

The permanent maxillary right first molar is moved distally (A). The permanent maxillary left first molar is rotated and moved mesially with an elastic extending from a button on the palatal side of the mesiopalatal cusp to the U-loop (B).

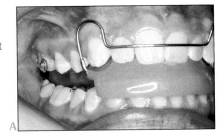
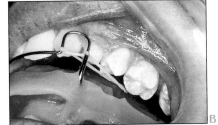

FIGURE 10-32

The permanent mandibular first molars are moved mesially with elastics at hooks embedded in the activator, which also contains tubes for a parietal headgear. Two buttons on each molar limit the tipping (A, B).

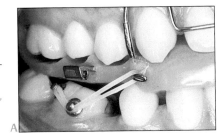
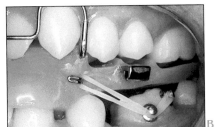

FIGURE 10-33

The mesial movement of mandibular molars is accomplished with elastics attached at the lingual and buccal sides to hooks in a plate that is firmly anchored with resin composite undercuts for the clasps (A, B).

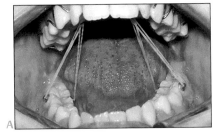
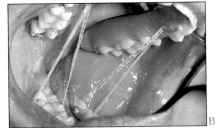

FIGURE 10-34

On this headgear-activator, elastics are placed at the headgear bows where they enter the acrylic resin. The elastics run crosswise to the brackets at the mandibular canines to close the diastemata in the mandibular anterior region, where two incisors are missing (A). The space should be closed without moving the anterior teeth lingually (B). The retention of the headgear-activator is increased by partial coverage of the maxillary teeth with acrylic resin and by the torquing springs at the maxillary central incisors (C, D).

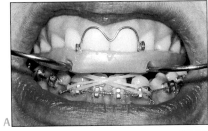
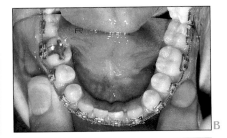
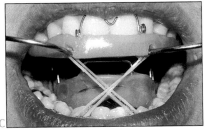
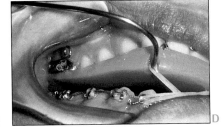

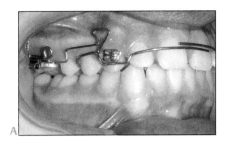

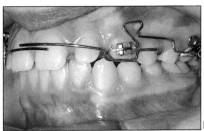

FIGURE 10-35

Canines can be moved distally and uprighted with sectional archwires, while labial arches and the acrylic resin margin of the plate provide guidance. At the same time, the position of the incisors can be improved with the labial arches (A, B).

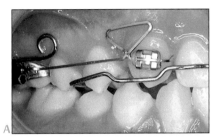

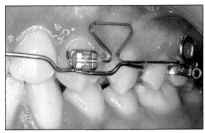

FIGURE 10-36

The labial bow should be located some distance away from the bracket when the canine has to be extruded (A). When the canine should not erupt further, the labial bow should be in contact with the bracket (B).

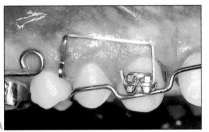

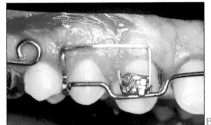

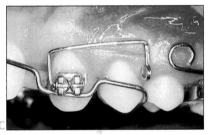

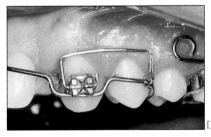

FIGURE 10-37

The acrylic resin covers the mesial side of the canines to block their mesial movement. The spring should be activated slightly (A). At the corners, the edgewise wire is twisted 90 degrees so that the widest side of the archwire is parallel to the mucosa. This twisting also facilitates bending the hook at the end and attaching it to the labial arch (B). On the left side, only the most distal section is twisted (C). The reaction force transmitted by the labial bow prevents extrusion of the canine (D).

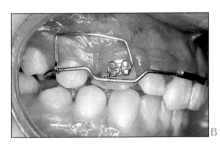

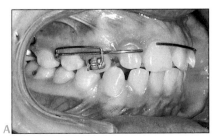

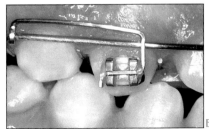

FIGURE 10-38

When the canine has to be extruded, the labial arch must be free of the bracket (A, B). Bending steps in the wire for that purpose is much simpler in divided labial arches than in a continuous labial arch with U-loops.

FIGURE 10-39

In patients with a buccal sulcus of little depth and low-extending mucosal bands, shallower extensions should be used (A). The pigtail spring that is embedded in acrylic resin supports the canine at the mesial side (B).

FIGURE 10-40

Two adjacent teeth, the apices of which have to be displaced in the same direction, can be moved simultaneously with extensions, as in this case, where the maxillary right second premolar was missing (A, B). In the preceding distal movement of the first premolar and canine, both teeth were tipped distally. One extension was placed at the cervical side of the bracket, and one extension was placed on the occlusal side. The labial arch had to be modified to neutralize the extruding component at the canine and the intruding component at the first premolar (C). The labial arch should be adapted when it shifts as an extension is attached (D). Prior to the attachment of the extensions, the labial arch should be in contact with the brackets (E). After the extensions are attached, the labial arches should be close together and run parallel in the anterior region (F). Most of the intended changes were realized after 2 months (G). The labial arch had become free of the mesial wing of the bracket at the canine (H). Two months later, the first premolar had been tipped too far, and a diastema had developed at its mesial side (I, J). Another 2 months later, an acceptable situation was reached. The position of the incisors was also improved. However, the canine was overextruded slightly, which was compensated for by grinding of the cusp tip (K, L). Without the use of complete fixed appliances, a compromised result was obtained in this case, which was complicated by the absence of the maxillary left central incisor.

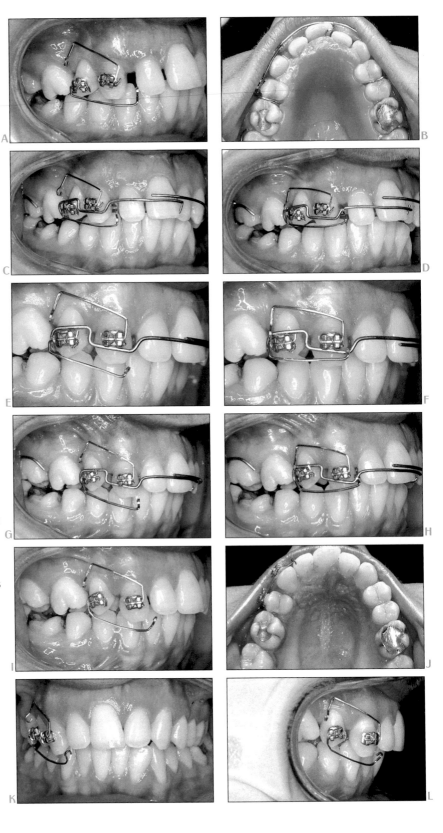

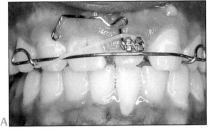

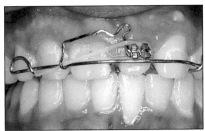

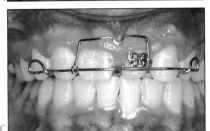

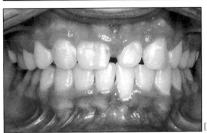

Figure 10-41

After the left lateral incisor was moved mesially over some distance, a bracket with an extension was placed for uprighting, while an elastic provided a mesially directed force (A, B). However, the elastic was not worn as directed, and the lateral incisor became positioned too far distally (C, D). A V-notch in the extension was created to preserve the frenum. Extensions should have a size and shape that avoids irritation of the gingiva and mucosa.

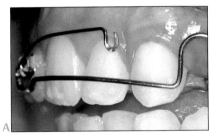

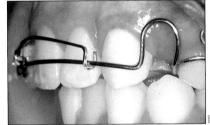

Figure 10-42

A V-notch does not have to be created to avert damage to the frenum when the height of the extension is kept small (A, B) or when the labial sulcus is deep.

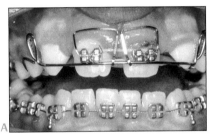

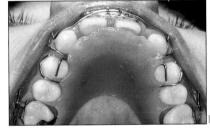

Figure 10-43

Two adjacent teeth can be uprighted in the opposite direction at the same time (A, B). A figure-eight ligature will prevent the teeth from moving apart, and an elastic can move them closer together.

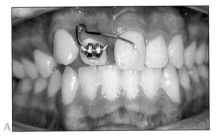

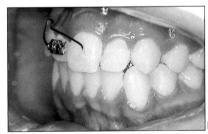

Figure 10-44

When a patient returns to the office because he or she has lost a plate, the extension can be bonded to the labial surface until a new plate can be placed (A, B).

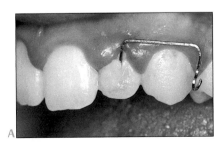

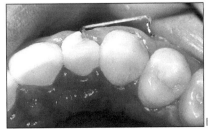

Figure 10-45

Sometimes it is desirable not to use a bracket but rather to bond the extension directly to the labial surface of the tooth that has to be uprighted (A, B).

Figure 10-46

A girl with a Class II division 2 malocclusion had lost her maxillary left central incisor in an accident (A). A removable plate was used to move the left lateral incisor mesially. Subsequently, the pigtail spring was embedded in the acrylic resin, and the two labial bows were soldered together (B). A bracket with an extension was placed on the left lateral incisor and a resin composite buildup was placed on the right central incisor cervical to the labial arch (C, D). With these additions, the lateral incisor was uprighted and the central incisor was intruded and torqued (E, F). The torquing effect was provided by the application of a caudally directed force anterior to the point of rotation. This force was exerted by the labial arch, which also prevented the crown from moving labially. With this construction, complicated tooth movements that facilitated the subsequent complete fixed appliance treatment were accomplished. The results of the fixed appliance treatment provided a good basis for transforming the appearance of the left lateral incisor into that of a central incisor (G, H).

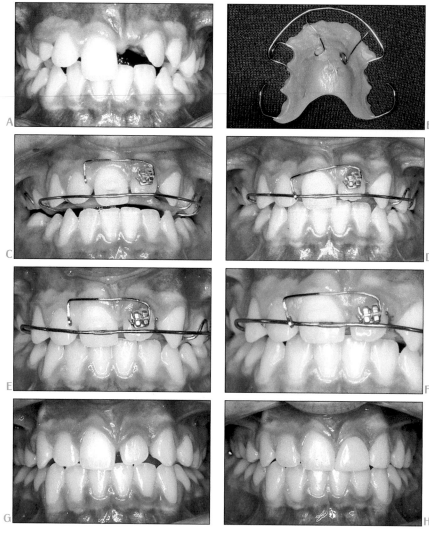

The combinations of removable and fixed appliances demonstrated in the preceding pages require some insight into, and feeling for, the mode of operation of the constructions shown. The patient should understand the system and have sufficient dexterity to release and fasten the hooks and to replace elastics daily. Furthermore, maintaining good oral hygiene becomes more troublesome. On the other hand, plates supplemented with extensions and elastics remain in place and do not move up and down.

With the demonstrated constructions, complex tooth movements can be performed in a relatively simple, well-controlled manner. That applies specifically to movement of impacted maxillary canines to the correct location in the dental arch, as will be clarified in the next chapter.

Treatment of Impacted Canines

After third molars, permanent maxillary canines are the most frequently impacted teeth, with a prevalence of 1.5% to 2.0% in the Western European population.[47, 196] The treatment of impacted canines is complex and lengthy. However, it is easy to detect abnormally positioned canines prior to emergence, and, even more important, their impaction can be prevented in the majority of patients by timely extraction of their predecessor 1 to 2 years prior to the anticipated emergence.

Normally, the crowns of permanent maxillary canines can be palpated buccally in the vestibule. The same applies to the mandible, where impaction is rare. A canine that cannot be palpated at the buccal side usually can be felt at the palatal side. Normally located, unerupted maxillary canines are visible as a prominence in intraoral photographs or color slides. Unerupted permanent canines often can also be observed and felt on plaster casts. In case of doubt, radiographs will provide the required additional information.

It is the task of the practitioner who is in charge of the dental condition of a child to check the position of unerupted permanent canines and to undertake the appropriate steps when impaction is detected or suspected. Timely interception will not only redirect the eruption path of the canine but also reduce the risk of root resorption in the adjacent incisors. This root resorption associated with canine impaction occurs more frequently than the 12% that has been observed in radiographic examinations.[61] Recent computed tomographic investigations have ascertained that the roots of the incisors are resorbed in about 50% of patients with impacted maxillary canines. However, as a rule, this resorption does not start before the child is 10 years of age.[60, 63, 64]

Not all canines that are in a deviating position at a young age become impacted. Sometimes the situation improves; mostly it worsens, however, so regular reexamination is necessary. How to manage impacted canines that were not prevented by timely extraction of their predecessors is shown in seven patients with various complications. How impacted canines can be moved effectively and brought to the correct position in the dental arch, through the use of a plate and elastics and a controlled magnitude and direction of force, is demonstrated. How the extra space needed in the dental arch can be gained simultaneously is also explained. However, the subsequent additional orthodontic treatment is not discussed in detail.

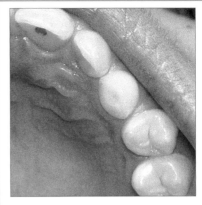
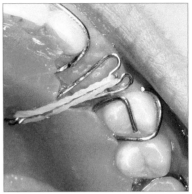
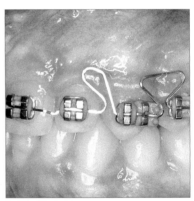
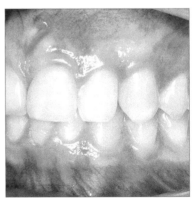

Orthodontic Concepts and Strategies

11

FIGURE 11-1

The distribution of the 46 impacted canines in the prospective study by Ericson and Kurol,[62] based on the medial position of the crown in five sections in the anterior plane, is derived from panoramic radiographs (A). The position of the crown of the impacted canine in relation to the incisors in the transverse plane is derived from axial-vertex radiographs (B). The mean mesial inclination of the canines to the midline (α) and the mean distance (d1) to the occlusal line (OL) are derived from measurements made in the anterior plane on the panoramic radiographs (C). In 91% of patients in whom the canine overlapped the lateral incisor by less than half of its root at the start of treatment, the position of the permanent canine normalized after extraction of the primary canine. When the canine overlapped the lateral incisor by more than half its root, normalization occurred in 64% of patients (D). (Reprinted with permission from Ericson and Kurol.[62])

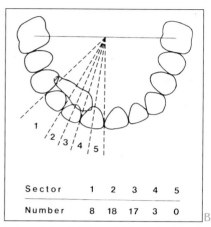
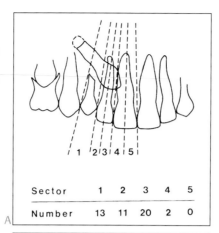

Sector	1	2	3	4	5
Number	13	11	20	2	0

A

Sector	1	2	3	4	5
Number	8	18	17	3	0

B

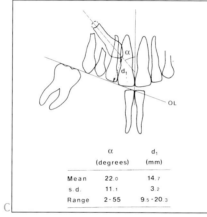
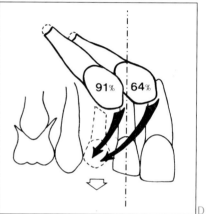

	α (degrees)	d1 (mm)
Mean	22.0	14.7
S.d.	11.1	3.2
Range	2-55	9.5-20.3

C

D

Rarely, there is no clear cause for the permanent canines not to emerge. Neither palpation nor radiographs demonstrate an abnormality, and adequate space might be available in the dental arch. Sometimes the eruption of the canines is retarded.

Impaction can be caused by ankylosis, which can only be ascertained by percussion after the canine has been surgically exposed. A consequence of ankylosis is that orthodontic movement of the affected tooth is impossible.

More than 60 years ago, in 1943, Berger[19] recommended the timely extraction of primary canines when impaction of permanent canines was anticipated. He also recommended the creation of more space in the dental arch when needed.[19]

In 1988, Ericson and Kurol[62] published a prospective study on the effect of extraction of primary canines in 46 patients without crowding, in whom the permanent maxillary canines could not be palpated (Fig 11-1, A to C).

In 10 (22%) of these 46 patients, no improvement was noticed after the extraction of the primary canines. In 36 patients (78%), the position of the permanent canines had normalized and attained a good position after emergence. The improvement was realized completely in nine patients after 6 months, in 13 after 12 months, and in 14 after 18 months.

The prognosis seemed to depend largely on the extent to which the canine overlapped the root of the lateral incisor. Of the 22 canines that overlapped the lateral incisors by more than half, 14 (64%) had normalized. Of the 24 canines that overlapped the lateral incisors by less than half, 22 (91%) had normalized (Fig 11-1, D). The axial inclination of the canine, and the distance from its cusp tip to the line of occlusion, did not seem to be relevant for the prognosis.[62] However, the chance of improvement after extraction of the primary canine is smaller when crowding is present in the dental arch than when sufficient space is available.[163]

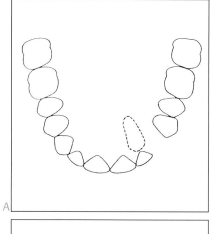

A

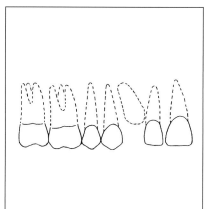

B

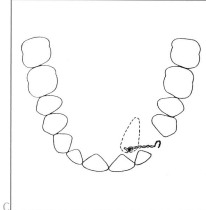

C

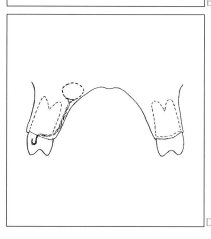

D

FIGURE 11-2

When the crown of an impacted canine is positioned close to the surface of the palate, and its axial inclination does not deviate much, removal of the covering mucoperiosteum and overlying bone will suffice. Application of periodontal packing prevents re-covering of the canine, so that eruption takes place. When the periodontal packing is lost, the patient can replace it with sugarless chewing gum (A, B).[205] Surgical exposure of the crown is needed when the canine is located far from its normal position in the arch and when its inclination is unfavorable. After exposure, an eyelet is bonded to the crown, and a soft 0.014-inch stainless steel ligature is threaded through. The free ends of the ligature are twisted loosely around each other a couple of times, after which the ligature is placed between the bone and the mucoperiosteum. The twisted end should protrude in the mouth at the position where the canine has to approach. The free end of the ligature is turned around an adjacent tooth to reduce the discomfort for the patient (C, D).

An impacted canine must be diagnosed and the primary canine must be extracted before the end of the second transitional period. Earlier extraction is not indicated, because spontaneous improvement can still occur. The patient should be told that if the extraction of the primary canine does not result in a correction, surgical exposure, ligation, and controlled movement of the impacted canine will be needed subsequently.

The axial position of permanent maxillary canines changes prior to emergence. The mesial angulation increases initially but decreases later. This change in angulation is related to the spatial alterations within the jaw associated with the eruption of the lateral incisor. Initially unfavorable canine angulations can worsen but also can improve.[68]

When a primary canine is extracted to improve the position of its successor, extraction of the primary canine on the other side has to be considered to prevent a midline deviation. Severely deviating impacted canines, and particularly those that are horizontally situated, do not improve in position after extraction of their predecessor. When no improvement has been observed after 12 months, another 6 months of observation is recommended, unless the permanent canine has approached the lateral incisor so closely that root resorption might occur. When that is the case, immediate action should be undertaken; an eyelet with a ligature is placed on the canine crown, and the impacted tooth is moved to the proper place.[17]

The timely extraction of primary canines is one of the few preventive measures in orthodontics. It spares the patient a lengthy and uncomfortable treatment phase and saves the parents the associated costs.

Impacted canines rarely emerge spontaneously later. Depending on their position, they have to be surgically exposed and provided with an eyelet and ligature (Fig 11-2). The subsequent treatment is elucidated with clinical examples (Figs 11-3 to 11-11).

Figure 11-3

A girl who was 14 years 10 months of age, with an attractive dentition and a moderate disto-occlusion, still retained her primary maxillary canines and primary maxillary left second molar. The primary maxillary canines were in contact with the adjacent teeth. The permanent maxillary canines were positioned palatally, close to the inferior surface of the palate, and were detectable by inspection and palpation. Space had to be gained in the dental arch for the larger permanent canines (A–D). The impacted maxillary canines were positioned favorably. Removal of the covering mucoperiosteum and prevention of its regrowth was sufficient treatment. For esthetic reasons, the maxillary primary canines were maintained as long as possible. A cervical headgear at the maxillary first molars was used to correct the disto-occlusion and to gain space in the dental arch (E). The left first premolar was moved distally with a sectional archwire in a bracket. After sufficient space had been created, buttons were bonded to the palatal surfaces of the canines, and a plate with a continuous labial arch was placed. Hooks were welded at this sturdy labial arch to apply elastics for the movement of the canines to the proper locations. Furthermore, posterior bite planes served to provide the clearance to move the canines buccally without occlusal interference (F–I). In that way, the canines could be moved to the proper positions, but they were not rotated sufficiently (J–L). Brackets with sectional archwires were used to rotate the canines and to improve their angulation and inclination.

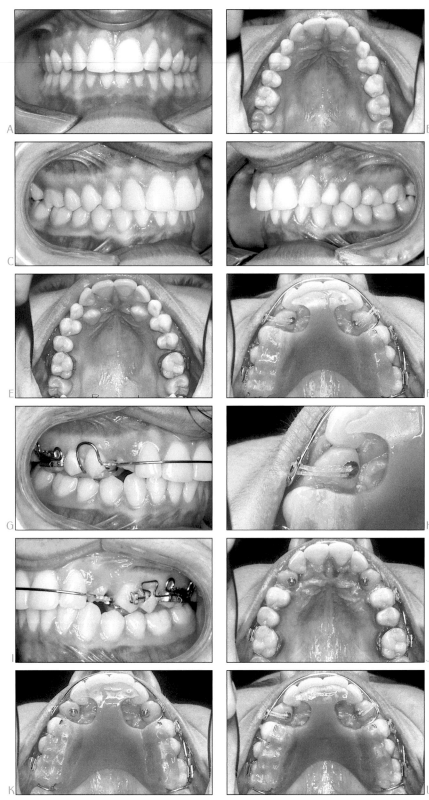

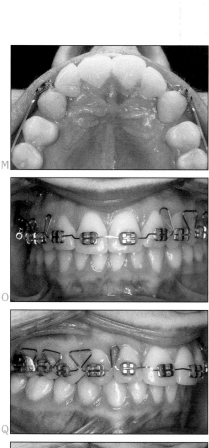

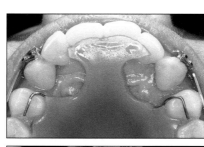

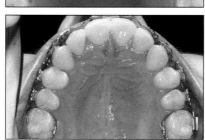

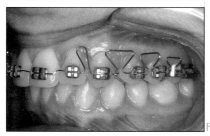

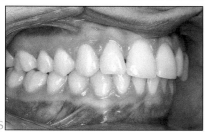

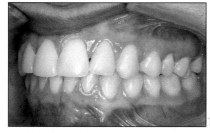

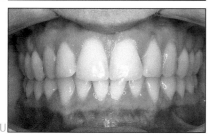

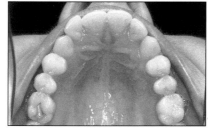

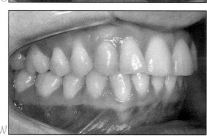

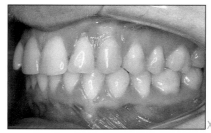

Treatment of Impacted Canines

FIGURE 11-4

The ligature used to move the canine to the proper place and to attach the elastic is of 0.014-inch soft stainless steel wire. The pieces of wire, which extend between the bone and mucoperiosteum, are turned slightly around each other and enter the oral cavity at the site where the canine has to be located (A). The strength required to attach an elastic is obtained by twisting the protruding section tightly. With a small mosquito pliers, the ligature is stretched carefully, so it will extend further (B). Subsequently, a second mosquito pliers is placed at the ligature in contact with the gingiva, and the ligature is twisted with the first pliers (C). Afterward, the excess is removed (D). Subsequently, the end is shaped to a hook with a ligature director (E, F). During the whole process, the second mosquito pliers has to be held firmly against the gingiva to prevent the movement of the ligature under the mucoperiosteum, which would cause pain to the patient.

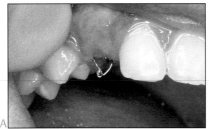
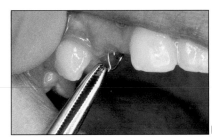
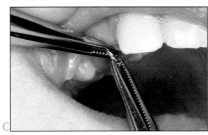
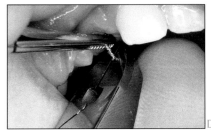
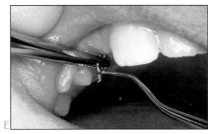
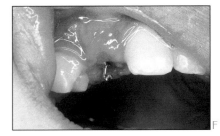
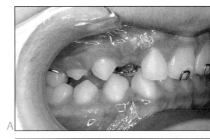
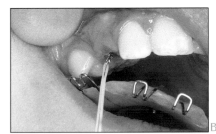

FIGURE 11-5

A guiding fork is embedded in the plate to orient the elastic. The direction of the force should be perpendicular to the occlusal plane. The elastic is placed at the ligature hook after the plate is slightly lifted (A, B). Subsequently, the elastic is laid in the fork and attached to the hook at the plate (C). Sometimes it is necessary to bend the fork slightly to prevent the patient from biting on it. This bending away is done in the patient's mouth, while the plate is held in place with a finger (D). In that way, a force that is well controlled in both magnitude and direction can be applied to the ligature at the canine. The exerted force should be about 30 g (E, F).

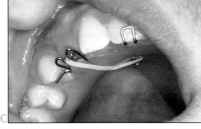
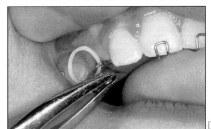
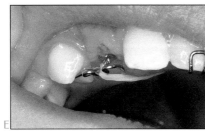
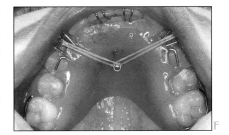

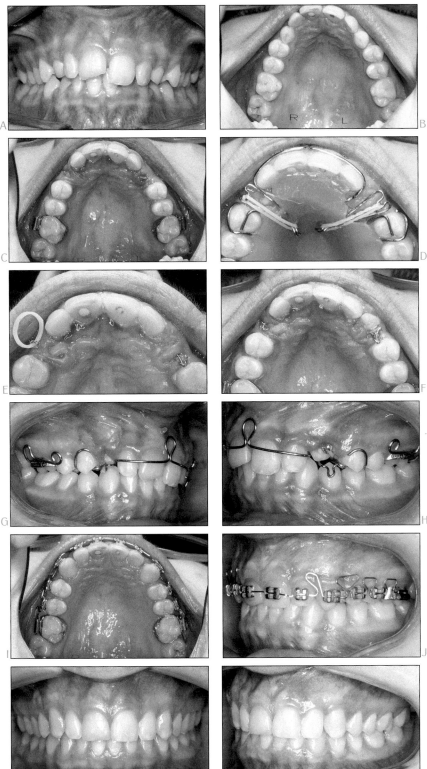

FIGURE 11-6

A girl 13 years 8 months of age had a moderate Class II division 1 malocclusion in which all primary teeth had been replaced except the primary maxillary canines (A, B). The permanent maxillary canines were impacted and positioned unfavorably, so surgical exposure and placement of an eyelet and ligature were needed. A cervical headgear was used to correct the disto-occlusion and to gain more space in the dental arch for the canines (C). A plate with guiding forks and elastics was applied to move the canines to the proper positions (D). The patient was examined every 5 weeks, and each time the end of the ligature extended 2 to 3 mm more than at the previous appoint-ment. Therefore, the protruding section was twisted further, shortened, and bent to a new hook. After 5 months, the right canine had emerged (E). Five weeks later, the left canine emerged, while the right canine had moved buccally in the mean-time (F). The eyelet at the left canine was removed, and a button was bonded to the buccal surface. The guiding forks were adjusted to maintain the correct direction of forces (G, H). In a way comparable to that used for the patient shown in Fig 11-5, the deep bite was corrected with the plate, and complete fixed appliances were used for 6 months in the maxilla only (I, J). The active treatment lasted a total of 1 year 8 months and was completed at the age of 15 years 5 months. Active treat-ment was followed by a retention period of 6 months. Five years later, at the age of 22 years 1 month, the patient exhibited a well-arranged dentition, correctly posi-tioned maxillary canines, and a healthy periodontium (K, L).

FIGURE 11-7

A girl who was 11 years 10 months of age had a Class II division 2 malocclusion with crowding in both dental arches. All primary teeth except the maxillary canines were replaced already. The four maxillary incisors were rotated, and the crowns of the lateral incisors were small and peg shaped (A–D). When primary maxillary canines persist in a well-aligned dental arch without diastemata, too little space is available for the permanent canines. Sometimes the extra space needed can be gained with a headgear, as shown in Figs 11-3 and 11-6. The space available for bringing the canines into position must be slightly larger than their mesiodistal width; otherwise, there is insufficient space to maneuver the canines. When crowding already exists in the dental arch, more local expansion is needed. The Crefcoeur appliance, as used in this patient, is well suited for this task. First, space was gained on the right side, after which the separation was filled with quick-curing acrylic resin. Subsequently, the plate was cut at the left canine area (E, F). In that way, the expansion of the dental arch and the movement of the canines could be achieved simultaneously, which shortened the treatment time. Essential for a controlled use of a Crefcoeur appliance are the firm anchorage of the two segments of the plate and a sturdy support with wire components resting against the teeth adjacent to the separation. Occlusal rests on the premolars are necessary for additional resistance against the reaction forces of the elastics, which tend to move the appliance in the cranial direction.

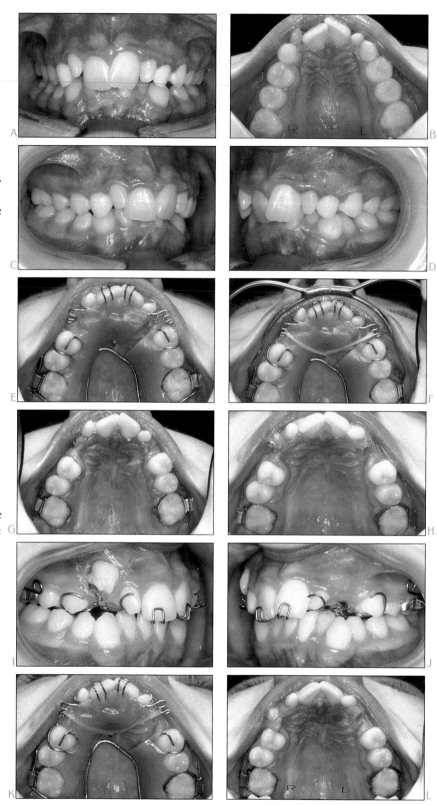

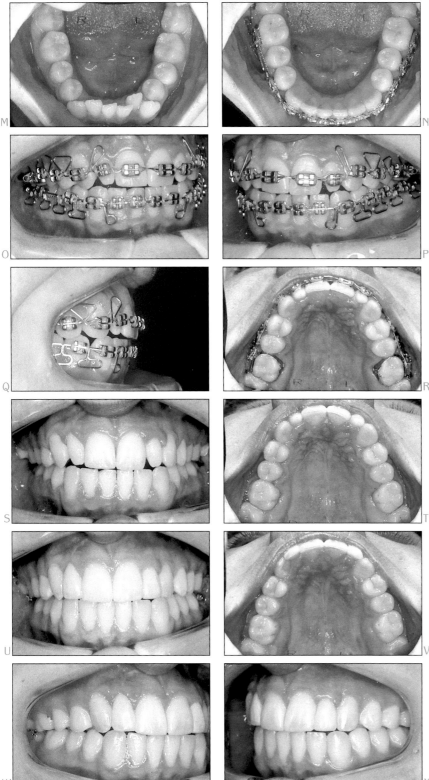

FIGURE 11-7 (CONTINUED)

After 10 months of treatment, sufficient space was gained on the right side but not on the left side (G). Four months later, sufficient space was gained on the left side, and the right canine had emerged. Indeed, extra space was needed to maneuver canines in the dental arch (H). The plate served well not only to provide an increase in space in the dental arch, first on the right side and then on the left side, but also to provide the correct direction for the forces exerted by the elastics. In addition, with the anterior bite plane, which was regularly increased in height, the deep bite was reduced and the curve of Spee was leveled. Meanwhile, the mandibular incisors were able to attain better positions, because the contact with the palatally tipped maxillary incisors was eliminated. In this procedure, the claw clasps at the maxillary incisors are essential (I, J), as explained in chapter 3. When claws are not applied, the anterior margin of the plate will be occluded into the mucosa, which causes irritation and hypertrophy of the gingiva. That is not the case when claws are used for vertical support and the patient maintains good oral hygiene (K, L). Fixed appliances were placed in the mandible during the last phase of repositioning the maxillary canines in the dental arch. The plate supported the mandibular incisors vertically and prevented occlusal interferences from hindering the improvement in the position of the mandibular posterior teeth (M, N). Subsequently, fixed appliances were placed in the maxilla (O–R). At the age of 16 years 11 months, all appliances were removed, and retention was started (S, T). Later, the maxillary lateral incisors were built up with resin composite. Five years later, the maxillary right canine was rotated slightly (U–X).

FIGURE 11-8

A girl aged 13 years 1 month had a Class II division 1 malocclusion with agenesis of the permanent maxillary lateral incisors and of the mandibular left second premolar; the maxillary canines were impacted. These canines had to be exposed and extruded with ligatures and elastics. More than enough space was available in the maxillary dental arch, which had a large central diastema (A–D). A cervical headgear was placed, the maxillary canines were exposed, and eyelets and ligatures were attached. Two weeks later, the plate with elastics was inserted. Occlusal rests were placed on the central incisors and first premolars. A hook was soldered to the cervical headgear to move the permanent mandibular left first molar mesially with an elastic (E, F). Ten months after the start of treatment, the right canine, to which a button had been bonded, had erupted extensively. The guiding fork was transformed to a hook to exert a distal force with the elastic (G). On the left side, the canine was close to emerging (H). Ten weeks later, the eyelet at the left canine was visible, and the right canine had moved slightly distally (I, J). Fixed appliances were placed in the mandible, and a few months later in the maxilla, to complete the treatment. Five years later, at the age of 20 years 6 months, little was lost of the result (K, L).

In this patient, the maxillary canines could not be palpated before the start of treatment at the buccal side or at the palatal side. Their crowns were near the roots of the central incisors. When that is the case, the canines must be extruded to the dental arch without delay, in view of the risk of root resorption in the incisors.

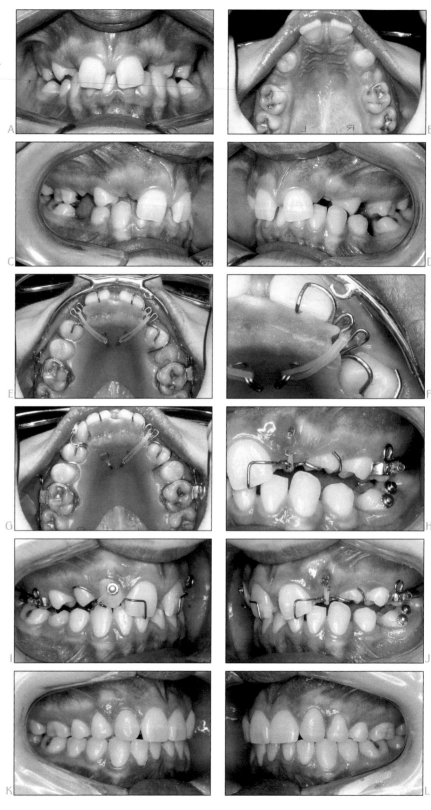

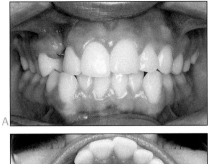

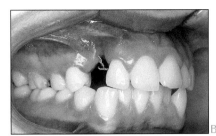

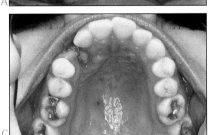

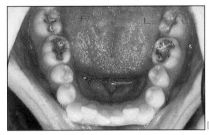

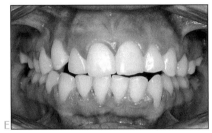

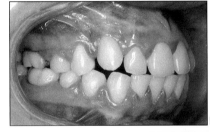

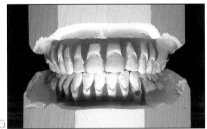

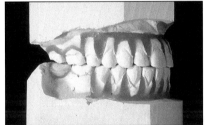

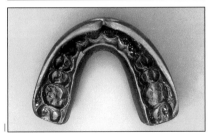

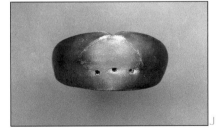

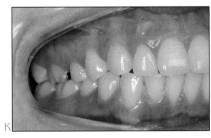

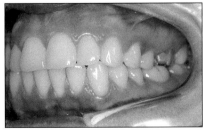

FIGURE 11-9

A girl aged 16 years 2 months had a Class I malocclusion with mandibular anterior crowding and a palatally located impacted maxillary right canine. This canine was moved to the correct place in the dental arch with an elastic attached to a ligature over a period of 8 months (A–D). The patient agreed to wear fixed appliances in the mandible but not in the maxilla. At the age of 18 years 6 months, the approximal surfaces of the mandibular incisors and the mesial surfaces of the canines were stripped. It took 7 months to align the mandibular dental arch. With a removable plate that was used for 2 years 10 months, the maxillary right canine was moved between the adjacent teeth. The occlusion in the posterior regions had been acceptable since the start of treatment, but the maxillary anterior region required further correction (E, F). A positioner based on a diagnostic setup with ideal arrangement was used to improve the position of the anterior teeth (G–J). Two months' intensive use of the positioner, 4 to 6 hours during the day as well as all night, resulted in the planned improvements. A retention wire was bonded lingually to the mandibular canines, and a Van der Linden retainer was placed in the maxilla (see chapter 18). This removable retainer was worn day and night for 6 months and during sleeping hours only for the following 3 years. Five years after treatment, at the age of 27 years 7 months, little of the result was lost (K, L). The retention wire was to remain in place until the patient reached 30 years of age, on the assumption that the alignment of the mandibular anterior teeth would not deteriorate subsequently; the large, flat contact areas created during treatment provided additional support to ensure stability.

Figure 11-10

A girl who was 13 years 5 months of age had a Class I malocclusion with impacted maxillary canines (A–D). The canines had caused severe root resorption of the permanent lateral incisors, which had become mobile. The radiographs revealed that the canines were close to the central incisors, and the risk of resorption of their roots did not permit any delay in the start of treatment (E, F). The maxillary primary canines were extracted, as were the permanent lateral incisors, the roots of which were almost completely resorbed (G, H). The impacted canines were exposed surgically and provided with eyelets and ligatures to extrude them to the dental arch with a plate, guiding forks, and elastics. Six months after the start of treatment, labially bonded buttons replaced the eyelets. The treatment was complicated: The neutro-occlusion in the posterior regions had to be altered to a disto-occlusion, because extractions in the ideally arranged mandibular arch, in which diastemata were already present, were considered inappropriate. Furthermore, the profile and facial appearance did not justify the extraction of two mandibular teeth. By means of a plate, ligatures, guiding forks, and elastics, the canines were extruded to the dental arch but not fully to the occlusal level, particularly not on the right side (I–L). This phase of the treatment was not completed, because preference was given to starting the use of the fixed appliances to alter the neutro-occlusion into a disto-occlusion. At the age of 14 years 5 months, 0.022 × 0.028-inch edgewise appliances were placed in the maxilla, and a 0.016 × 0.022-inch Sentalloy nickel-titanium wire (GAC International, Bohemia, New York) was inserted to move the canines to the proper places (M, N).

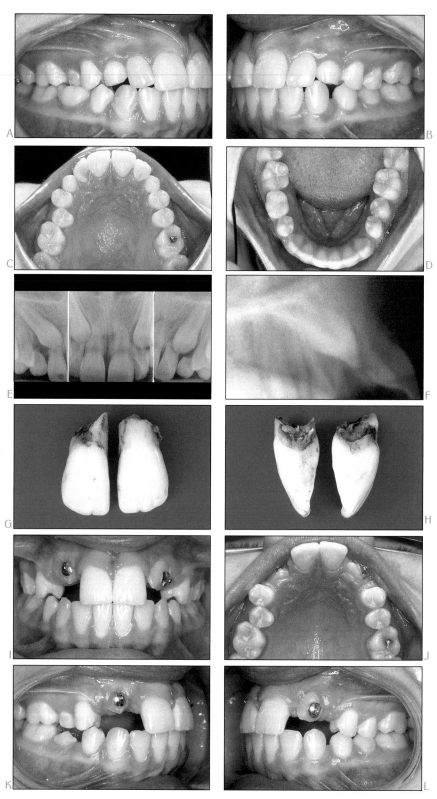

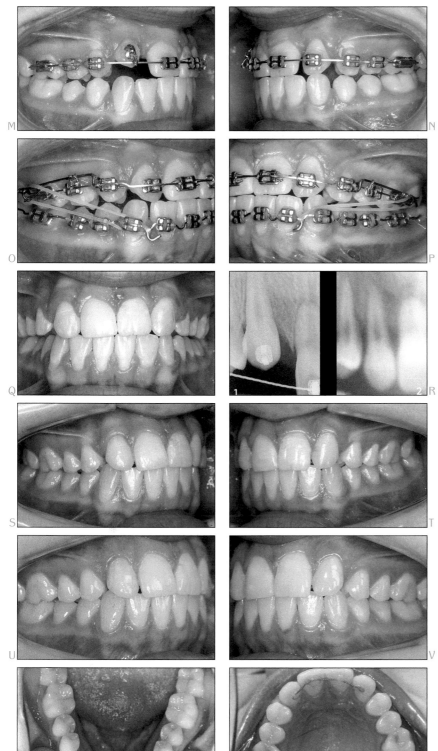

FIGURE 11-10 (CONTINUED)

Subsequently, fixed appliances were placed in the mandible, and a 0.0175-inch braided wire was inserted. This wire was replaced later by a 0.016 × 0.025-inch stainless steel wire, on which hooks for Class III elastics were soldered, mesial to the canines. The elastics were attached to sliding jigs in the maxilla, which were shifted on the archwire, and transmitted mesially directed forces against the brackets at the first premolars. A sliding jig consists of a sturdy piece of heavy rectangular wire with closed, round loops at the ends. One loop rests against the tooth on which the force has to be exerted. The other loop is located about 3 mm away from the bracket or tube to avoid contact with that attachment when the planned movement takes place. At that loop, a hook is soldered or bent to attach the elastic (O, P). At the age of 14 years 11 months, after an active treatment period of 1 year 6 months, all appliances were removed (Q). The maxillary canines were positioned as planned. The root apices of the maxillary central incisors were resorbed (R: RIGHT), but that was already the case when the fixed appliances were placed (R: LEFT). For retention, a 0.0175-inch dead-soft braided wire was bonded to the lingual surfaces of the maxillary central incisors and canines. No retention was used in the mandible (S, T). Eight years later, at the age of 22 years 7 months, the result was stable, although small diastemata had developed distal of the maxillary canines; this movement could have been prevented by including the first premolars in the retention wire (U–X). The previously made suggestion to alter the crowns of the maxillary canines by grinding and with resin composite buildups, to simulate lateral incisors, was rejected by the patient again at the last visit.

Treatment of Impacted Canines

FIGURE 11-11

A boy 10 years 1 month of age had a Class II division 2 malocclusion with regular dental arches. The primary molars were still present, but the primary canines were only present in the maxilla. The permanent mandibular canines had emerged already (A–D). At the initial investigation and in the analysis of the collected records, the absence of prominences at the buccal sides of the alveolar processes high in the vestibule, which indicates that the permanent canines are positioned properly within the jaw, was overlooked. In hindsight, it was realized that the incorrect positioning of the permanent canines could have been detected on the intraoral photographs (A–D) and on the dental casts made before treatment started (E, F). The latter also applies to the dental casts collected 1 year later (G, H). Regrettably, the primary maxillary canines were not extracted before the start of treatment. The radiographs obtained at that time did not reveal a distinct deviation in the position of the maxillary canines (I) as was the case 1 year later (J). Had the maxillary primary canines been extracted early, as recommended at the beginning of this chapter, the permanent maxillary canines probably would have spontaneously attained a good position. The use of a headgear-activator combination in the first phase of the treatment might have resulted in a worsening of the situation, while the maxillary incisors were intruded (K, L). Intrusion of maxillary incisors prior to the emergence of permanent canines can lead to displacement of the latter when the roots of the lateral incisors are near the crowns of the canines. Consequently, impaction or a reduction in the chance for spontaneous improvement can result. This aspect is of particular relevance when fixed appliances are used in crowded dental arches. Indeed, after 1 year of treatment, impaction of the maxillary canines was confirmed. The canines were surgically exposed, and eyelets and ligatures were placed (M, N).

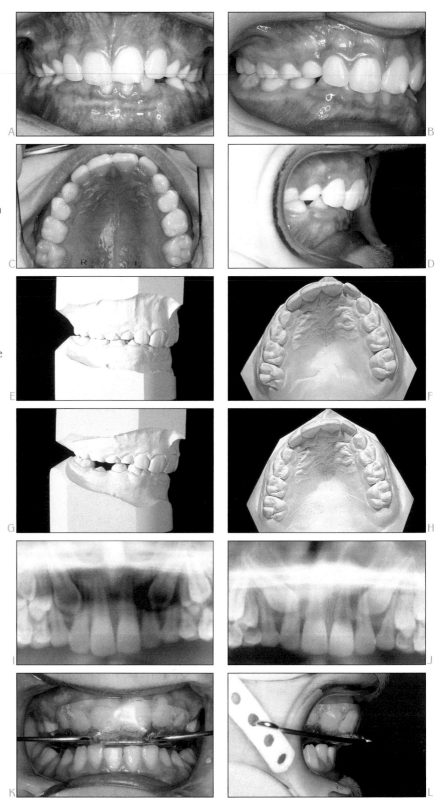

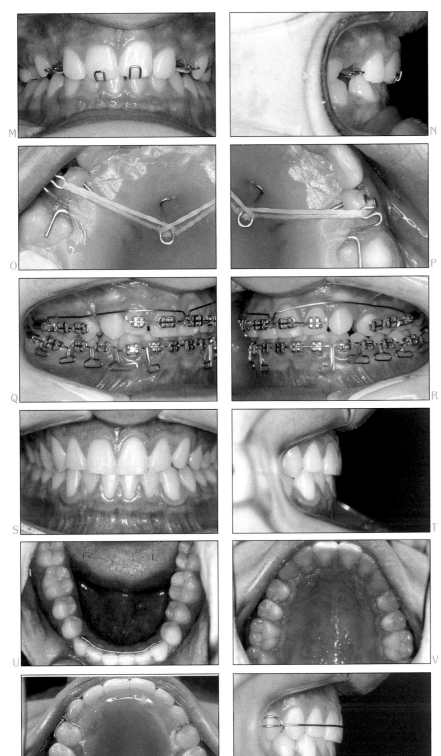

FIGURE 11-11 (CONTINUED)

In 4 months' time, the canines had moved almost completely to their correct position (O, P). At the same time, while the plate with guiding forks and elastics brought the canines to the dental arch, the deep bite was corrected and the curve of Spee was leveled by increasing the height of the bite plane regularly. The lower anterior facial height also was increased, which meant an improvement in this patient with a Class II division 2 malocclusion. Furthermore, the maxillary incisors were covered less by the lower lip, reducing its unfavorable influence on these teeth. Fixed appliances were placed in the mandible, and all planned improvements were realized before fixed appliances were placed in the maxilla. Initially, no brackets were placed at the maxillary canines, which were moved to their correct positions through the rather simple technique recommended in this chapter. A sectional archwire was inserted in the maxillary incisor brackets, and a basic intrusion arch, coming from the first molars, was tied to the middle of that sectional archwire. Sectional archwires in the posterior regions prevented the reaction force of the basic intrusion arch from leading to distal tipping of the first molars (Q, R). At the age of 15 years 1 month, all appliances were removed (S, T). A Van der Linden retainer was placed in the maxilla, and a wire was bonded to the mandibular canines to stabilize the mandibular anterior teeth. In the 3 years following, little had changed (U, V). The Van der Linden retainer[220] was used in a modified form, because the labial arch could not pass between the lateral incisors and canines, but enough space was available distal to the canines. In that design, the clasp function in the anterior region is placed at the first premolars (W, X) (see chapter 18).

The method described and illustrated here for moving impacted canines to their place in the dental arch causes relatively little discomfort to the patient. The elastics keep the plate in place and the patient will always wear it, because otherwise the end of the ligature will irritate the mouth. An important advantage of this method is that the reaction force does not impact the adjacent teeth alone, as is the case when complete fixed appliances without additional provisions are used to move impacted canines to the proper place. With the recommended method, the reaction force is absorbed not only by all teeth encompassed by the plate but also by the palate. Another important advantage of this method is that, with a Crefcoeur spring, the space in the dental arch can be increased simultaneously with the extrusion of the canine.

Two weeks after the eyelets and ligatures are placed, an impression can be taken for a dental cast. Before that time, there is still swelling and the tissues are too sensitive, although the extension of the ligature is tied around the first premolar or lateral incisor. The first time, the placement of an elastic is somewhat painful, as the ligature is stretched and shifts under the mucoperiosteum. From one recall visit to the next, the section of the ligature that protrudes becomes larger. The increase in the extent that the ligature protrudes is a measurement of the movement that has occurred since the last appointment. The absence of an increase in the length of the extension could be a sign of ankylosis and requires further exploration. Indeed, when the canine is ankylosed, removal is indicated; when sufficient space is available in the dental arch, transplantation to the proper place is an option.

A healthy periodontium and a good clinical crown height result when impacted canines are moved into correct positioning as recommended. In addition, after treatment, the canines tend to stay in place, probably because the extrusion and correct positioning are completed before the periodontal tissues mature.

The preservation of well-aligned primary canines with little or no root resorption can be considered when no other orthodontic abnormalities exist, especially when the impacted canine is in a severely deviating position. When they are located far cranially and away from the roots of the incisors, leaving them in place can be the best choice but requires a radiographic examination every 2 years. When the primary canines are lost in later years, a fixed partial denture or an implant with a crown can replace them.

Finally, when the lateral incisor is missing adjacent to an impacted canine, the placement of the canine in contact with the central incisor and first premolar is recommended. Comprehensive treatment is required anyway, so closure of the remaining diastemata, resulting in a continuous dental arch, does not require extra effort. Creation of space for a fixed partial denture or an implant is not a good solution in these patients. Furthermore, it is unlikely, and never has been proved, that a canine at the location of the lateral incisor has disadvantages in the long term.[149, 168]

Treatment of Class II Division 2 Malocclusions

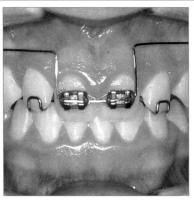

For many years, Class II division 2 malocclusions and Class I malocclusions with symptoms of Class II division 2 malocclusion—together denoted as coverbite (Deckbiss in the German language)—have been considered difficult to treat and prone to relapse.

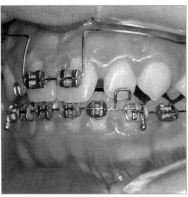

Recently it has become clear that coverbites are caused by only one, well-defined factor: the excessive labial coverage of the maxillary incisors by the lower lip. As such, coverbites are an exception in orthodontics. Not only the etiology but also the development of coverbites is specific. Because the etiology is evident, treatment can be directed to eliminate the cause from the very beginning; when that is accomplished, spontaneous corrections occur. Not only will the apices of the maxillary incisors move palatally, but secondary aspects, such as crowding in the maxillary and mandibular dental arch, will also improve.

In contrast to Class II division 1 malocclusions, coverbites are not considered initially as malocclusions when the maxillary incisors are well aligned.

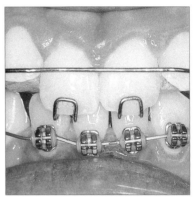

Lack of knowledge regarding the cause and development of coverbites leads to faulty diagnostic conclusions and incorrect treatment plans. When the cause is not eliminated, the treatment result will not be stable.

First, two patients who were treated in the early 1960s are shown. In the first patient, the coverbite returned completely. In the second patient, the treatment result was stable. Some years later it became evident why in, the long term, the first treatment failed and the second treatment was successful.

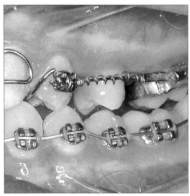

Subsequently, the specific development of coverbites is presented. In addition, the variation encountered in the arrangement of the maxillary anterior teeth in relation to the spatial conditions is explained, and three different types of arrangements are distinguished.

To emphasize the importance of the etiology, a patient is shown who was treated for a Class II division 1 malocclusion, but altered in an extreme coverbite after treatment, while the neutro-occlusion was maintained.

Finally, successfully treated coverbite patients are shown, and the recommended treatment strategy, including the technical details, is elucidated.

Orthodontic Concepts and Strategies

12

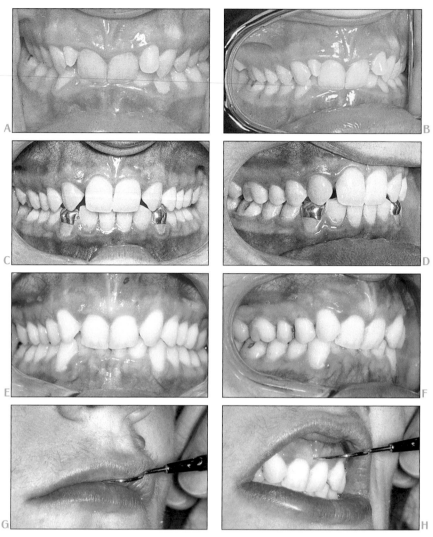

FIGURE 12-1

A girl who was 13 years 6 months of age had a Class II division 2 malocclusion with a disto-occlusion of one premolar crown width (A, B). She was treated with a cervical headgear with a Kahn spur and complete fixed appliances. The disto-occlusion could not be changed to a neutro-occlusion, even with the prolonged use of Class II elastics. Therefore, the maxillary lateral incisors were extracted, partly because the right one was peg shaped. At the age of 16 years 1 month, the appliances were removed, and retention was started (C, D). To that end, a classic canine bar was placed in the mandible, and a retention plate was placed in the maxilla. Three years later, at the removal of the canine bar, the maxillary central incisors had already tipped slightly palatally. In the following years, the maxillary central incisors attained a more upright position, and the coverbite returned completely, as shown in the photographs collected at 29 years 7 months of age (E, F). The lower lip covered the maxillary incisors excessively, which was the cause of the relapse (G, H).

The general opinion has been that coverbites are associated with a typical facial pattern: a large nose, a prominent chin, and a small lower anterior facial height. However, a study of the skeletal morphology of adults with a Class II division 2 malocclusion revealed that coverbites are found in a large variation of facial configurations.[186] Nevertheless, many have a small lower anterior facial height.[155]

The first publication that pointed to a relationship between the excessive coverage of the maxillary incisors by the lower lip and Class II division 2 malocclusions was authored by Nicol[146] and appeared in the English literature in 1963. A few years later Fränkel and Falck[71] followed in the German literature and Kolf[106] in the French.

This information was not available when the patients presented in Figs 12-1 and 12-2 were treated. Afterward it became clear why the coverbite had returned in the first patient and not in the second patient. The girl shown in Fig 12-1 did not grow during treatment. The maxillomandibular relationship could not be influenced anymore, and the lower anterior facial height did not increase. At the end of treatment, the lower lip still covered the maxillary incisors excessively, which led again to the palatal tipping of the maxillary incisors after retention was concluded. Secondarily, the overbite increased, and, with the palatal tipping of the maxillary incisors, the mandibular incisors tipped lingually and became crowded.

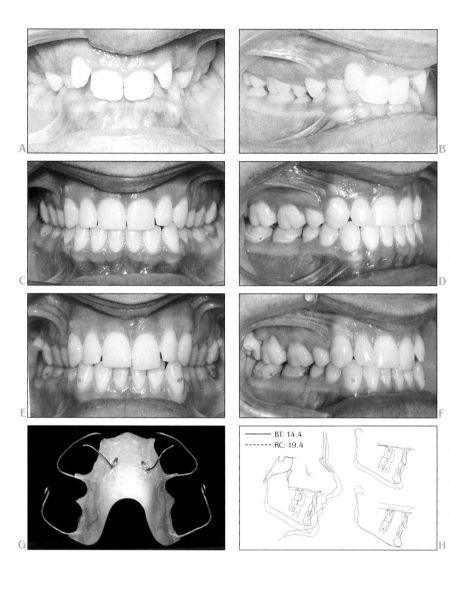

FIGURE 12-2

The maxillary first premolars were extracted from a boy aged 14 years 4 months who had a Class II division 2 malocclusion and a disto-occlusion of one premolar crown width (A, B). A cervical headgear was placed, and a few weeks later a plate was added to distalize the canines and align the lateral incisors. The treatment was completed with fixed appliances and lasted a total of 1 year 5 months. A retention plate was used in the maxilla for 2 years; in the last year, it was worn only during sleep. A canine bar was placed in the mandible and removed at the age of 19 years 4 months (C, D). Five years later, at the age of 24 years 4 months, some irregularities had developed in the maxillary anterior region, but the coverbite had not returned (E, F). The plate that was used to distalize the canines and align the lateral incisors had also corrected the deep bite (G). Together with the cervical headgear, the raising of the bite through the plate had resulted in a substantial increase in the lower facial height and a change in the relationship between the lower lip and the maxillary incisors (H). These records were collected at the beginning of treatment (BT) and at the completion of retention (RC).

On the other hand, the boy presented in Fig 12-2 still had much growth to experience when the orthodontic treatment was started. The removable plate that was used to distalize the maxillary canines and align the lateral incisors without causing unwanted reaction forces on the adjacent teeth—as happens when fixed appliances are used—stimulated an increase in lower anterior facial height through the bite plane used to reduce the overbite. In addition, the cervical headgear placed on the permanent maxillary first molars contributed to the increase in lower facial height. The spontaneous improvement in the inclination of the maxillary central incisors, which occurred in the meantime, was striking. However, at that time, the author did not realize the relationship between this improvement and the position of the lower lip.[207] In this patient, the reduction in the coverage of the maxillary incisors by the lower lip had the effect that the coverbite did not return (Fig 12-2, H). However, this alteration was not pursued in the treatment, and the favorable effect was not realized until some years later. Indeed, in the meantime it has become clear that the increase in lower facial height had resulted in a descent of stomion. The same effect is reached immediately when the distance between the nose and the chin is enlarged with an anterior bite plane.

FIGURE 12-3

In a normal situation, the permanent maxillary central incisors are formed within the jaw in a labially inclined position (A). Six months later, the permanent maxillary central incisors have erupted further, and the bone at their labial side is thinner (B). Seven months thereafter, their predecessors are still present, and the unemerged permanent incisors have erupted further, without a change in angulation, while the bone at the labial side has been resorbed (C). Eighteen months later, the permanent maxillary central incisors as well as the mandibular incisors have erupted completely and reached incisal contact. The lower lip lies against the incisal edges of the maxillary incisors and covers their labial surfaces only for a small extent (D). The inclination of the maxillary central incisors has exhibited little or no change during the whole eruption process. The developing part of roots of the incisors remained at the same location. (Reprinted with permission from Falck and Fränkel.[65])

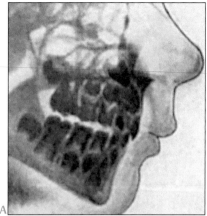
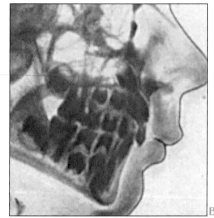
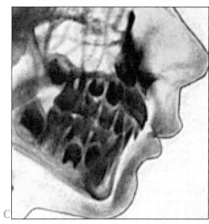
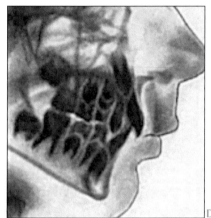

The relationship between stomion and the anterior teeth and the extent of coverage of the maxillary incisors by the lower lip also can be altered by intrusion of the maxillary incisors. However, this procedure leads to less favorable results, as will be explained later.

The transition of the maxillary incisors and their changes in inclination during normal development are illustrated in Fig 12-3; the same stages during development of coverbite are shown in Fig 12-4. The most important difference between the two forms of development is the extent of coverage of the maxillary primary and permanent incisors by the lower lip. In addition, the child with the coverbite has thicker and larger lips than the child without a malocclusion. With voluminous lips, stomion is positioned more superiorly. Another important factor is the length of the upper lip, in which a large variation exists. In individuals with a short upper lip and a competent lip seal, the lower lip tends to cover the maxillary incisors excessively, and a coverbite can develop.

Longitudinal investigations have revealed that, in normal development, the inclination of the maxillary central incisors changes only slightly or remains unchanged during their eruption. In Class II division 1 malocclusions, the labial inclination increases after emergence. In Class II division 2 malocclusions, the central incisors start to tip palatally prior to emergence, when the crown is covered not by bone anymore but by the mucosa only. After emergence, the palatal tipping continues, and the maxillary incisors attain an upright position.[113]

With the palatal tipping of the maxillary incisors, the mandibular anterior teeth will move lingually after contact in the anterior region has been reached. If large spaces exist in the mandibular anterior region, the incisors can tip lingually without the occurrence of crowding. However, in the absence of excess space, the lingual tipping will lead to overlapping of the mandibular anterior teeth.

The sagittal relationship of the jaws, and particularly that of the anterior sections of the alveolar processes, is another determinant in the degree of lingual tipping of the mandibular incisors. Contact between the maxillary and mandibular incisors is established at an earlier stage in a neutro-occlusion than in a disto-occlusion, in which lingual tipping and crowding will not happen as soon and will be less severe.

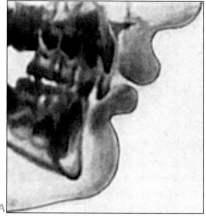
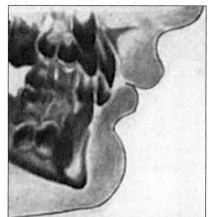
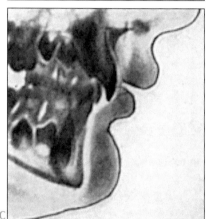
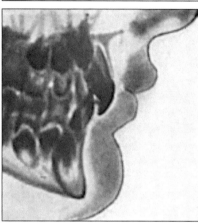

FIGURE 12-4

In a developing coverbite, the maxillary primary incisors are covered excessively by the lower lip, and the permanent maxillary incisors are in a more upright position than normal prior to emergence (A). Seven months later, the permanent maxillary incisors are more labially and occlusally positioned, and their predecessors are ready to be exfoliated (B). Six months thereafter, the permanent maxillary central incisors have emerged and are covered by the lower lip for about half their crown height (C). Eighteen months later, incisal contact has been established, and the lower lip completely covers the crowns of the permanent maxillary central incisors (D). These sections from lateral cephalograms demonstrate that the initially somewhat steeply inclined maxillary central incisors first move labially but tip palatally after emergence. Furthermore, in this individual, an angle between the long axis of the crown and the long axis of the root resulted, the so-called column angle of Andresen. (Reprinted with permission from Falck and Fränkel.[65])

It is not clear why the developing part of the root of the palatally tipping maxillary central permanent incisors in some cases moves labially and in other cases maintains its original location. When the developing part of the root is not displaced, a curved root results (Figs 12-4, D, and 12-5, D). The angle between the long axes of the crown and the root found in coverbite patients is caused by this phenomenon. Consequently, the alveolar process in the apical region will not be expanded anteriorly, as will happen when the developing part of the root moves labially. In the latter case, the roots can tip so far labially that they are not covered by bone at their labial surfaces (Fig 12-7, E).

Indeed, the labial movement of the developing parts of the maxillary incisors leads to forced anterior growth of the alveolar process. An assessment of the anterior position of the maxilla, derived from a cephalogram by means of point A (the most posterior point on the curvature between the anterior nasal spine and prosthion), is misleading in coverbite patients in whom the maxillary central of the incisors did not deform. Indeed, when the apices of the incisors are not moved labially, point A will be located more posteriorly.[209]

Likewise, an assessment of a dental cast to determine the position of the anterior border of the maxillary apical area will be misleading, when the forced expansion of the alveolar process is not taken into account. Both methods of assessment have consequences for the estimation of the sagittal maxillomandibular relationship and for the evaluation of the size of the apical area in the maxilla.

The development of a coverbite is shown in a Class II division 2 malocclusion in Fig 12-5, and in a Class I malocclusion in Fig 12-6, in which, as could be expected, severe crowding appeared in the mandibular dental arch. The alveolar process at point A has not been expanded anteriorly in the Class II division 2 dentition, where column angles developed, as illustrated in Fig 12-4, D. However, in the Class I malocclusion, the maxillary central incisors were not deformed, and the alveolar process grew anteriorly.

FIGURE 12-5

In a child of 7 years 10 months with a disto-occlusion, the permanent maxillary central incisors had emerged and the primary lateral incisors had exfoliated. The posterior teeth were in a disto-occlusion of one premolar crown width. Sufficient space was available in both dental arches (A, B, G). One year later, the permanent maxillary central incisors had erupted further and tipped palatally. In the meantime, the maxillary lateral incisors had emerged and were positioned steeply also. The posterior regions had changed little (C, D). At the age of 11 years 10 months, the maxillary incisors had tipped further, the overbite had increased, and the permanent canines had emerged. In the mandible, all primary molars were replaced by their successors, without a shortage of space. In the maxilla, the primary right second molar was still present; sufficient space was available in the dental arch. After the replacement of the primary maxillary right second molar by the smaller premolar, the permanent maxillary right first molar will migrate mesially and arrive in a disto-occlusion of one premolar crown width (E, F, H).

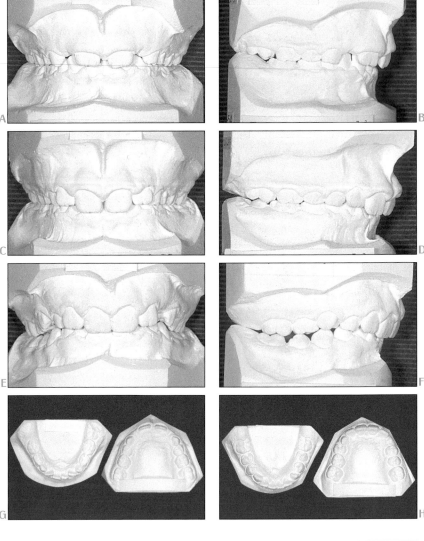

FIGURE 12-6

In a child aged 6 years 7 months with a neutro-occlusion, the permanent maxillary central incisors were present in the mouth. The right incisor had erupted farther than the left incisor and was tipped more palatally. The primary lateral incisors were still present, and there was sufficient space in both dental arches. The posterior teeth were in neutro-occlusion, so this case demonstrated the development of a coverbite in a Class I situation (A, B, M).

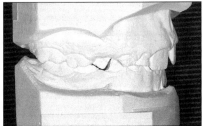
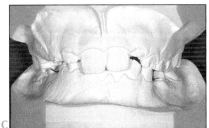
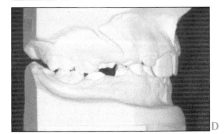
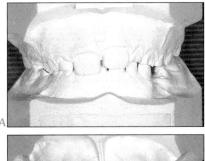

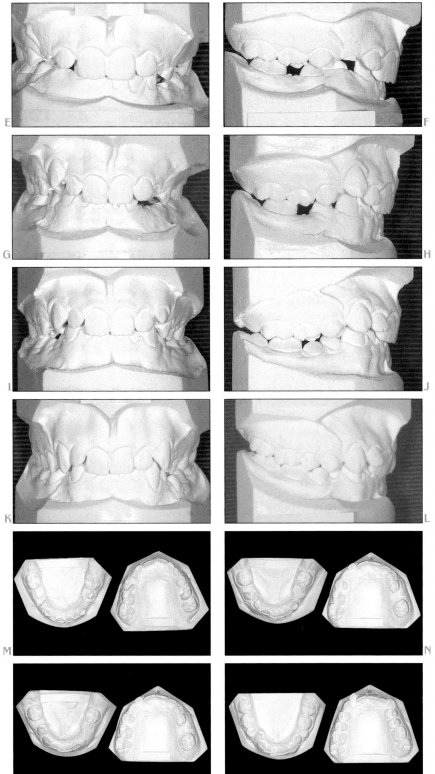

FIGURE 12-6 (CONTINUED)

One year later, the maxillary left central incisor had reached the same level as the right incisor and had tipped palatally accordingly. Some time before, the permanent maxillary lateral incisors had emerged in a normal inclination. The mandibular central incisors were in contact with the maxillary central incisors (C, D). Again 1 year later, the maxillary central incisors had erupted further, and the overbite had increased. The maxillary left lateral incisor had tipped palatally and the right lateral incisor labially. The permanent first molars were in neutro-occlusion with a solid intercuspation and seemed not to have migrated mesially, despite the fact that the primary molars were lost prematurely. Nevertheless, the space available for the mandibular premolars had become insufficient. This deficiency was caused primarily by the distal movement of the mesially located teeth as a result of the pressure exerted by the maxillary incisors on the mandibular anterior teeth (E, F, N). At the age of 9 years 8 months, only the primary maxillary right second molar and a remnant of the primary mandibular left second molar were still present. All permanent canines had emerged. Sufficient space was available in the maxillary dental arch, but in the mandible too little space was left for the premolars (G, H, O). One year later, the maxillary right lateral incisor had tipped more labially, while the primary maxillary right second molar was not yet lost. The permanent first molars were still in neutro-occlusion (I, J). At the age of 13 years 7 months, crowding had developed in the maxillary dental arch, while the crowding in the mandible had increased. The maxillary central incisors and the left lateral incisor were tipped extremely palatally, while the right lateral incisor had become more labially tipped. The maxillary left canine was positioned too far buccally. The crowding in the mandible was concentrated at the first premolars, which were both in endo-occlusion (K, L, P).

FIGURE 12-7

Normally, maxillary incisors are labially inclined and their roots are covered by bone. A posteriorly directed concavity is present between the anterior nasal spine and the cervical margins at the maxillary incisors (A, B). In a coverbite, the crowns become palatally displaced and the apices are labially displaced, while bone is deposited at the labial surface of the alveolar process to keep the roots covered. Consequently, the anterior border at the apical region is expanded anteriorly and the concavity is filled (C, D). However, the potential to deposit bone at the labial surface is limited and is insufficient when the roots are moved far outside their normal boundaries. In extreme situations, the labial surfaces of the roots become denuded of bone (E, F). When a column angle develops, the roots will not protrude and penetrate the bone, because the developing part of the tooth and the apex do not become displaced.

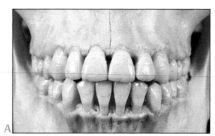
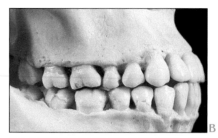
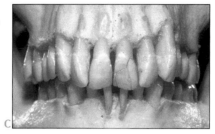
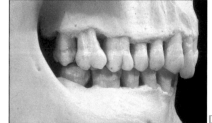
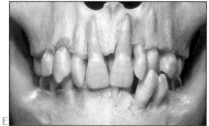
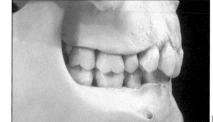

FIGURE 12-8

The alveolar process adapts to the presence of the roots, especially in the maxillary anterior region, where the range of variation in root location is relatively large (A). Consequently, the validity of point A in determining the anterior position of the maxilla is limited (B).[209]

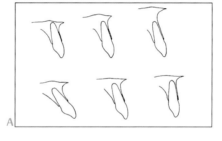
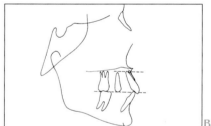

FIGURE 12-9

When a coverbite develops in an individual with a neutro-occlusion, a Class I malocclusion with symptoms of a Class II division 2 arrangement will result. The mandibular anterior teeth will tip further lingually and excessive crowding will develop in the mandibular dental arch (A, B).

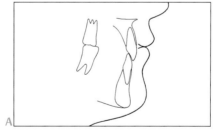
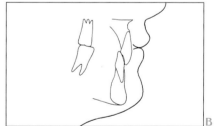

The anterior expansion of the alveolar process in response to a coverbite is shown on skulls (Fig 12-7). It is also obvious on lateral cephalograms and tracing made from these radiographs (Fig 12-8). The severe lingual tipping of the mandibular anterior teeth when a coverbite develops in a Class I situation is also visible on tracings (Fig 12-9). Coverbites arise as the permanent maxillary incisors become excessively covered by the lower lip, independent of the occlusion. That means that coverbites are superimposed on already existing malocclusions. Initially present crowding will increase. When mandibular teeth are missing, the mandibular anterior teeth will become retruded further, and the maxillary incisors will tip further palatally. Furthermore, the risk of injuries to the mucosa palatal to the maxillary incisors and labial to the mandibular incisors increases.

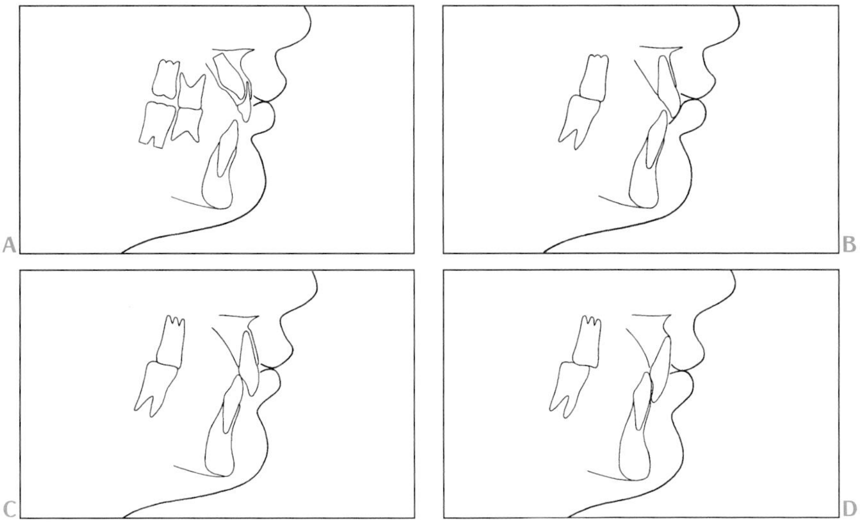

FIGURE 12-10

Normally, the primary incisors are inclined about perpendicular to the occlusal plane, even when a coverbite will develop. Only the complete coverage of the maxillary primary incisors by the lower lip indicates that a coverbite will develop (A). Prior to emergence, the inclination of the maxillary incisors starts to change. After emergence, excessive contact with the lower lip leads to their gradual palatal tipping and overeruption (B, C). The contact with the maxillary incisors leads to lingual tipping of the mandibular incisors and a further increase of the deep bite (D).

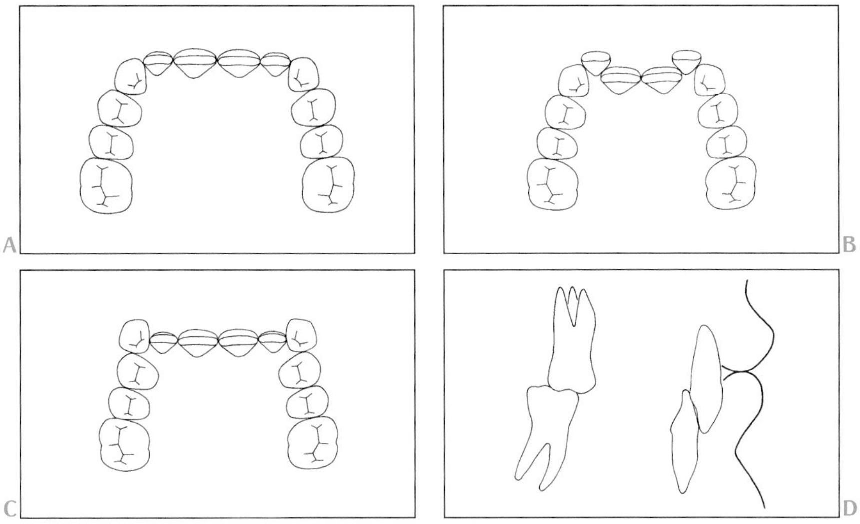

FIGURE 12-11

The type of coverbite that develops depends on the spatial conditions in the maxillary anterior region (D). Type A: With extra space, all four incisors tip palatally and become arranged more or less in a straight line (A). Type B: Without extra space, the palatal tipping of the central incisors will lead to lack of space for the lateral incisors, which will tip labially, and the lower lip will become located at their palatal side, which will lead to a further increase in their labial tipping (B). Type C: With crowding, the primary maxillary canines will be lost prematurely and their successors will erupt outside the dental arch (C).[212]

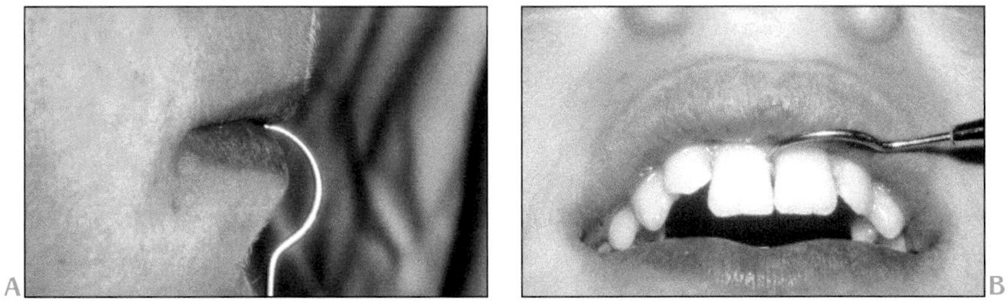

FIGURE 12-12

An unexpected lifting of the upper lip in an individual at rest will reveal the extent of coverage of the maxillary incisors by the lower lip. A more accurate assessment can be made with an explorer or, preferably, a periodontal probe.

The change in inclination that occurs in coverbites before and after emergence of the maxillary central incisors is illustrated in Fig 12-10. The spatial conditions in the dental arch mainly determine which type of coverbite will develop (Fig 12-11).

The extent of coverage of the maxillary incisors by the lower lip can easily be assessed (Fig 12-12). Such an assessment should be carried out regularly in all orthodontic patients, particularly those with Class II division 1 malocclusions. Neglecting this aspect can lead to the development of a coverbite in a patient with a seemingly adequately treated Class II division 1 malocclusion (Fig 12-13).

The treatment of a Class I malocclusion with a type A coverbite, in which the lip coverage was given appropriate attention, is presented in Fig 12-14.

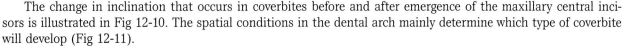

Figure 12-13

A boy aged 10 years 4 months had a Class II division 1 malocclusion with a disto-occlusion of one premolar width. His lower lip was positioned palatal to the maxillary incisors, which were overerupted. The mandibular incisors were tipped lingually (A, B). He was treated with a headgear, a maxillary plate, and a lip bumper in the mandible. However, the appliances were worn irregularly and mistreated. More than once, molar bands became loose; the plate was broken often; and its wires were frequently deformed. Furthermore, oral hygiene was inadequate. Therefore, a less vulnerable approach was preferred, and the plate and lip bumper were replaced by an activator. The headgear was maintained and worn together with the activator. With these limited means, a seemingly acceptable result with a neutro-occlusion was obtained after 2 years of treatment. However, the maxillary incisors were too upright and the bite was too deep (C, D). At the end of treatment, it was not realized that the lower lip covered the maxillary incisors excessively, just as it was overlooked in the initial diagnosis that the maxillary incisors were overerupted. The treatment was not followed by a retention period, and after 1 year the maxillary central incisors were more palatally inclined, and the overbite had increased (E, F). At that time, the excessive coverage of the maxillary incisors by the lower lip was verified (G, H). Photographs taken 2 years 6 months later revealed that the maxillary incisors, except the right lateral incisor, had tipped further palatally, and the overbite had increased more. Concomitantly, the mandibular incisors had tipped lingually, and crowding had developed in the mandibular anterior region. However, the solid intercuspation in neutro-occlusion was maintained (I, J). Three years later, at the age of 18 years 10 months, the situation was even worse (K, L).[215]

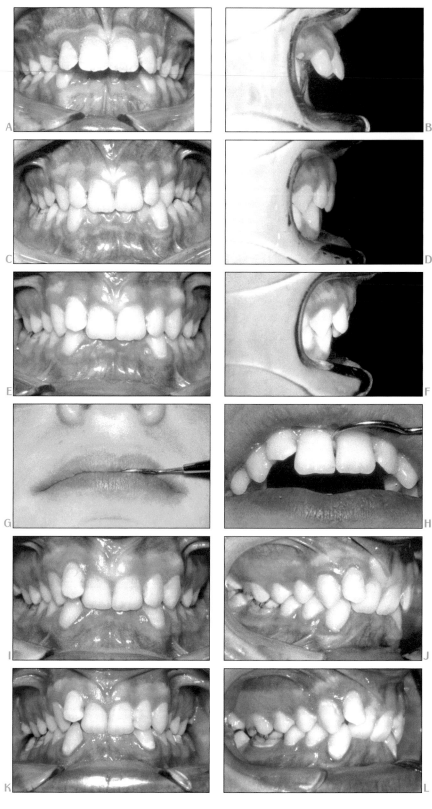

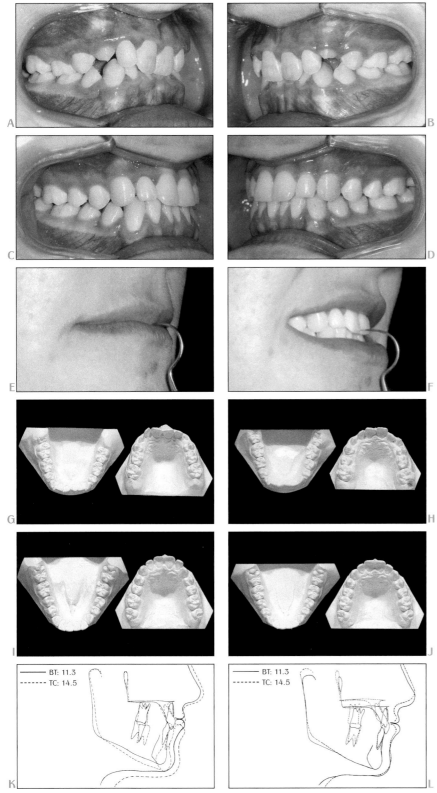

FIGURE 12-14

A girl aged 11 years 3 months had a Class I malocclusion with a coverbite, in which the maxillary central incisors and the left lateral incisor were tipped palatally. The mandibular incisors were tipped lingually and crowded (A, B, G). A cervical headgear was placed to exert an extruding force on the permanent maxillary first molars and to increase the lower facial height. A maxillary plate with an anterior bite plane and claw clasps on the three palatally tipped incisors was used to prevent the lower lip from contacting the labial surfaces of the maxillary incisors and to reduce the deep bite. Later, fixed appliances were placed in the mandible; the mandibular anterior teeth already had improved spontaneously in position, because the bite plane had provided the freedom for them to migrate labially. Furthermore, the deep bite had been eliminated, and the curve of Spee had been leveled. Therefore, in the mandible, only minor corrections had to be carried out by the fixed appliances. Fixed appliances were not placed in the maxilla until all mandibular teeth were aligned. Fortunately, the maxillary incisors did not have to be torqued any further. Because the lower lip had been restricted from contacting the labial surfaces of the maxillary incisors, their apices had moved spontaneously in the palatal direction, and the teeth had attained correct inclinations (H). However, they still had to be intruded slightly. After 3 years of treatment, a fine result was obtained (C, D, I). Stomion was positioned correctly (E, F). The dental casts made before the treatment started (G), prior to the placement of fixed appliances in the mandible (H), at the end of active treatment (I), and 2 years later (J) showed that the dental arches were sufficiently large to contain all teeth. The most notable of the spontaneous corrections that occurred during treatment with the headgear and the maxillary plate was the change in inclination of the maxillary incisors (G, H, K, L). These records were collected at the beginning of treatment (BT) and at the completion of treatment (TC).

12-15

A boy 13 years 6 months of age had a Class II division 2 malocclusion, type B coverbite, a disto-occlusion of one premolar crown width, and a deep bite. The arch length discrepancy was –4 mm in the mandible and –3 mm in the maxilla (A, B). After 2 years 2 months of treatment with a cervical headgear, a bite plate, and fixed appliances, a good result was obtained. For retention, a plate was used in the maxilla and a canine bar in the mandible. The retention plate was worn day and night for 6 months and only during sleep for 3 more years. At the age of 18 years 2 months, the retention was concluded, and the canine bar in the mandible was removed (C, D). Five years later, at the age of 23 years 2 months, the occlusion was still perfect, and the position and inclination of the incisors had not changed noticeably (E, F). The stability of the result was related to the improvement in the position of stomion, because the maxillary incisors were not covered excessively by the lower lip (G, H). Seventeen years after the end of retention, when the patient was aged 35 years 4 months, the occlusion exhibited little or no change (I, J).

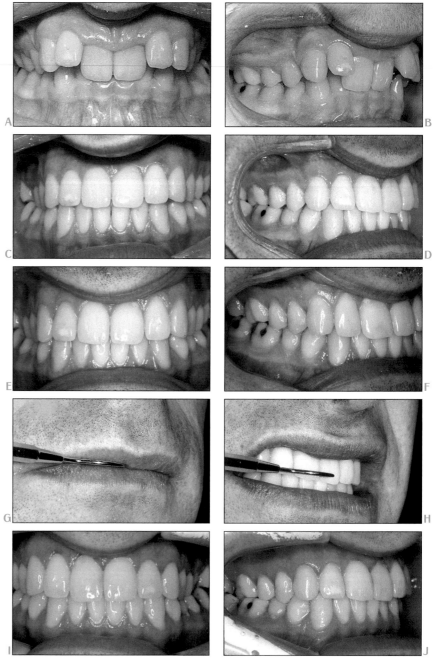

Fig 12-15 shows the treatment of a Class II division 2 malocclusion with a type B coverbite. As in all coverbites, the long-term results of treatment depended primarily on the position of stomion in relation to the maxillary incisors at the end of treatment.

Indeed, the aim should be to eliminate the cause, the excessive coverage of the maxillary incisors by the lower lip, right from the beginning and 24 hours a day. The best appliance for that purpose is a maxillary plate with a bite plane, which should be removed only for cleaning. At the same time, the maxillary central incisors can be intruded if needed. After the mandibular teeth have been aligned with fixed appliances, they can serve as an occlusal template for the proper positioning of the maxillary teeth.

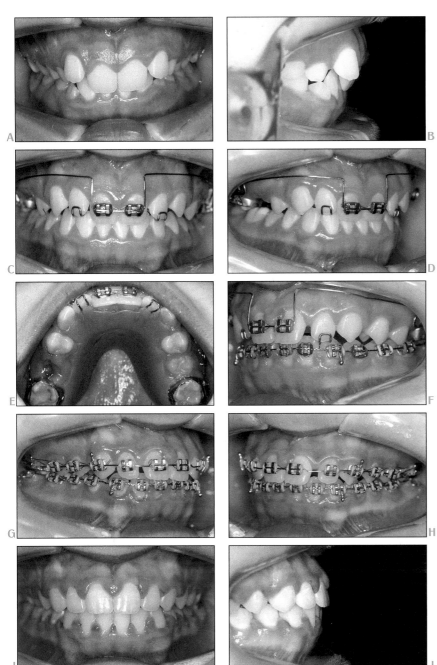

FIGURE 12-16
A girl aged 10 years 2 months had a Class II division 2 malocclusion, type B coverbite, and a disto-occlusion of one premolar crown width (A, B). A cervical headgear was placed to improve the occlusion and to stimulate the vertical development of the lower face. In addition, a plate with claw clasps was placed at the maxillary lateral incisors. A few months later, brackets were bonded to the maxillary central incisors, and a light rectangular archwire was inserted to protrude and intrude these teeth (C, D). The plate was anchored with clasps at the permanent first molars, while the claws provided firm retention, because of the artificial resin composite undercuts at the labial surfaces (SEE FIGS 3-11 AND 3-12). This approach had several additional advantages: It allowed the "rail" mechanism to work; the plate could be used while the primary molars were replaced; and the plate caused little discomfort (E). Furthermore, the incisal contact was relieved, and the mandibular teeth were able to migrate spontaneously over the bite plane to better positions. During the correction of the remaining irregularities in the mandibular arch with fixed appliances, the bite plane provided vertical support to the anterior teeth and relieved the occlusion of the posterior teeth (F). Fixed appliances in the maxilla were needed only for a short period of time (G, H). The goals of treatment were met (I, J).

In Fig 12-16, the treatment of a Class II division 2 malocclusion is shown. The causal factor had been eliminated right from the beginning, and the dentition benefited in an optimal way from spontaneous corrections. A bite plane on the maxillary plate provides the freedom for the mandibular incisors to migrate labially and for the spontaneous improvement of malaligned teeth. In addition, the curve of Spee is leveled before fixed appliances are placed to arrive at an ideally arranged mandibular dental arch. When the bite plane is retained during that phase of treatment, the eruption of the mandibular incisors is blocked, and the interference of occlusal contacts with corrections in the posterior regions is hindered. Furthermore, the bite plane can prevent the maxillary incisors from contacting the brackets on the mandibular teeth.

FIGURE 12-17

A boy 16 years 6 months of age had a Class II division 2 malocclusion with a type B coverbite. It was decided not to use a cervical headgear but to extract the permanent maxillary second molars and distalize the first molars with partial fixed appliances. A maxillary plate was used for anchorage and to keep the lower lip from contacting the labial surfaces of the maxillary incisors. The claw clasps at the central incisors and the retention arch with clasp functions at the canines kept the plate firmly in place. After some time, fixed appliances were placed in the mandible (A–D). The maxillary first molars were distalized with Sentalloy coil springs (GAC International, Bohemia, New York) on rectangular wire sections. The plate was tightly in contact with the anterior teeth and first premolars, but the second premolars were free to drift distally along the acrylic resin margin of the plate. Indeed, the second premolars migrated spontaneously in the distal direction (E, F).

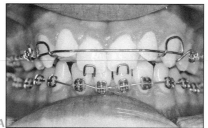

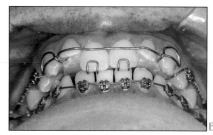

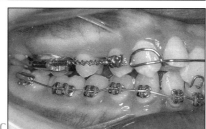

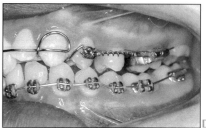

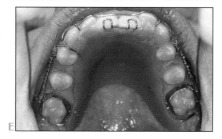

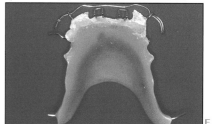

In patients treated without facial orthopedic support, in whom the occlusion is changed by moving teeth within the dental arches, the same considerations and rules for treatment of coverbite apply. The same holds true for patients in whom maxillary premolars are extracted (Fig 12-2) and permanent maxillary first molars are distalized to arrive at a neutro-occlusion, with or without preceding extraction of the permanent maxillary second molars (Fig 12-17). When a coverbite is combined with impacted maxillary canines that have to be moved into the dental arch, the treatment can follow the same concept and principles (Fig 12-18).

Coverbites cannot be prevented. Early treatment makes little sense, because the treatment cannot be finished before the transition is completed and the posterior teeth occlude well. Premature action leads to lengthy treatments with all their associated disadvantages. Certainly, treatment should be started before facial growth is completed; otherwise, attempts to stimulate the vertical development of the lower face will have little effect. Furthermore, in Class II division 2 malocclusions, treatment should be started before the primary second molars are lost, so that the leeway space can be used for the correction of the disto-occlusion.

The risk that treatment will be started too late to influence facial growth is limited in boys, even when the transition of the posterior teeth is completed (Fig 12-2). However, in girls this can happen easily, because they experience the adolescence growth spurt, on average, 2 years earlier than boys. Therefore, the risk of starting treatment too late in girls should not be underestimated (Fig 12-1). Furthermore, the age of onset of puberty and the adolescence growth spurt has lowered gradually over the last 50 years in both sexes.

The fact that facial growth continues considerably longer in boys than in girls is of relevance for the retention strategy. As explained in chapter 8, girls have completed their facial growth at 15 years of age or earlier. Indeed, facial orthopedic improvements in girls will not erode after facial growth is completed. However, in boys, facial growth can continue until 20 years of age or even later, and an increase in lower facial height can be partially lost when retention is not applied.

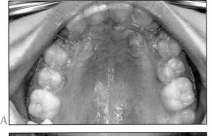
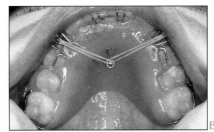
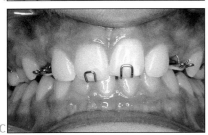
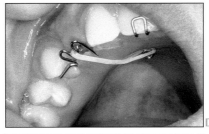
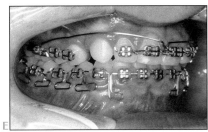
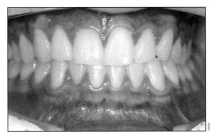

FIGURE 12-18

In coverbite patients with impacted canines, the plate can be utilized to move these teeth to their places in the dental arch, as is described in detail in chapter 11. When this procedure is followed, occlusal rests should be placed on the first premolars, and the margins of the acrylic resin plate should be well adapted for control of the reaction forces (A–D). In this patient, the maxillary incisors were intruded with a basic intrusion arch, tied to the middle of the sectional wire, which was placed in the brackets of the four incisors. To prevent distal tipping of the permanent first molars, sectional wires were placed in the posterior regions (E). With the subsequent addition of fixed appliances to the maxillary canines and to the mandibular teeth, a good result was obtained (F).

Hence, boys should continue to wear a retention plate with a bite plane during sleeping hours until facial growth is completed. Experience has revealed that wearing a retention plate during the night for many years is well accepted by most patients, provided that the plate fits well and is not uncomfortable. A well-designed, well-manufactured, and well-adapted retention plate can function for many years and does not have to be reexamined more than once a year (see chapter 18). The retention period should be especially lengthy in patients with a small lower anterior facial height and a horizontally directed growth pattern (Fig 12-19).

With the maturation of the face and with aging, the upper lip becomes longer and stomion descends.[144, 232] In patients in whom the lower lip covers the labial surfaces of the maxillary incisors too extensively at the end of treatment, a prolonged use of the retention plate can improve the stability in the long term.

The canine bar in the mandible should not be removed before the patient is 30 years of age, provided that good oral hygiene is maintained.[41] When a solid intercuspation has not been established, premolars can become lingually or buccally displaced, so they should be incorporated in the bonded retention wire.

A special point of concern in the treatment of coverbites is how much of the maxillary anterior teeth will be visible later during speaking and laughing. The intrusion of maxillary incisors can lead to a reduction of facial animation, charm, and attractiveness, because the visibility of these teeth plays a large role in that respect (Fig 12-20). This is one of the reasons that an increase in the lower facial height is preferred for the alteration of the position of stomion over the intrusion of the maxillary incisors. As indicated earlier, a cervical headgear and a plate with a bite plane are excellent means to reach that goal.

Great forces are not needed to move teeth. A continuous force of 5 g is sufficient, provided that the movement is not hindered.[234] Coverbites also develop in individuals with weak facial musculature. However, individuals with strong and voluminous facial musculature, a small lower facial height, a short upper lip, and a horizontal growth pattern are more apt to develop a coverbite.

FIGURE 12-19

Especially in patients with a small anterior facial height and a horizontal mandibular inferior border, a retention plate with an anterior bite plane should be worn during sleep until facial growth is completed (A). This means until about 15 years of age in girls but much longer, sometimes even until 22 years of age, in boys (B, C). The mandibular retention wire or canine bar should be maintained longer and preferably should not be removed before the patient is 30 years of age (D).

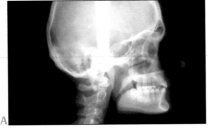
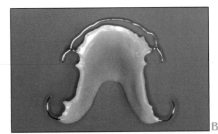
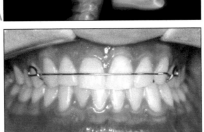
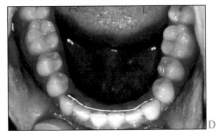

FIGURE 12-20

Intrusion of the maxillary incisors involves the risk that the anterior teeth will not be sufficiently visible when the patient is speaking and laughing posttreatment. Thus, after treatment, the face could become less attractive than it was at the start of treatment (A, B). This problem particularly affects patients with a short upper lip in whom the lower facial height could not be increased. Indeed, the dentition may look attractive at the end of treatment, and stomion may be positioned correctly, but the overall result will not be completely satisfying (C, D).

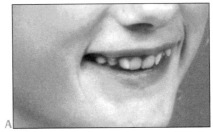
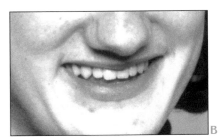
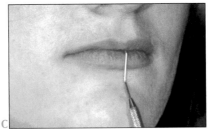
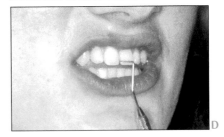

Many spontaneous corrections take place when the cause of the coverbite—the excessive coverage of the maxillary incisors by the lower lip—is eliminated right from the beginning. When this approach is followed, torquing of the maxillary incisors is often not needed. This is an important advantage, because when torque is applied to maxillary incisors that are covered by the lower lip, the pressure of the lower lip will counteract the torquing force. This will lead to mobility of these teeth, with the associated increased risk of root resorption.

Finally, in patients with coverbites, extraction of mandibular teeth mesial to the permanent first molars should be avoided, even in situations with seemingly severe crowding. This crowding usually is entirely, or in large part, a secondary effect of the coverbite, caused by the lingual tipping of the mandibular anterior teeth.

Treatment of Asymmetries

An asymmetry in the dentition can be caused by differences between the left and right sides of the facial skeleton, by differences in the positioning of teeth, or by a combination of both. Severe asymmetries of the facial skeleton can only be corrected by surgery and by distraction osteogenesis.[79, 93, 125] However, a mild asymmetry of the face is usually not disturbing. An asymmetry in the position of teeth can be camouflaged by the movement of teeth within the dental arches.

Asymmetries in the positioning of teeth are due to differences in locations where teeth are formed, migrations caused by premature loss of primary teeth, and agenesis or extraction of permanent teeth. Asymmetries in tooth positioning are combined sometimes with lateral forced bites (shifts).

In general, surgical correction of an asymmetry has to wait until the growth of the facial skeleton is completed, but distraction osteogenesis can be carried out earlier. Correction of asymmetries within the dental arches preferably should be started before the transition of the posterior teeth is completed. In this way, differences in crown size between primary molars and premolars can be exploited for the correction. In addition, the migration of permanent first molars can still be controlled. A delay until all permanent teeth, except the third molars, have erupted completely makes the treatment more complex.

The orthodontic treatment is facilitated when asymmetric positioning of teeth is corrected first. For that purpose, asymmetric headgears, removable plates, palatal arches, and lip bumpers can be used. The Crefcoeur appliance is particularly suited for shifting groups of teeth and for gaining space locally in the dental arch.

First, a theoretical discourse regarding the different causes of asymmetries and how asymmetric malocclusions can be corrected is given. Various situations and treatment strategies are presented. The treatment of severe asymmetries of the facial skeleton, which requires surgical correction or distraction osteogenesis, is not discussed.

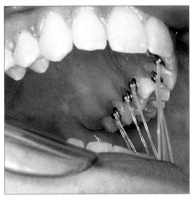
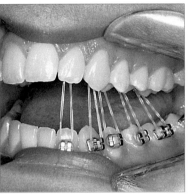
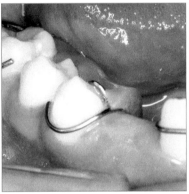
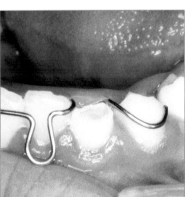

Orthodontic Concepts and Strategies

13

Treatment of Asymmetries

FIGURE 13-1

In most humans, the facial skeleton is slightly asymmetric,[173] and muscles and other soft tissues often differ on the left and right sides. The mandible can be positioned asymmetrically because the locations of the temporal fossae do not correspond. In addition, the mandible itself can be asymmetric (A). An asymmetry of the face and the maxilla is usually associated with some asymmetry of the mandible (B). In an asymmetry of the lower part of the face, both the size and the shape of the two sides of the mandible are usually different (C). Asymmetries of the face are visible in anterior views (D). The positions of the teeth adjust to the asymmetry of the facial skeleton. The dentoalveolar compensatory mechanism can compensate for skeletal asymmetries.

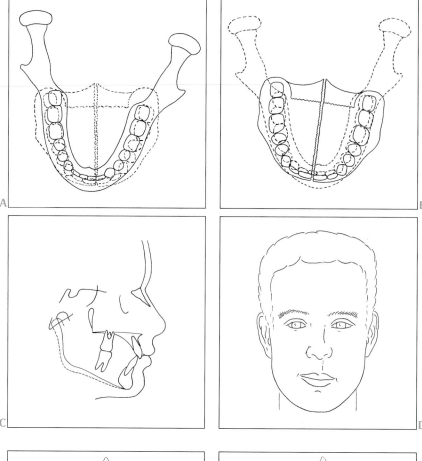

FIGURE 13-2

A schematic representation of an ideal situation is shown (A). An asymmetry in jaw size or position can lead to deviations in the occlusion, such as a Class II division 1 subdivision (B), a Class II division 2 subdivision (C), or a Class III subdivision (D). The midlines of the two dental arches also can deviate without asymmetry of the jaws or the posterior occlusion.

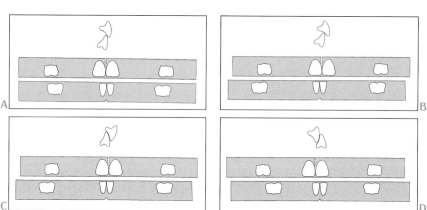

Asymmetries in the facial skeleton are most frequently caused by a deviation of the mandible (Fig 13-1). Asymmetries in the dentition, resulting from deviating positions in the locations where teeth are formed, occur in many variations (Fig 13-2). Combinations of both are encountered quite often.[22, 96] An asymmetry in the dental arches can develop secondarily to, or be increased by, loss of primary teeth (Fig 13-3). The same applies to agenesis and extraction of permanent teeth (Fig 13-4).

In nonextraction cases, there are distinct advantages to correcting asymmetries in the positions of teeth before complete fixed appliances are applied. A Crefcoeur appliance, with its heavy spring of 1.2-mm stainless steel wire, is particularly suited for that purpose.

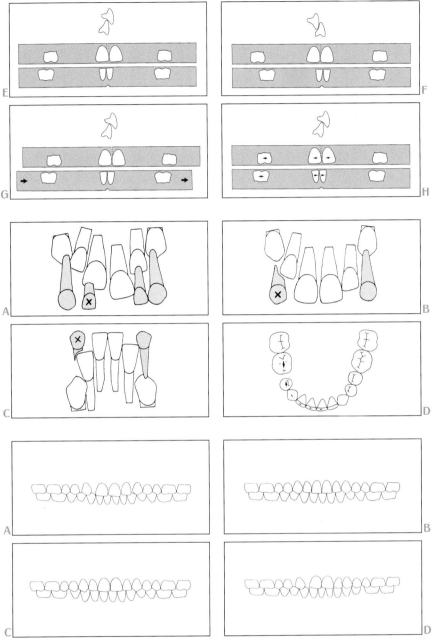

FIGURE 13-2 (CONTINUED)

Such an asymmetry can result from the position of the mandibular or maxillary anterior teeth, or of a combination of both. When the molars are also positioned asymmetrically, a Class II subdivision (E) or a Class III subdivision will result (F). When an asymmetry is surgically corrected, tooth movements can be limited (G). In less severe cases, tooth movements, possibly supported by efforts to influence facial growth, can lead to acceptable results (H).

FIGURE 13-3

Premature loss of primary anterior teeth is usually a sign of crowding. A primary maxillary lateral incisor can resorb when the permanent central incisor erupts (A) and a primary canine when the permanent lateral incisor erupts (B). The latter occurs more often in the mandible than in the maxilla (C).[87] Premature loss of primary molars—usually a result of caries—can lead to migrations and result in asymmetry of the occlusion (D).

FIGURE 13-4

A missing permanent maxillary right lateral incisor will result in a tipping of the other three incisors to the right side, but the roots will not pass the median suture (A). However, in the mandible an incisor can pass the median plane (B). Agenesis of a mandibular second premolar leads to migration from both sides (C). Agenesis of both a maxillary right lateral incisor and a mandibular left second premolar has a cumulative effect on the deviation of the midlines (D).

As was explained in chapter 3, with the heavy spring of the Crefcoeur appliance, dental arch segments can be pushed away from each other over quite a distance. However, that requires firm anchorage of the plate. If artificial undercuts of resin composite are placed on the buccal surfaces of crowns, three-quarter clasps can provide rigid fixation.

Occlusal rests will provide support for the plate and prevent pressure on the mucosa. Firm retention and support of the teeth adjacent to the separation in the plate is essential, because the forces are exerted primarily on these teeth. However, the forces should be transmitted to all teeth in the segments encompassed by the plate, necessitating a good overall fit and anchorage of the appliance. The heavy 1.2-mm wire should be far enough away from the acrylic resin and the palate, or the mucosa in the mandible, to allow activation and change in shape without causing irritations or soft tissue lesions.

FIGURE 13-5

When a disto-occlusion of half a premolar crown width is present only on one side and the maxillary third molar is also present on that side, extraction of the maxillary second molar and distalization of the first molar and the other teeth mesial to that molar can be a good solution, particularly when the dental arches show few abnormalities (A, B). In a Class II division 1 malocclusion, a cervical headgear can be used to distalize the permanent first molar on the extraction side and to influence facial growth at the same time. It is not necessary to make the headgear asymmetric, but the force should not be too great. The molar on the nonextraction side will exhibit little or no distal movement. In a dentition with unilateral crowding in the canine region, and a disto-occlusion of more than one premolar crown width on that side, extraction of a maxillary first premolar is a good choice (C, D).

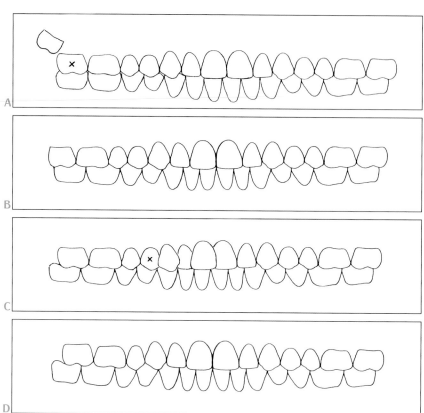

Furthermore, the loops at the posterior side of the plate should be sufficiently free of acrylic resin to allow activation of the heavy spring. In the mandible, the wire is located inferior to the acrylic resin and at some distance from the lingual mucosa. With a well-fitted and activated Crefcoeur appliance, 1 to 2 mm of space can be gained in a period of 6 weeks. The widening of the separation reflects the increase in dental arch length (Fig 13-9, G).

With a Crefcoeur appliance, space can be gained at every location in the dental arch. Furthermore, with the same appliance, space can be gained first at one place and subsequently at another place, provided that the construction and especially the metal parts of the appliance have been designed for that purpose. To change the location of activity, the widened separation should be filled with quick-curing acrylic resin, and subsequently a new separation should be created at the other place where space gain is needed. Indeed, the anchorage of the Crefcoeur plate is a matter of concern, but the activation is not simple either.

If a palatal bar is placed on the permanent maxillary molars, one of these teeth can be moved distally and rotated. That applies to first molars as well as second molars (Fig 13-17).

After extraction of a permanent maxillary second molar, the adjacent permanent first molar can be moved farther distally with a cervical headgear than the first molar on the other side. As explained in chapter 4, a larger distal force can be exerted on one side than the other side, by bending away the outer bow from the cheek on that side and shortening the outer bow on the other side. However, the molar that receives the greater distal force will also absorb a force in the palatal direction (Fig 13-18).

A lip bumper can be used in the maxilla but works better in the mandible. However, it cannot provide an asymmetric distal force. A unilateral movement will occur only when space is available distal to the molar on one side only.

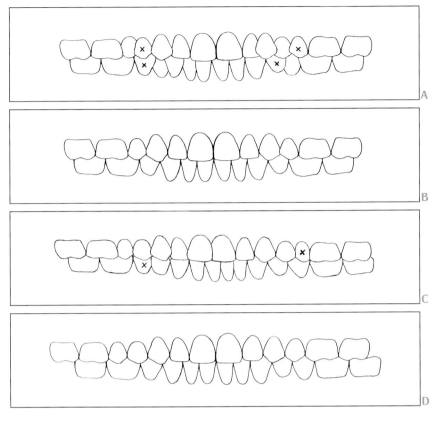

FIGURE 13-6

In patients with severe crowding, deviations of midlines can be corrected more easily by asymmetric extractions. For example, on the left side a second premolar can be extracted from the maxilla and a first premolar from the mandible, and on the right side the opposite can be done (A, B). There are distinct advantages to extracting first on the side where the teeth have to move mesially and later on the other side. In situations with a large deviation of the midlines, extraction of a maxillary premolar on one side and a mandibular premolar on the other side can be a good solution. That particularly applies when the mandibular incisors have to move in the opposite direction from the maxillary incisors (C, D). Sometimes the extraction of a mandibular incisor is an acceptable solution in situations with a midline deviation, but extraction of a maxillary incisor is not appropriate.

When lip bumpers or 0.045-inch archwires are used in both arches, a Class II elastic can be placed between them on one side and a Class III elastic on the other side to produce asymmetric effects.

Most asymmetries are combined with crowding in the dental arches. When extractions are part of the treatment plan, the correction of the asymmetry can be facilitated by strategic planning of the extractions at different times.

For an asymmetric occlusion in the posterior regions, in the presence of well-formed and situated third molars, extraction of the permanent maxillary second molar on one side is a good solution, particularly when the adjacent third molar will not have enough space to erupt. Subsequently, this third molar will move and tip anteriorly before emergence and arrive without further guidance at the correct place in the dental arch (Fig 13-5, A and B). Extraction of a permanent mandibular second molar to correct an asymmetric occlusion is seldom indicated and requires complex treatment. Unlike maxillary third molars, third molars in the mandible seldom attain a good position in the dental arch after extraction of permanent second molars. Furthermore, in Class II malocclusions, extraction of only mandibular teeth is mostly unwarranted. When the asymmetry is located in the anterior region, unilateral extraction of one premolar can lead to good results. Depending on the degree of asymmetry, the first or the second premolar will be the tooth to be sacrificed. When the first premolar is extracted, the angulation of the anterior teeth, which are moved distally, requires special attention (Fig 13-5, C and D). In asymmetries with severe crowding in both dental arches, and in which extraction in all four quadrants is indicated, asymmetric extraction is a good solution (Fig 13-6, A and B). In an oppositely directed asymmetry in the dental arches, the extraction of one tooth on one side in the mandible and one tooth on the other side in the maxilla can be the best approach (Fig 13-6, C and D). To further elucidate the strategies described, various treatment procedures are demonstrated in patients (Fig 13-7 to 13-16).

FIGURE 13-7

A girl 16 years 4 months of age had a Class I malocclusion with a crossbite of all teeth on the left side, except the central incisors. The lateral forced bite and the deviating transverse occlusion had affected the inclination of the teeth in crossbite. The solid intercuspation had led to labial and buccal tipping of the mandibular teeth and to palatal tipping of the maxillary teeth (A–D). To correct the teeth in crossbite, brackets and a tube were bonded to the involved mandibular teeth, and buttons were attached palatally on the maxillary teeth (E, F). Elastics were placed between these attachments at the corresponding teeth (G, H). The elastics were worn all the time, except during toothcleaning. After 4 weeks, the lateral incisors and premolars had moved sufficiently, and the wearing of elastics was continued only at the canines and molars. Four weeks later, these teeth were corrected and the attachments were removed. More than 18 months later, at the age of 17 years 1 month, the occlusion had improved the intercuspation and inclination of the posterior teeth (I, J). Retention was not applied, because the occlusion guaranteed the stability of the result. Five years later, at the age of 22 years 0 months, the situation was still excellent (K, L).

In crossbites without a good intercuspation, which is often the case, the prognosis for treatment is poor. In patients in whom the tongue is positioned between the teeth at rest, the associated narrow maxillary dental arch is mostly due to lack of stimulation of widening by the occlusion. As a rule, these patients do not have a forced bite with a lateral shift.

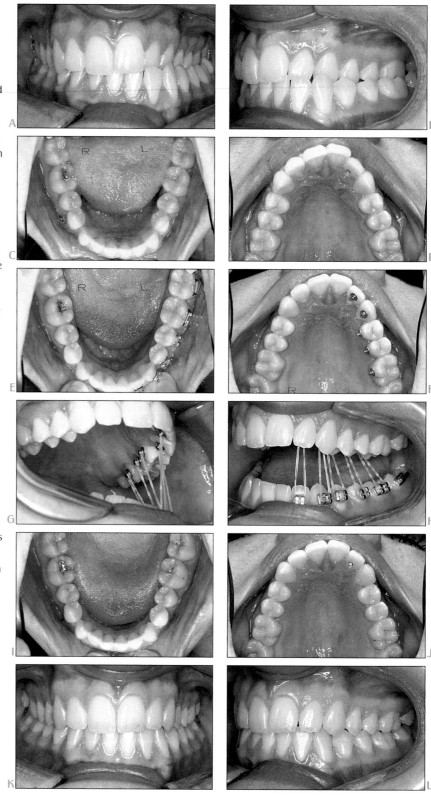

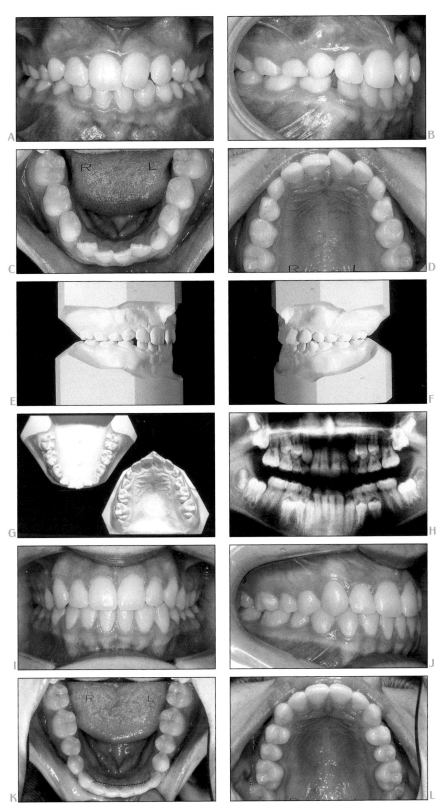

FIGURE 13-8

A girl aged 12 years 2 months, with a Class I malocclusion, had lost her primary mandibular right canine prematurely, and the incisors had migrated to the right side. There was not enough space for the maxillary anterior teeth, which had migrated slightly to the left side (A–G). To correct the asymmetry, the primary mandibular left canine and the primary maxillary right canine were extracted. Some time later, partial fixed appliances were placed in the maxilla to intrude the incisors and move them labially. Two months later, the same was done in the mandible. Sufficient space became available in the mandibular dental arch, but the permanent first molars rotated distolingually, and the permanent second molars emerged mesiolingually rotated. At the start of treatment it was not realized that the posterior sections of the apical area in the mandible were small and that the permanent second molars were positioned partially in the mandibular ramus (H). Consequently, these molars would emerge in a rotated position and not align before the length of the mandibular corpus had increased sufficiently to allow them to arrive at a better position in the dental arch.[124] When, in these situations, a distally directed force is placed on the buccal surfaces of the permanent mandibular first molars, their distal sides will move lingually. Correction of such malpositionings is not simple and is best carried out by removing the tubes from the first molars and bonding (mini) tubes to the second molars. Through the placement of a compressed coil spring on a straight wire between these tubes and the brackets on the second premolars, the needed space can be gained. Through this action, the second molar will derotate, and the first molar will spontaneously attain the correct position when sufficient space has become available (see Fig 16-2). The treatment in this patient lasted longer than needed, and it took 3 years before the end result was obtained (I–L). Some years later, the third molars were removed.

Treatment of Asymmetries

FIGURE 13-9

A boy aged 13 years 6 months had a Class II division 1 malocclusion with tongue interpositioning in the anterior and posterior regions. The mandibular dental arch was almost normal, but the maxilla showed extensive crowding in the anterior region. Insufficient space was available for the already emerged canines, particularly on the left side (A–E). The treatment was started with a cervical headgear. Six weeks later, a Crefcoeur appliance was placed in the maxilla (F). The 1.2-mm hard stainless steel wire spring at the palate was used to generate a force to increase the space between the lateral incisor and first premolar, first on the right side and later on the left side (G). As already explained, strict demands have to be met regarding the anchorage and activation of a Crefcoeur appliance. The direction of force has to be parallel to the dental arch, and the two segments of the plate should be aligned with each other, before and after activation. A twisting of the two segments and a too forceful activation should be avoided. After activation, the appliance should be inspected and controlled on the dental cast on which the plate was made. Modified three-quarter clasps on top of the tubes of the molar bands were used to anchor the appliance. In addition, three-quarter clasps at the first premolars, which had artificial undercuts of resin composite, provided optimal retention (G, H). The same applies to the labial arch at the lateral incisors, which were also built up with resin composite (I, J). Combined with the extra space that became available after the primary second molars were replaced by the premolars, the space generated by the appliance provided sufficient arch length. The deviation of the midlines was fully corrected with the Crefcoeur appliance (K, L). Subsequently, complete fixed appliances were used to conclude the treatment.

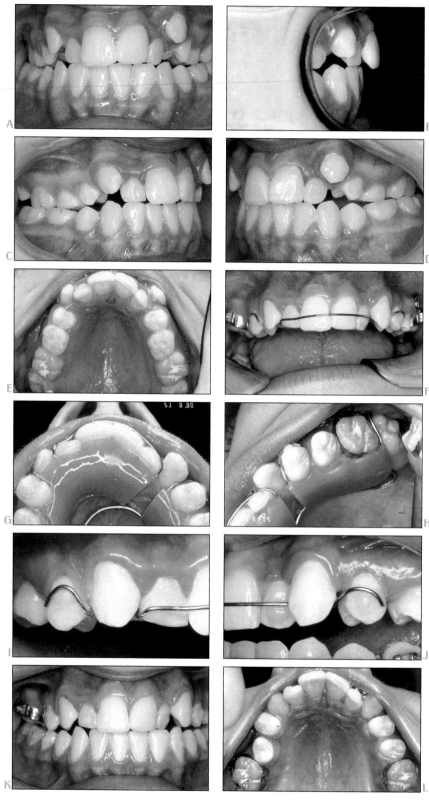

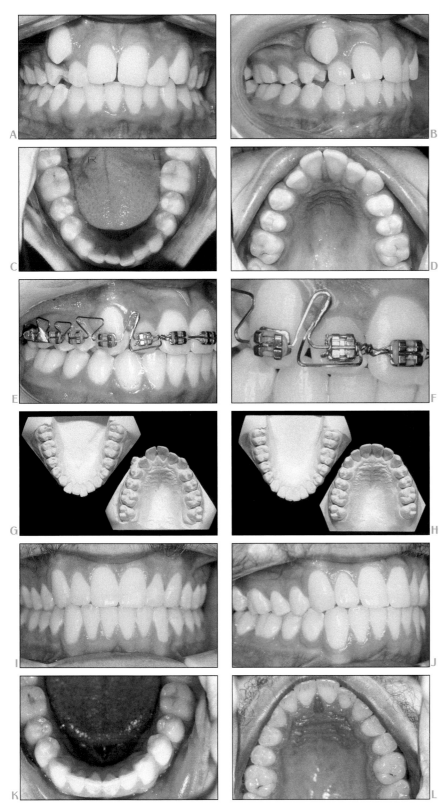

FIGURE 13-10

In a boy 11 years 7 months of age, with a mild disto-occlusion, the maxillary right primary canine was lost prematurely, and the incisors had migrated to the right side. The maxillary right lateral incisor was positioned too far palatally and in crossbite. The mandibular anterior teeth were malaligned and in contact with the opposing teeth (A–D). First a cervical headgear was placed; shortly thereafter a Crefcoeur appliance, comparable to the plate used in the patient shown in Fig 13-9, was added. With these appliances, the space for the maxillary right canine was gained, and the midline deviation was corrected. Subsequently, complete fixed appliances were placed in the maxilla. An auxiliary spring was welded and soldered to the multipurpose archwire, to move the apex of the right incisor labially (E, F). Had this lateral incisor not been torqued, its crown most likely would have returned to the palatal position. Such a relapse should be expected not only for initially palatally positioned maxillary incisors but also for initially lingually positioned mandibular lateral incisors, which are encountered more often. Orthodontic appliances were not used in the mandibular dental arch. Nevertheless, an ideal arrangement resulted. With the correction of the maxillary anterior teeth, the occlusal contacts altered, and the mandibular incisors aligned spontaneously. The mandibular right canine, initially in contact with the palatally positioned maxillary lateral incisor, moved spontaneously to the correct position in the dental arch after the treatment was concluded (G, H). The active treatment continued for 1 year 3 months. Subsequently, a Van der Linden retainer was worn for another 1 year 6 months. Five years after the end of retention, little had changed (I–L).

Treatment of Asymmetries

FIGURE 13-11

A boy 9 years 0 months of age had a Class II division 1 malocclusion in which the mandibular right primary canine was lost prematurely. The mandibular incisors had moved to the right side, and the midlines had deviated accordingly (A, B). As explained in chapter 3, the use of removable appliances in the mandible is difficult and cumbersome. A horizontal plane that provides vertical support, such as the palate, is missing. The lingual mucosa is sensitive, and the space available to embed the clasps and other metal parts in acrylic resin is limited. Furthermore, the buccal contour and the inclination of the mandibular posterior teeth offer few or no undercuts for clasp functions. However, with the introduction of resin composites, artificial undercuts can be placed, providing excellent retention and making it possible to place the clasps away from the cervical borders. Standard three-quarter clasps have the tendency to creep in an apical direction, with many detrimental effects. On the other hand, three quarter claps have the advantage that the patient does not have to occlude on metal parts. Indeed, occluding on metal parts makes removable appliances unnecessarily uncomfortable and makes it difficult to keep them in the mouth, particularly during meals. Not only secure anchorage of the plate on both sides of the separation, but also the full adaptation of the acrylic resin to the teeth, is essential. A great force is placed on the teeth on the side with the separation, which should be transmitted to all teeth in both segments. Once again, a good fit and firm fixation are of the utmost importance (C–F). After 10 months, sufficient space had been gained in the mandibular dental arch, and the midline deviation was corrected (G, H). The separation in the plate was filled with quick-curing acrylic resin, and the appliance was worn subsequently only during sleeping hours (I). Several other corrections were realized with the headgear and maxillary plate, as was revealed by the records collected at 11 years 5 months of age (J–L). The treatment was concluded with a complete fixed appliance.

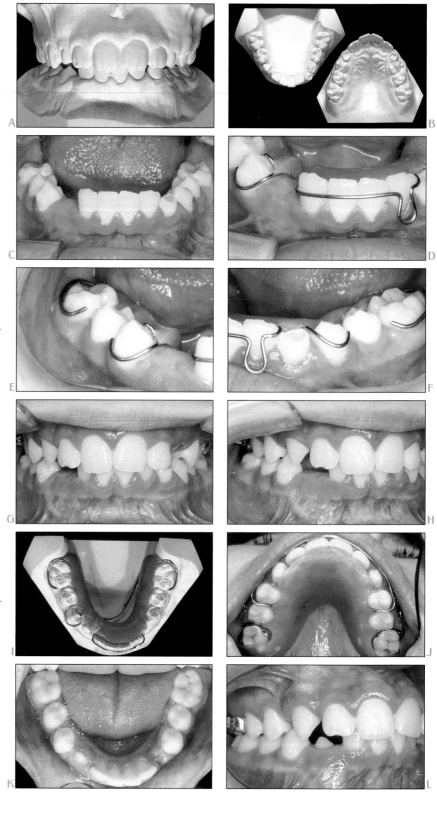

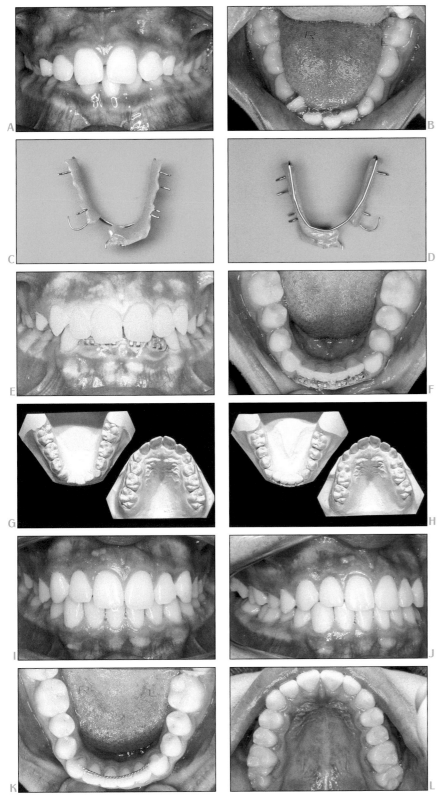

FIGURE 13-12

A boy who was 10 years 7 months of age had a Class I malocclusion in which the primary mandibular right canine was lost prematurely. The adjacent permanent lateral incisor had migrated distally and was rotated 90 degrees (A, B). The Crefcoeur appliance used in the mandible was designed to put the expansion force between the primary right first molar and the permanent right central incisor (C, D). Purposely, the right lateral incisor was not incorporated in the system, because this tooth had to be moved mesially and rotated. To that end, a button was bonded on the lingual surface of the right lateral incisor, on which an elastic was hooked. The elastic ran labial to the right central incisor and extended to a button at the labial surface of the left central incisor. The acrylic resin at the lingual side of the three incisors prevented their movement. Adequate anchorage was achieved with occlusal rests, a three-quarter clasp supported with a resin composite undercut at the first premolar near the separation, and a small clasp on the right central incisor. In addition, the elastic provided a good fixation of the plate in the anterior region. After sufficient space was gained, the midline deviation was corrected, and the right lateral incisor was positioned properly, brackets and a sectional stabilizing arch were placed on the four incisors. The incisors were tied together with a soft 0.008-inch ligature (E, F). With this approach, the mandibular arch was normalized in a period of 12 months, before the second transitional period was completed (G, H). After the maxillary second premolars had emerged, a short treatment with complete fixed appliances led to a satisfactory result (I–L). In this patient, as well as in the one in Fig 13-11, sufficient space was created locally in the dental arch without disturbing the position of the posterior teeth. Such a disturbance can easily happen when a lip bumper or fixed appliances are used for expansion.

Treatment of Asymmetries

FIGURE 13-13

A boy 10 years 11 months of age had a Class II division 2 malocclusion with a disto-occlusion of one premolar crown width on the right and half a premolar crown width on the left. Both dental arches showed mild crowding. A complicating factor was the agenesis of the mandibular right second premolar, because a complete set of mandibular teeth is important in the correction of Class II division 2 malocclusions. Both primary mandibular second molars were ankylosed (A–D). The treatment conformed to the protocol for the correction of Class II division 2 malocclusions, presented in the previous chapter. First a cervical headgear was placed, and 1 month later a maxillary removable appliance with claw clasps on the incisors was added. With the increase in lower facial height by the bite plane, the lip was kept away from the labial surfaces of the maxillary incisors, and the overbite was reduced. To prevent distal migration of the mandibular teeth mesial to the ankylosed primary right second molar, only its distal half was removed after endodontic treatment.[214] The adjacent permanent mandibular first molar migrated spontaneously to the mesial, as the records collected at 11 years 11 months of age showed. These records also demonstrated the improvement in the disto-occlusion, the deep bite, and the inclination of the maxillary incisors (E–H). Shortly thereafter, the maxillary right second premolar was extracted, and slightly later the remaining mesial half of the primary mandibular right molar was removed. The cervical headgear and plate were replaced by a parietal headgear that was attached to a Bass plate (see Fig 5-19). The plate was trimmed mesial to the permanent maxillary right molar, so that this tooth could migrate mesially. Finally, complete fixed appliances were used for 1 year 6 months, and a pleasing end result was reached (I–L). One of the goals in the treatment of this patient was to prevent lingual movement of the mandibular anterior teeth. The maxillary right second premolar was extracted as a compensatory effort, to arrive at a good occlusion. The midlines of both dental arches shifted only slightly to the right side, which was not conspicuous or disturbing when the patient was laughing and speaking.

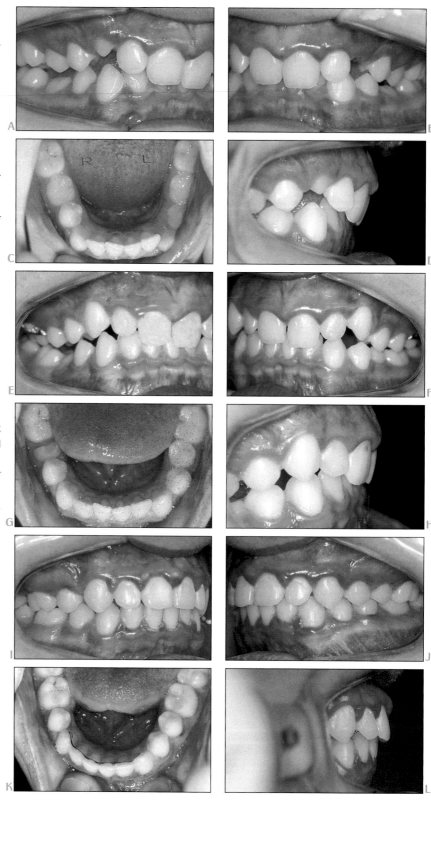

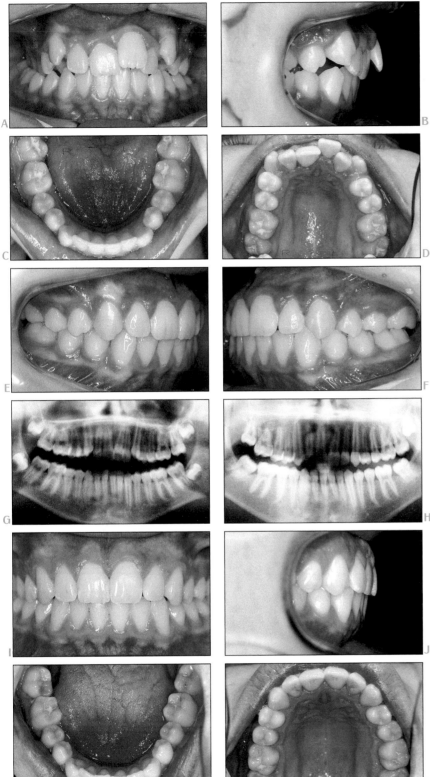

FIGURE 13-14

A boy 11 years 9 months of age had a Class II division 2 subdivision with a neutro-occlusion of the permanent left first molars and a disto-occlusion of one half a premolar crown width on the right. The arch length discrepancy was –7 mm in the maxilla and –2 mm in the mandible. The midline of the mandibular dental arch deviated 3 mm to the right in relation to the maxillary midline (A–D). All third molars were present and well formed. The decision was made to preserve the permanent maxillary left second molar and to extract the other three second molars. With a palatal bar and a cervical headgear, the maxillary first molars were rotated and the right first molar was moved distally. In addition, the maxillary dental arch was expanded to correct the crossbite on the right side. After sufficient space was gained in the maxillary dental arch, the canines and left central incisor were moved palatally with elastics extending from buttons on these teeth to hooks on the palatal bar. The extraction of the mandibular second molars was followed by a distal migration of the other posterior teeth. They aligned spontaneously, as did the anterior teeth. A comparable, but less extensive, improvement had occurred in the maxilla. After 1 year 3 months of treatment without the use of fixed appliances, a positioner was utilized for 8 weeks for further detailing (E, F). Subsequently, a Van der Linden retainer was used for a period of 12 months. The panoramic radiographs made before (G) and after (H) treatment demonstrated that the mandibular third molars erupted well but the right molar was tipped mesially. The maxillary left third molar was to be removed after it emerged. When the patient was aged 20 years 10 months, 5 years after the end of retention, the mandibular third molars were well aligned in the dental arch; however, the right one was still tipped too far mesially (I–L). This treatment is a fine example of the result that can be reached without fixed appliances.

FIGURE 13-15

A girl aged 11 years 8 months had a Class II division 1 malocclusion in which the primary mandibular right molars were lost prematurely and no space remained in the dental arch for the impacted second premolar. There was also some crowding in the other regions of the mandibular dental arch but not in the maxilla (A–D). The treatment was started with a cervical headgear and a removable plate in the maxilla. A lip bumper was placed in the mandible to gain space, but that was not effective, and the impacted second premolar was removed. Subsequently, the lip bumper was replaced by a lingual arch to carry out the needed corrections in the mandible. Finally, the four maxillary incisors were aligned with partial fixed appliances. After treatment, the midlines of the two dental arches did not coincide, and the mandibular posterior regions as well as the occlusion differed on the left and right sides (E, F). However, there was good intercuspation, with a mesio-occlusion on the right side and a neutro-occlusion on the left side. That was also the case some years after the treatment was completed (G, I, J).

A deviation of the midlines of the dental arches is usually not disturbing and certainly not when the teeth are well aligned. It is important that the maxillary anterior teeth be in the middle of the face, particularly when these teeth are fully visible in laughing and speaking. However, a deviation of up to 2 mm does not catch the eye when the contact area between the central incisors is not angulated and is parallel to the median plane of the face. When little is shown of the maxillary anterior teeth, their position in the face is less relevant. There is nothing wrong with an asymmetric occlusion in the posterior regions, because it does not have to be visually disturbing and can function well (H, K, L).

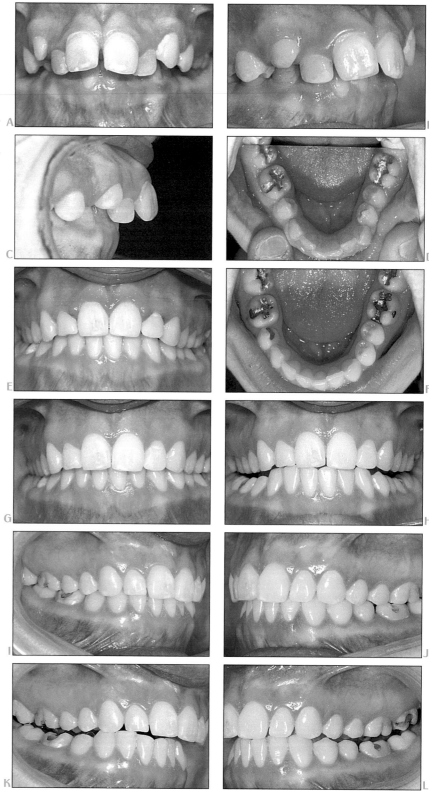

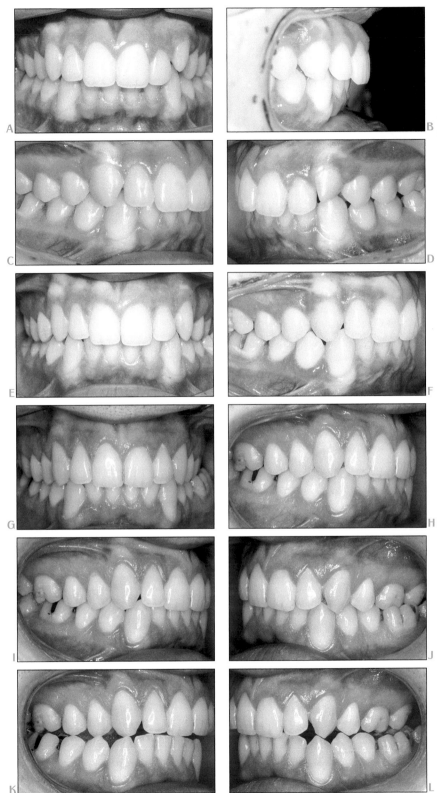

FIGURE 13-16

A boy aged 14 years 3 months of age had a Class II division 1 malocclusion with a neutro-occlusion on the right side and a disto-occlusion of three-quarters of a premolar crown width at the left side. In addition, a crossbite existed on the left side, with the permanent maxillary first and second molars in endo-occlusion. The mandibular dental arch and the right side of the maxillary dental arch were almost normal. On the maxillary left side, crowding existed in the canine region, and the permanent molars were positioned too far palatally. The midlines of the dental arches deviated 2 mm. In relation to the upper lip and nose, the maxillary anterior teeth were positioned too far to the right. The deviation of the midlines was clearly due to the position of the maxillary teeth (A–D). It was decided not to treat the mandibular dental arch but rather to maintain the crossbite, extract the maxillary left first premolar, and move the canine and incisors toward the extraction side. By allowing the teeth posterior to the extraction site to migrate mesially, a disto-occlusion of one premolar crown width was realized on the left side, with a good intercuspation in the mesiodistal direction. An acceptable result was reached after 18 months (E, F). Ten years later, at 25 years of age, little had changed (G, H). The lateral and anterior excursive movements were undisturbed. In excursions to the right, there was occlusal guidance between canines, premolars, and molars (I, K). In excursions to the left, the molars that were in crossbite lost contact, while the remainder of the teeth in that region continued to have occlusal guidance (J, L). Indeed, molars in crossbite lose contact during lateral excursions. The same applies to premolars in crossbite. Crossbites of permanent molars and second premolars are not esthetically disturbing. However, crossbites of first premolars are rarely acceptable, because the dental arch will have an inward step distal to the canine, which is visible during speaking and laughing.

FIGURE 13-17

With a palatal bar, molars can be rotated and moved distally (A). That applies to first molars as well as to permanent second molars. When the bar is placed at the first molars, a second molar can be moved distally with a sectional wire after a band with a tube is placed on the second molar (A, D) or a tube is bonded (B, C). When a palatal bar is used together with a headgear, the forces applied by the two appliances should be coordinated.

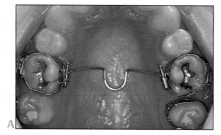
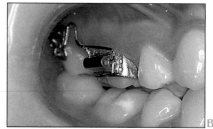
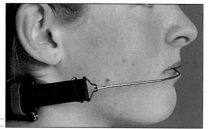
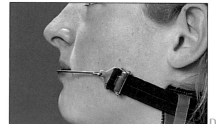

FIGURE 13-18

An asymmetric force can be exerted by a cervical headgear if the long outer bow is bent away from the cheek on the side where the greater force is needed and the outer bow on the other side is shortened (A–D). However, the molar that is exposed to the greater force will also receive a force in the palatal direction, which can be controlled by a removable plate (SEE FIG 5-2).[80] This control can also be provided by a palatal bar, which has the additional potential to exert rotational and distalizing forces and to offer control over the inclination and angulation of the molars.

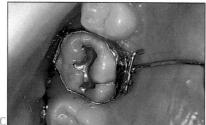
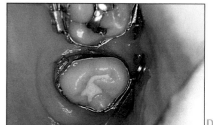
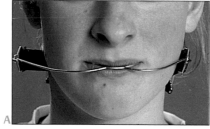
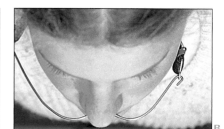

The correction of midline deviations in the last phase of a fixed appliance treatment is difficult. Patients find the wearing of anterior diagonal (oblique) elastics to be annoying. Furthermore, at the end of treatment, the endurance and compliance of patients are no longer optimal. These problems are avoided when asymmetries are eliminated at the start of treatment.

When a solid intercuspation is not reached at the end of treatment, and a tongue interpositioning has not disappeared, the treatment result will be unstable. For the treatment and retention of open bites and non-occlusions, special rules apply; these are elaborated in the next chapter.

Treatment of Open Bites and Non-occlusions

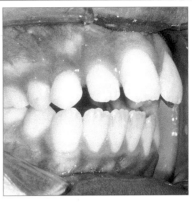

In the teaching of dentistry, and in textbooks of operative and prosthetic dentistry, maximal occlusal contact is taken for granted. However, that by no means applies to all individuals. Open bites, and particularly non-occlusions, in which opposing teeth overlap each other without making any or complete contact, occur often. Open bites and non-occlusions are caused by disturbances in eruption, ankylosis, or other factors that hinder eruption. Digit sucking, whether or not it is combined with positioning of the tongue between the teeth at rest, is the common cause in children. In adults, tongue interpositioning is usually the cause. With the growth and maturation of the face, the tongue interpositioning disappears in about half of the affected children.

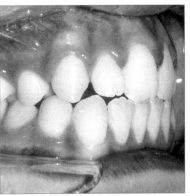

Open bites and non-occlusions occur in Class I, Class II division 1, Class II division 2, and Class III malocclusions. Most abnormalities in the dental arches also occur in open bites and non-occlusions. Open bites and non-occlusions in individuals with well-aligned anterior teeth are not esthetically disturbing. Patients and others in their social environments often are not aware that "something is wrong." Furthermore, open bites and non-occlusions rarely present functional problems.

Open bites and non-occlusions caused by tongue interpositioning are difficult to treat. Attempts to realize an ideal occlusion are by no means always successful. Painstakingly obtained results often partially deteriorate after treatment. Indeed, the goal and strategy for treatment and retention should be adapted to the prevailing specific functional conditions.

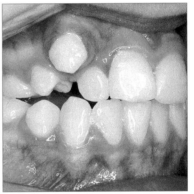

First, various types of open bites and non-occlusions are distinguished, and the difference between dental and skeletal open bites is explained. Attention is paid to the diagnosis of open bites and particularly of non-occlusions in the posterior regions.

Subsequently, treated patients are shown. To emphasize the genetic aspect involved, the records of two patients will be presented with those of a parent. Finally, a patient in whom facial disfiguration was corrected surgically and further improved with esthetic dentistry is shown.

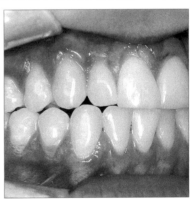

14

Orthodontic Concepts and Strategies

FIGURE 14-1

In a Class I situation, the incisors overlap each other with contact in the anterior region (A1). In a non-occlusion, the anterior teeth overlap but do not contact each other; there is some space between them (A2). Only when there is no overlap is the term open bite used (A3). In a Class II division 1 malocclusion, there can be a large space between opposing teeth, while they still overlap each other: non-occlusion (B3). The same applies to Class II division 2 malocclusions (C2, C3). In Class III malocclusions, anterior non-occlusions are rare (D2) and open bites are often large (D3).

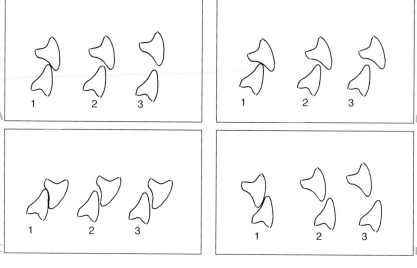

FIGURE 14-2

Normally, the posterior teeth occlude maximally in a solid intercuspation (A). However, opposing teeth can contact each other partially or completely without overlapping, in one or both posterior regions: non-occlusion (B). Open bites in the posterior region also can be partial (C) or complete. Sometimes, a non-occlusion is found between all teeth, with or without a local open bite (D).

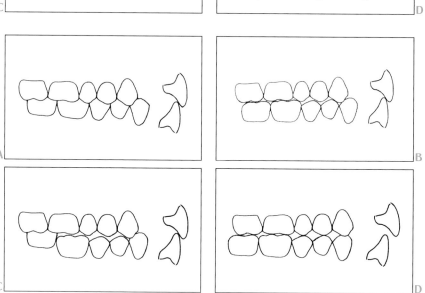

In open bites, the opposing mandibular and maxillary teeth do not overlap each other in the anterior region (anterior open bite) or in the posterior region (posterior open bite). An open bite can involve only a few teeth, as in intensive pipe smokers, or more, as in digit suckers, or can involve a larger area, as caused by tongue interpositioning (dental open bite). An open bite can be caused by a divergence of the skeletal structures of the face (skeletal open bite or apertognathia).

In non-occlusions, maximal contact does not exist in habitual occlusion. Non-occlusions, like open bites, are caused by disturbances in eruption or by factors that interfere with the eruption, such as digit sucking and tongue interpositioning. Depending on the location and extent, a distinction is made among anterior, posterior, and total non-occlusions.

In an anterior non-occlusion, the teeth overlap each other to some extent, as is often seen in Class II division 1 malocclusions (Fig 14-1, B2 and B3).

In a posterior non-occlusion, the premolars and/or molars are not in maximal contact. Posterior non-occlusions can vary considerably in the number of teeth and occlusal contacts involved (Fig 14-2, B).

In a total non-occlusion, there is no maximal occlusal contact anywhere in the posterior regions, and a non-occlusion or open bite is present in the anterior region (Fig 14-2, D). In a total non-occlusion, the tongue is positioned between all opposing teeth at rest.

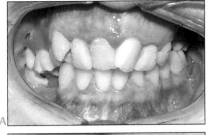
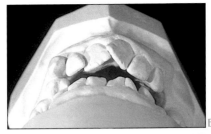

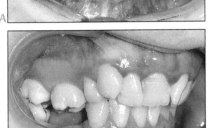
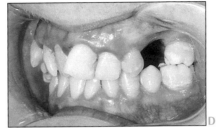

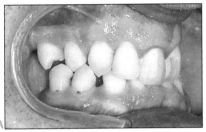
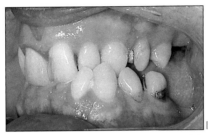

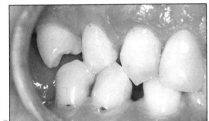
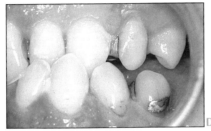

FIGURE 14-3
Anterior open bites do not occur in Class II division 2 malocclusions; however, coverbites are sometimes combined with an anterior non-occlusion (A–D). In these cases, the tongue is kept at rest between the mandibular anterior teeth and the palate. Then there are two deviating functional conditions: a tongue interpositioning, which causes the non-occlusion, and the excessive overlapping of the labial surfaces of the maxillary incisors by the lower lip, which causes their palatal tipping.

FIGURE 14-4
Even when an excess of space is available for the tongue, as in this 60-year-old man with agenesis of all permanent molars, a lateral open bite and non-occlusion can occur. There is an open bite between all premolars on the left side (B) but only between the second premolars on the right side (A, C). The short dental arches, the coverbite, and the reversed overbite of the lateral incisors and canines on the left side (D) have not led to functional disturbances of speech or chewing or to temporomandibular joint complaints.

The differentiation between open bites and non-occlusions is arbitrary. The changeover point is where the overlap begins. Whether or not an overlap exists in borderline situations is irrelevant for the therapy and the subsequent development.[142]

As already mentioned, open bites and non-occlusions occur in combination with all types of malocclusions as well as in coverbites (Figs 14-3 and 14-4). They are found in all countries worldwide, and frequently in the Netherlands. A large Dutch epidemiologic study, published in 1990, revealed that the mandibular incisors were not in contact with the maxillary incisors in 40% of the 2,273 examined individuals between 15 and 70 years of age. This was even more common in adolescents (between 15 and 20 years of age), among whom 59% of 525 examined individuals did not have anterior contact. For the posterior regions, the percentages for open bites and non-occlusions combined were 10% and 18% for the study group as a whole and adolescents, respectively. These data indicate that open bites and non-occlusions occur more frequently in adolescents than in adults.[51, 72] Based on these findings and information from other studies, it can be concluded that open bites disappear spontaneously in about half of children between 8 and 15 years of age and in about one third of adolescents.[78, 86]

In most cases, the mainly genetically determined tongue interpositioning plays a major role. The transition to another tongue position in the growing and maturing face is related to changes in size and in relationships among the various structures as well as to a genetically determined tongue position at an older age.

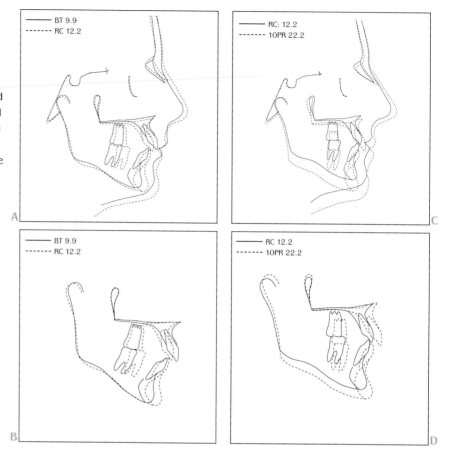

FIGURE 14-5

Superimposed tracings of a girl with a Class II division 1 malocclusion and an anterior non-occlusion, shown in Fig 14-13. At the start of treatment, the lower anterior facial height was rather large, and a parietal headgear was applied to control the vertical development of the lower face and improve the sagittal maxillomandibular relationship (A). Further eruption of the permanent maxillary first molars was prevented, and the distance between the anterior nasal plane and the lower border of the mandible did not increase (B). Facial growth continued after the conclusion of the treatment, at the age of 12 years 2 months. Without a change in the sagittal maxillomandibular relationship, the height of the lower face increased markedly, and the permanent maxillary first molars overerupted (C). In addition, the occlusal contact between the incisors was lost, so the anterior non-occlusion relapsed (D). However, in the adult stage, the facial configuration and dental situation were satisfying. These records were collected at the beginning of treatment (BT), at the completion of retention (RC), and 10 years postretention (10PR).

When feasible, the dental situation of the parents should be considered (Figs 14-9 to 14-12), but siblings should also be examined for comparison.

As already explained, open bites can be caused by local factors (dental open bites), and by a deviation in the skeletal configuration (skeletal open bites).

Figure 14-5 shows superimposed tracings illustrating the changes during treatment and the subsequent observation period of a patient with an anterior non-occlusion. The skeletal configuration was not obviously deviating. The treatment and subsequent development followed as could be expected in a patient with an anterior non-occlusion (Fig 14-13).

The patient presented in Figs 14-6 and 14-14 had a skeletal open bite, with an excessively long face. The internal functional components dominated the external ones, which led to the development in a caudal direction (see chapter 4). As previously stated, skeletal alterations realized through facial orthopedic means largely relapse after treatment; relapse can be prevented by continuation of the facial orthopedic guidance in the retention phase until growth is completed. That stage is reached in girls at about 15 years of age and in boys at 20 years of age or later. However, it is not realistic to assume that teenagers are willing to wear a parietal headgear or even a bite block for years during sleep. That applies particularly to boys, in whom retention can be needed for many years. In this respect girls have the advantage that their adolescent growth spurt occurs earlier; however, it does not last as long as growth in boys.

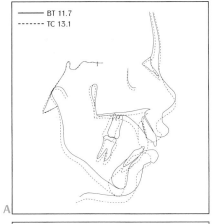

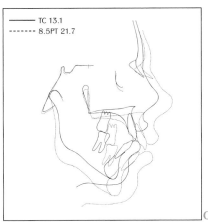

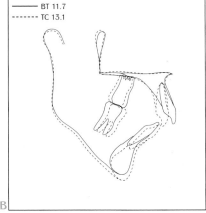

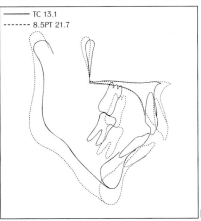

FIGURE 14-6

Superimposed tracings of a boy with a Class II division 1 malocclusion and an anterior open bite, shown in Fig 14-14. He was treated with a parietal headgear to restrict the vertical development of the lower face. During treatment, the height of the face increased, but that was mainly due to a lengthening of the midface (A). Although the maxillary first molars seemed not to have erupted further, the distance between the nasal plane and the lower border of the mandible increased slightly (B). The face grew substantially after the conclusion of the treatment, at the age of 13 years 1 month. The height of the midface, but particularly of the lower face, increased excessively. After growth was completed, he had a disfiguring facial configuration (C, D). These records were collected at the beginning of treatment (BT), at the completion of treatment (TC), and 8.5 years posttreatment (8.5PT). Surgical correction was recommended but was considered unnecessary by the patient and his parents.

A distinction has to be made between patients with a skeletal open bite who have a facial configuration that is acceptable to the patient and the surrounding social environment and patients in whom that is not the case. For the latter, surgical correction after growth is completed can solve the problem.

Skeletal open bites also have a dental open bite component, as a result of tongue interpositioning. After surgical correction, the improvement in the facial appearance will be maintained to a large extent. However, that does not always apply to the correction of the dental component of the open bite. When the tongue interpositioning persists after the surgical correction, the affected teeth will intrude. That can also happen when subsequently the teeth are built up and lengthened with resin composite or other means (Fig 14-17).

The tongue movement during swallowing in individuals with an anterior open bite or non-occlusion is different from that of individuals in whom the anterior teeth are in contact in habitual occlusion.[76] Individuals with open bite move their tongue anteriorly to close off the space between the teeth in swallowing. It is incorrect to consider this typical tongue movement in swallowing (tongue thrust) as the cause of the open bite. Indeed, the tongue movement adapts to the anatomic situation and not the other way around. The position of the tongue at rest, and particularly during sleep, is the essential determinant in the location of the teeth. The many swallowing acts performed over a period of 24 hours result in no more than 15 to 20 minutes of cumulative, potent pressure on the teeth. These 15 to 20 minutes are too few to have an effect on the position of teeth, for which at least 6 hours would be required.

FIGURE 14-7

An anterior open bite and tongue inter-positioning become visible when the lips are moved apart rapidly (A, B). An anterior non-occlusion is difficult to detect by inspection when the distance between the mandibular and maxillary incisors is small. The evidence can be obtained if the patient occludes on a cellophane strip or a soft piece of wax. Posterior open bites are easy to detect, but some posterior non-occlusions are difficult to ascertain (C, D). Posterior tongue interpositionings are difficult to detect, because patients tend to withdraw the tongue when the lips are touched. However, an interpositioned tongue can usually be observed when the lips are carefully separated with two blunt instruments at the corner of the mouth (E, F).

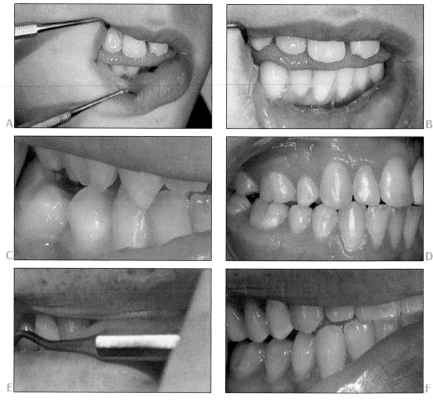

Anterior open bites and posterior open bites can be easily detected, although non-occlusions are not readily apparent. It is also difficult to determine the position of the tongue at rest, except when the lips are held apart, which is often the case in patients with open bite (Fig 14-7). Particularly in individuals with skeletal open bites, the lips are often too short for a competent lip seal. In addition, these patients frequently have difficulty in breathing adequately through the nose and have to keep their mouth open to let air pass.

Non-occlusions can be difficult to detect clinically but are easy to spot on a set of dental casts. Viewed from different sides and from the lingual direction, the casts can be examined carefully to determine if teeth are in maximal occlusion. As a rule, absence of maximal occlusion indicates tongue interpositioning. Another sign is a maxillary dental arch that is too narrow in relation to the mandibular dental arch. Normally, the erupting opposing posterior teeth are guided into maximal occlusion by the "cone-funnel" mechanism. With tongue interpositioning, this mechanism cannot function, and the maxillary posterior teeth will not be stimulated by the occlusion to move buccally. The mandibular posterior teeth will maintain the upright position in which they have emerged and not become inclined lingually. In a crossbite without tongue interpositioning, the cone-funnel mechanism can function, and maximal occlusion can develop; however, this is not often the case. Most crossbites are combined with tongue interpositioning and the associated non-occlusion.

Besides intraoral examination and the analysis of dental casts, other methods can be utilized to detect a non-occlusion. In individuals with a total non-occlusion, not one single pair of opposing teeth are in maximal occlusal contact. The tongue is positioned at rest between all teeth or parts of teeth. That also is the case during the swallowing act, in which the chewing muscles will not become contracted firmly, because nothing hard is met in biting. The fact that in a total non-occlusion the chewing muscles are contracted only slightly during swallowing can be detected by palpation of the temporalis and masseter muscles.

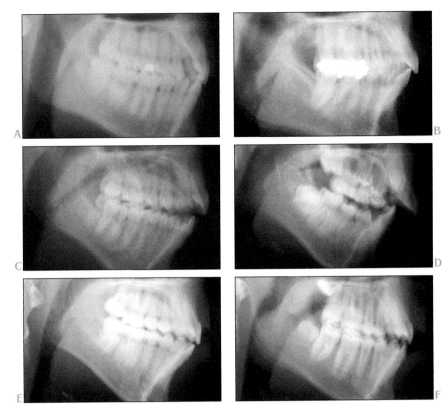

FIGURE 14-8
Lateral cephalograms made while the patient is in habitual occlusion can provide an insight into the overlapping of posterior teeth. In a symmetric situation, the corresponding teeth will be projected on top of each other, and the enamel of the intercuspating teeth will be visible as a light gray zone (A). In an asymmetric lower face, the light gray zone will not be even. However, radiopaque restorations interfere with the formation of an opinion (B). In large open bites (C) and in posterior open bites (D) the image is clear. A total non-occlusion is projected as a small, dark strip (E). In a bilateral posterior non-occlusion in an asymmetric lower face, two small, dark strips will appear (F).

Another way to detect a total non-occlusion is to ask the patient to close the mouth with a firm snap. If a hard click is not heard, only incidental contacts that do not provide a solid sound are being made.

Furthermore, lateral cephalograms, made with the patient in habitual occlusion, allow diagnosis of an open bite or non-occlusion in the posterior regions (Fig 14-8).

The fact that it is difficult to predict if an open bite and non-occlusion will disappear spontaneously with aging complicates matters. Even an open bite caused by digit sucking will not disappear completely when the tongue interpositioning persists after the patient breaks the habit.

A tongue that appears oversized at the start of treatment can become less dominant with continuing facial growth. Alterations in the neuromuscular control system also can result in a change in tongue positioning.

When it is unlikely that a solid intercuspation will develop in later years, expansion of the maxillary dental arch and coordination of the widths of the dental arches makes little sense. Rapid maxillary expansion will not be of much benefit either.

Attempts to completely eliminate an open bite or non-occlusion are often not successful. During attempts to obtain closure with vertical elastics in one area, an open bite or non-occlusion can develop in another area. Furthermore, these attempts can lead to excessive apical root resorption.[82] Even if complete closure is achieved, partial opening often occurs later.

Open bites and non-occlusions are encountered frequently in Class II division 1 malocclusions. Correction of the disto-occlusion with a parietal headgear limits the increase in lower facial height during treatment. However, subsequently, excessive vertical development occurs. When a cervical headgear is used, the reverse happens. It is questionable how far the use of a parietal headgear has advantages over the use of a cervical headgear, except when the treatment is carried out during the last phase of facial growth or the development of the face in vertical direction is controlled until facial growth is completed (see chapters 4 and 8).

FIGURE 14-9

A boy 13 years 7 months of age had a Class I malocclusion with a non-occlusion and an open bite at some locations in the posterior regions (A–D). The treatment was started with a cervical headgear and a Crefcoeur appliance to create space in the maxillary dental arch. The details of this treatment are presented in Fig 13-9 in the preceding chapter, which discussed the treatment of asymmetries. Fixed appliances were used in both arches to complete the treatment. However, it was impossible to obtain a solid intercuspation of the posterior teeth, despite lengthy use of vertical elastics. When the treatment was concluded at the age of 16 years 7 months, a non-occlusion was still present in the posterior regions (E, F). That was also the case 3 years later, when the maxillary dental arch had narrowed. The premolars and molars occluded in a transverse end-to-end position (G, H). In the years following, this situation did not alter noticeably.

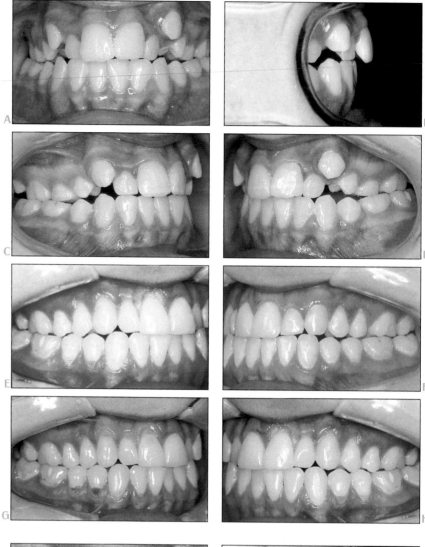

FIGURE 14-10

The boy shown in Fig 14-9 strongly resembled his father in appearance and behavior. The father had an anterior open bite, a non-occlusion in the left posterior region, and a solid intercuspation on the right side (A–D). The son had limited tongue interpositioning in both posterior regions, where the tongue was positioned at rest between the lingual cusps, not the buccal cusps. The father had this phenomenon only on the left side, but in addition had an anterior tongue interpositioning.

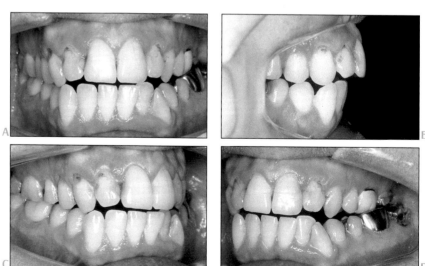

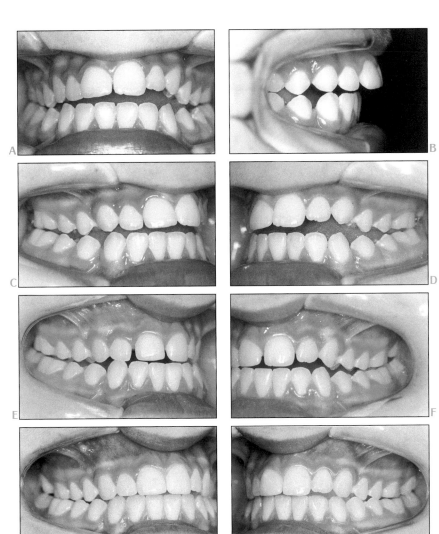

FIGURE 14-11

A girl aged 9 years 9 months had a Class II division 1 malocclusion with an anterior open bite and a posterior open bite at the left first and second premolars. The right side and the left molars were in non-occlusion (A–D). She had sucked her thumb until the day she was brought in for the first consultation. She was treated with a Lehman headgear-activator combination. After 13 months, the treatment was ended, and it was decided to await further development. The records collected at 11 years 0 months of age demonstrated that the disto-occlusion and the anterior open bite were corrected and the open bite between the left first premolars had decreased. However, there was a posterior non-occlusion on both sides, and the maxillary dental arch was too narrow to match the mandibular dental arch (E, F). At 13 years 2 months of age, the anterior open bite was limited to the left lateral incisors. The other anterior teeth and both posterior regions were in non-occlusion (G, H).

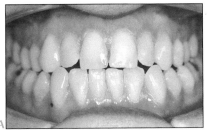

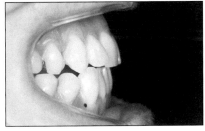

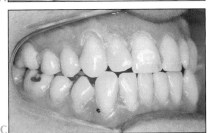

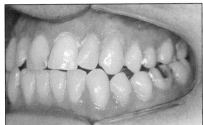

FIGURE 14-12

The girl presented in Fig 14-11 strongly resembled her mother, including a similar dentition. The mother had a comparable non-occlusion in the anterior and left posterior regions. Only the right second premolars and molars were in solid intercuspation and properly positioned in the transverse direction (A–D). Mother and daughter had comparable tongue interpositionings, which was of no concern to either of them. They were not disturbed by the occlusion and arrangement of the dentition. However, dentists often consider this condition to be inadequate.

FIGURE 14-13

A girl 9 years 9 months of age had a Class II division 1 malocclusion and an anterior non-occlusion, with only a slight overlapping of the incisors. Both dental arches showed considerable crowding. She did not have a history of digit sucking and could breathe well through the nose. At rest, she kept the anterior section of the tongue on top of the incisal edges of the mandibular anterior teeth (A–D). After extraction of the four first premolars, a parietal headgear was placed. In a later stage, fixed appliances were used in both arches, and a positioner was applied for finishing and retention. After a treatment of 1 year 8 months, an ideal result was obtained, as demonstrated by the records collected at 12 years 2 months of age (E, F). Two years later, a good, solid intercuspation still existed in the posterior regions (G, H). However, the incisors were not in contact anymore, and the tongue was again positioned on top of the incisal edges of the mandibular anterior teeth at rest (I, J). In the years following, little change took place. At the age of 27 years 11 months, the anterior non-occlusion and the increased overjet were still present (K, L). The superimposed tracings of this girl, shown in Fig 14-5, show that extensive growth took place after the conclusion of treatment. The treatment was carried out at a relatively young age, which was possible because the permanent canines and premolars erupted at an early age. It is unlikely that the occlusion will alter much with further aging of this patient.[116] In general, after an individual reaches 30 years of age, the changes occurring in the dentition are limited, and the intraoral functional conditions seem to alter little.

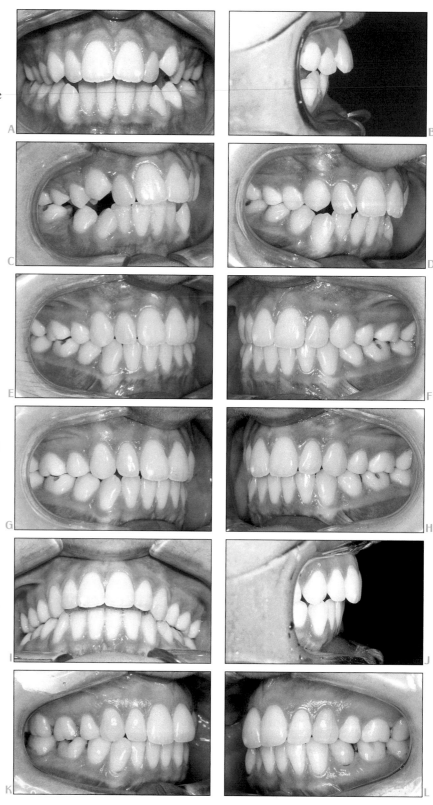

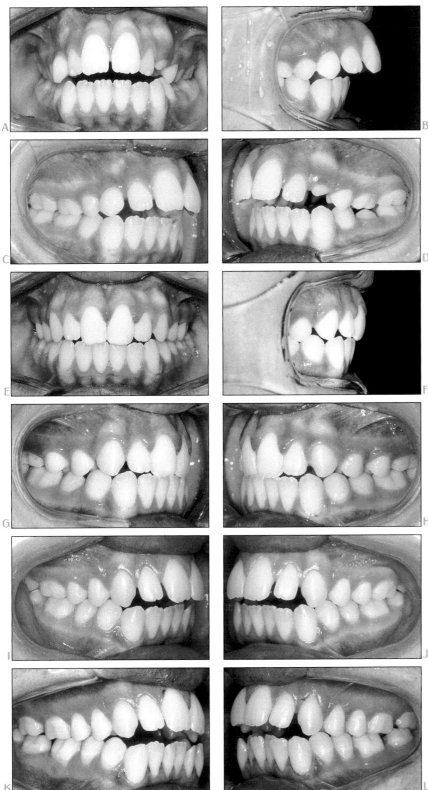

FIGURE 14-14

A boy aged 11 years 7 months had a Class II division 1 malocclusion with an anterior open bite. He had a long, narrow face, a large lower facial height, a receding chin, and a steeply oriented lower border of the mandible. At rest, his mouth was open and his tongue was positioned between the mandibular and maxillary incisors. His nasal passage was obstructed, and he breathed mainly through the mouth (A–D). He was treated with a parietal headgear and a removable appliance in the maxilla. After a treatment of 1 year 5 months, an acceptable result was obtained, but retention was not applied (E–H). At the age of 16 years 5 months— which was 3 years 4 months posttreatment—the occlusion in the posterior regions was stable because of the solid intercuspation. However, the anterior open bite had returned, and the functional conditions seemed not to have changed. He was still a mouth breather without a competent lip seal (I, J). At the age of 21 years 7 months, the anterior open bite had increased further and crowding had developed in the mandibular anterior region (K, L). After treatment, the face developed excessively in the vertical direction, as shown in the superimposed tracings of this patient in Fig 14-6. Certainly, it was a mistake not to apply retention. It cannot be expected that retruded anterior teeth will not relapse labially in an individual with an open mouth posture and especially in a patient with such a tongue interpositioning. Undoubtedly, he was a candidate for correction of the facial disfiguration by combined orthognathic surgical and orthodontic treatment at a later age.

FIGURE 14-15

A girl of 13 years 9 months had a Class I malocclusion with a non-occlusion of the permanent molars and an open bite mesial to these teeth. The maxillary right lateral incisor was not formed, and the left lateral incisor was peg shaped. She held her tongue between the teeth, which was clearly visible when she was speaking and laughing. The mandibular dental arch was broad and well aligned, but the posterior teeth were in a transverse upright position. The broad mandibular arch and the upright position of the posterior teeth was related to the low position of the tongue against the lingual surfaces of these teeth and the absence of intercuspation that would normally lead to a lingual inclination of the mandibular posterior teeth. The maxillary dental arch was too narrow, mainly for the same reasons (A–D). It was decided not to coordinate the width of the dental arches, because the tongue interpositioning was so dominant, and to correct only the abnormalities in the maxillary dental arch with fixed appliances. After 18 months, an acceptable result was obtained. However, the open bite had increased in the incisor region, although it had decreased slightly in the canine-premolar area (E–H). On the day that the fixed appliances were removed, a 0.0175-inch dead-soft braided wire was bonded to the palatal surfaces of the anterior teeth and to the occlusal surfaces of the first premolars. A few months later, the size and shape of the maxillary anterior teeth were improved by grinding and buildup with resin composite (I–L). Three years later, little had changed. However, the open bite seemed to have increased slightly after the anterior teeth were built up. The non-occlusion of the molars had not changed. The patient was pleased and satisfied with the result.

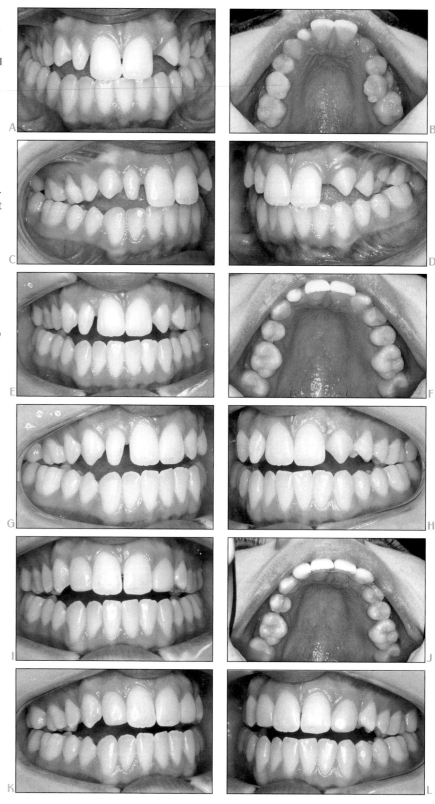

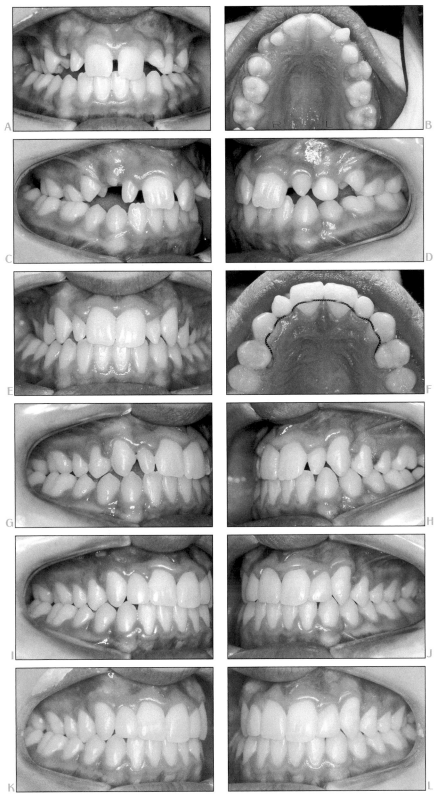

FIGURE 14-16

A boy 13 years 5 months of age, who happened to be a brother of the girl shown in Fig 14-15, had a Class I malocclusion comparable to that of his sister, albeit less severe. He also had a non-occlusion of the permanent molars but only on the right side. He did not have contact in the anterior region, but his incisors overlapped slightly. According to the definitions, he had not an anterior open bite but an anterior non-occlusion.[48] The first premolars had emerged recently, and the open bite between these teeth could be attributed to the incomplete eruption. Furthermore, the maxillary left lateral incisor was present, although it was peg shaped, like his sister's. His tongue interpositioning was less extensive and not as obvious as in his sister (A–D). Coordination of the widths of the dental arches was not attempted, and fixed appliances were only used in the maxilla. An acceptable result was obtained, as was apparent at the age of 16 years 11 months (E–H). A good occlusion was realized on the left side, and in the anterior region contact was reached. A non-occlusion still existed on the right side, where the maxillary teeth were positioned too far palatally in relation to their opposing teeth. Six months later, the maxillary incisors were built up, and an esthetically satisfying dentition was obtained. Furthermore, some intercuspation had come about on the right side (I, J). Eighteen months later, the intercuspation on the right side had improved further, so that the maxillary second premolar and first molars were in endo-occlusion (K, L).

FIGURE 14-17

A boy 11 years 5 months of age had a Class II division 1 malocclusion with a large open bite, which reached to the permanent first molars. He had a long, narrow face, a large lower facial height, and a receding chin (A, B). Because of amelogenesis imperfecta, the crowns of his teeth were abnormal in form, size, composition, and color (C, D). An activator was used for 2 years to improve the maxillomandibular relationship. Although the mandible attained a more anterior position in relation to the maxilla, the height of the lower face increased substantially. Six years later, at 19 years 8 months of age, little remained of the improvement in sagittal relationships. The lower facial height had increased even more, and the open bite now extended to the second molars (E–H). The patient did not like his facial appearance, consulted an oral surgeon, and asked what could be done. A Le Fort I operation was performed in three segments, and a chin correction was accomplished. The posterior segments of the maxilla were repositioned rather high, which resulted in an autorotation of the mandible and a substantial reduction of the lower facial height. The anterior lower facial height was reduced further by an osteotomy of the chin, which was carried out primarily to produce a chin prominence.

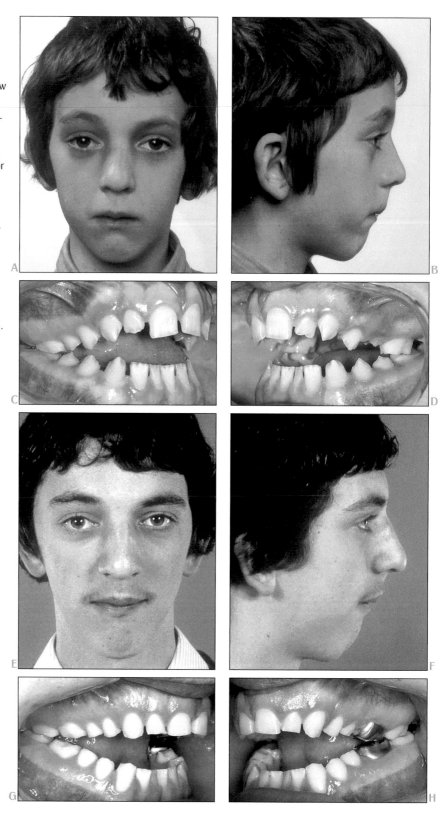

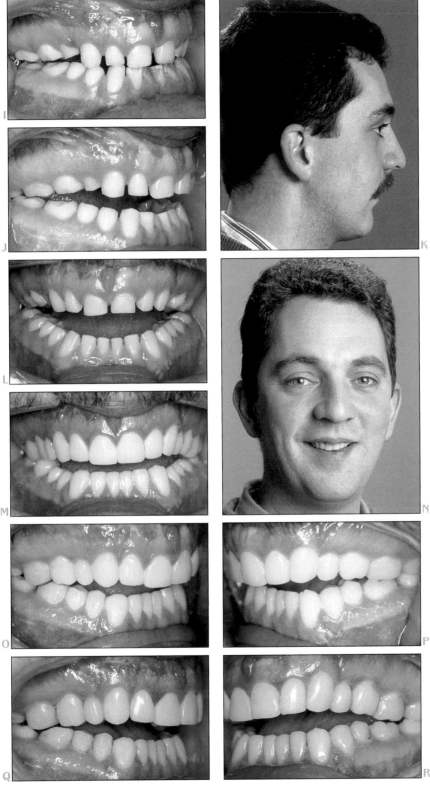

FIGURE 14-17 (CONTINUED)

Although orthodontic treatment had not preceded the surgery, the anterior teeth were in contact after the operation, and only a slight open bite existed in the posterior regions (I). Gradually, the bite opened again; by 3 years 6 months after surgery, only the last molars were in contact (J). At the age of 26 years 1 month, little was lost of the improvements realized by the surgery, which had resulted in good facial proportions and an acceptable profile (K). However, in the 3 preceding years, the open bite had increased (L). At the age of 27 years 8 months, the teeth were built up with resin composite to obtain an esthetically pleasing dentition as well as to close the open bite of the molars and reduce the open bite anterior to these teeth. The result was esthetically satisfying (M, N). However, in subsequent years, the open bite increased again, as was revealed by the records collected at the age of 28 years 1 month (O, P) and 33 years 11 months (Q, R). Again, only the last molars contacted each other. However, the esthetic improvement of the dentition had not diminished in the eyes of the patient or of individuals in his social environment.

FIGURE 14-17 (CONTINUED)

The superimposition of the tracings shows the improvement in the skeletal configuration achieved with the Le Fort I osteotomy in three segments and the surgical chin correction. The autorotation of the mandible following the repositioning of the posterior maxillary segments in cranial direction is evident, as is the effect of the chin operation (S). In the 3 years after the surgery, the anterior extending section of the mandible was resorbed, and the anterior border of the chin, the alveolar process, and the mandibular incisors moved posteriorly. In addition, the incisors in both jaws had intruded, as had the mandibular first molars (T).

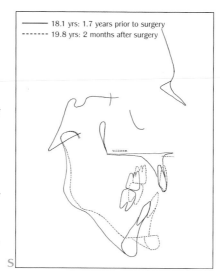

—— 18.1 yrs: 1.7 years prior to surgery
------ 19.8 yrs: 2 months after surgery

S

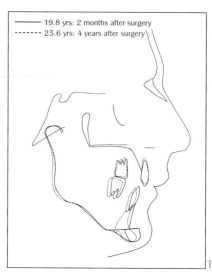

—— 19.8 yrs: 2 months after surgery
------ 23.6 yrs: 4 years after surgery

T

In patients with anterior open bites and non-occlusions, special attention has to be paid to the retention of corrected rotations and closed diastemata. Occlusal contacts, which normally contribute to stability, are lacking. Furthermore, the tongue is not positioned within the dental arches and can push the anterior teeth labially again. When the treatment has been carried out for esthetic reasons only, the improvements should be maintained with special care. To that end, a 0.0175-inch dead-soft braided wire, bonded to all anterior teeth and the first premolars, is preferred. When the first premolars are not incorporated in the retention wire, they can relapse palatally, and diastemata can re-form at their mesial sides. Depending on the occlusion, the retention wire can be bonded to the occlusal surface or can be attached at the palatal side of the first premolars (Fig 14-15, J and 14-16, F).

As has been explained earlier, open bites and non-occlusions are difficult to correct.[3] When obstructions in the nasal airway can be eliminated, and a competent lip seal can be established, the prognosis is favorable. Surgical reduction of the tongue will be of benefit only in extreme situations.

It is not realistic to expect much from myofunctional therapy.[190] It never has been proved that this type of therapy can eliminate tongue interpositioning at rest and tongue thrust during unconscious swallowing. The same applies to crib appliances and to pieces of wire with sharp ends, intended to change the position of the tongue. As long as these devices are worn, the tongue position is affected, but the question is whether the correction will persist after therapy is ended.

In general, the approach to the orthodontic treatment of open bites and non-occlusions should not be the same as that to the treatment of malocclusions with normal functional conditions, so the following strategy is recommended.

The clinician should begin by finding out what the real complaint is for the patient; in most instances, that is only the esthetically disturbing aspect. If this exclusively concerns the positioning of the teeth, then they should be aligned and the result should be permanently retained (Figs 14-15 and 14-16).

If the patient's concern is concentrated on an unacceptable facial disfiguration—and that applies to most skeletal Class III malocclusions with an open bite—the treatment should be postponed until facial growth is completed, and the facial disfiguration should be corrected by orthognathic surgery, supported by fixed orthodontic appliance therapy. When indicated, disturbances in tooth positions might be corrected and retained at a younger age.

Treatment of Missing Incisors

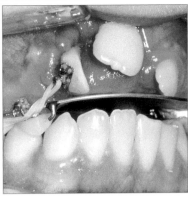

Agenesis of maxillary lateral incisors and loss of one or more anterior teeth to trauma occur rather often. Early detection of agenesis offers the possibility to guide the development of the dentition and thereby facilitate later treatment. The best solution is to close the diastemata and place the canines adjacent to the central incisors.[130] Problems caused through loss of permanent anterior teeth because of trauma are more difficult to solve, particularly when two central incisors are involved. However, in these cases too, the development of the dentition can be redirected when the loss occurred at an early age. Young children who have lost a permanent central incisor are often better off with space closure than with space maintenance and subsequent replacement of the lost tooth with a fixed partial denture or an implant. That also applies to older children in whom the development of the dentition and facial growth is not yet completed. In adults, the replacement of an anterior tooth with an implant or fixed partial denture is the preferred solution.

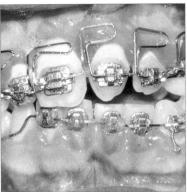

The introduction of resin composites has enhanced the potential to arrive at acceptable results without resorting to fixed partial dentures or implants. Maxillary canines can be reshaped to simulate lateral incisors, and lateral incisors can be altered to look like central incisors. Achievement of a good result after orthodontic treatment depends not only on the competence of the clinician who will perform the restorative treatment but also, and perhaps even more, on the position, inclination, and angulation of the involved teeth at the end of the orthodontic treatment and on the subsequent stability.

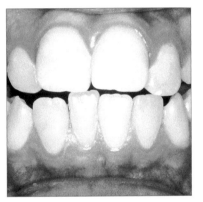

The indications and contraindications for orthodontic closure are discussed. The essential aspects of treatment and the requirements that have to be fulfilled to reach optimal results are presented and illustrated in detail. Subsequently, problems that can arise are discussed.

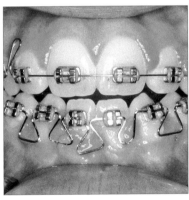

Little attention is paid to the shape and color of the labial surfaces of the substituting teeth. These aspects, and particularly the preferred position, angulation, and inclination of the teeth, have to be discussed, before orthodontic treatment, with the dentist who will carry out the esthetic treatment.

Patients are shown to illustrate misjudgments, mistakes, and failures, but satisfactory results are also shown. Advice is given to prevent disappointments.

Orthodontic Concepts and Strategies

15

FIGURE 15-1

In an ideal arrangement, maxillary central incisors are angulated 2 degrees, and lateral incisors are angulated 5 degrees. The highest point of the crown is located more distally on lateral incisors than on central incisors (A). With various techniques, crowns of lateral incisors can be built up to simulate central incisors (B). The cervical margins of the two teeth at the center should be at the same height (C). When they are not, gingivectomy can offer the solution (D). When the angulation is not altered sufficiently, the distance at the cervical level is too large (E). If the lateral incisor is placed with its mesial surface parallel to the median suture, this distance becomes shorter. The diastema at the mesial side of the lateral incisor has to be smaller than that at the distal side (F). The central papilla will not fill the intradental space completely when the contact area does not extend to the middle of the crown height. A broad canine at the location of the lateral incisor is not acceptable, particularly with a small lateral incisor on the other side (G). This discrepancy can be corrected by narrowing the canine and broadening the lateral incisor (H).

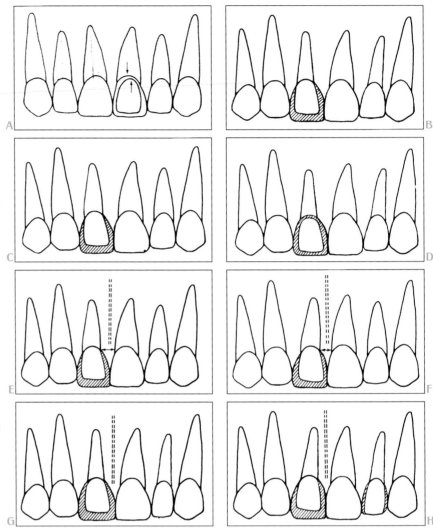

In Class II division 1 malocclusions, the maxillary anterior teeth are extra vulnerable and are prone to loss through trauma. When a child loses one incisor, the best solution is to close the space and extract a premolar from the other side of the arch. A partial disto-occlusion can be increased to a complete one to attain a good intercuspation and contact in the anterior region. Even a neutro-occlusion can be altered into a disto-occlusion, unilaterally or bilaterally, by orthodontic and facial orthopedic means.

The treatment of these cases is less complex, and the result is more stable, in dental arches with crowding than those with spacing. In patients with a neutro-occlusion and considerable crowding in both dental arches, extracting one dental unit in each quadrant is the preferred solution. As a rule, extractions from the mandible are contraindicated in patients with Class II division 1 malocclusions. In Class III patients in whom the dental arch relationship will not be corrected surgically, a solution without artificial replacement of missing maxillary anterior teeth by a fixed partial denture, implant, or partial prosthesis is rarely possible.

An attractive dentition is of great importance, particularly in adolescents and young adults.[2] Attainment of optimal results when permanent incisors are missing is difficult and depends on many factors.[241, 243] The positions of the teeth that serve as substitutes for lost incisors are critical and have to fulfill specific requirements. That applies particularly to the distances to the adjacent teeth, to inclinations, and to angulations. The height of the cervical margins is also of importance. This type of treatment requires a skillful handling of fixed appliances (Fig 15-1).

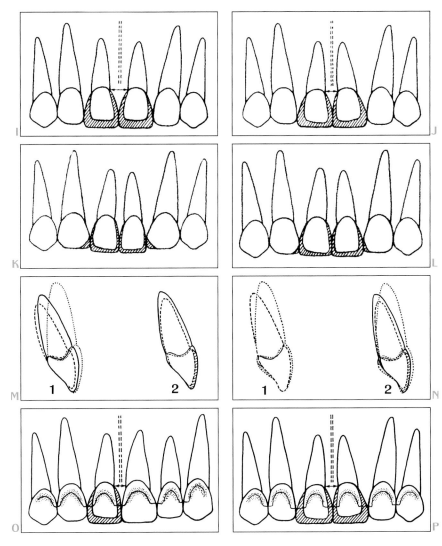

FIGURE 15-1 (CONTINUED)

When both central incisors are replaced with lateral incisors, the parallelism of the mesial surfaces is even more important (I, J). Large canines should not be broadened (K) but should be narrowed so that they will be narrower than the built-up lateral incisors (L). When the two incisors and the canine are superimposed at their palatal surfaces, the differences in inclination and crown thickness are obvious (M1). Consequently, a lateral incisor that substitutes for a central incisor should be uprighted (M2). A canine at the location of the lateral incisor should be ground palatally, and its apex should be moved palatally (N1). A lateral incisor in the location of a central incisor and a canine in the place of a lateral incisor should be adapted in shape and inclination (N2). Permanent retention is needed to maintain changes in angulation (O); this is of particular importance when two lateral incisors replace the central incisors (P). Furthermore, the retention wire should include the first premolars, to secure the angulation of the canines and to prevent the occurrence of diastemata distal of the canines.

The amount of the maxillary anterior teeth that is shown while the individual is speaking and laughing is essential. The incisal edges are always visible, but not the cervical margins. In an asymmetric arrangement of the maxillary anterior teeth, for example, when one lateral incisor is missing, the incisal edges should be in a straight line (Fig 15-16, B).

The course of the cervical margins is critical in patients with high smile lines but is of little relevance when the cervical margins are never shown.

Irregularities in the transverse direction usually do not catch the eye when the cervical margins and incisal edges are perceived as normal. Moderate midline deviations are not noticed when the contact plane between the two teeth in the center is parallel to the median plane of the face.[20, 97, 105, 134, 245] That applies even more when the incisal half of the crowns corresponds in shape and color to what the viewer expects to see.

In the labiopalatal direction, the thickness and shape of the crowns and the location of the cervical margins are important.[214] When occlusal contact exists between opposing anterior teeth, the palatal surfaces have to be adapted to the occlusion and excursive movements; this is not necessary if open bites or non-occlusions are expected to persist. A maxillary canine can be very thick labiopalatally, and this can be a disturbing factor when such a tooth is placed adjacent to a central incisor. A reduction in crown thickness and a palatal movement of the apex of the canine are indicated in such cases.

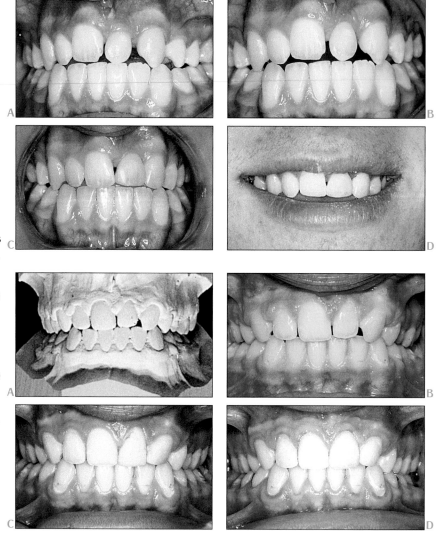

FIGURE 15-2

On the day the fixed appliances were removed, the maxillary left lateral incisor was displaced sufficiently to the mesial for an ideal distribution in width of the adjacent diastemata (A). However, 3 weeks later, on the day that retention was implemented, the tooth was located too far distally (B). With the buildup of the crown, an acceptable, but not optimal, result still could be achieved. However, the maxillary right central incisor, which had been uprighted in the mesiodistal direction, had lost this change in angulation (C). The central papilla did not fill the interdental space completely; the end of the contact area was inferior to the incisal half of the crowns (D).

FIGURE 15-3

After removal of the fixed appliances, the angulation of the substituting maxillary left lateral incisor and the distribution and size of the diastemata conformed to the criteria for replacements (A). On the same day, a maxillary retention plate was placed, but no retention wire was bonded to the palatal side. The distribution and size of the diastemata did not change, but the angulation of the left lateral incisor did (B). After this tooth was built up to look like a left central incisor, the angulation changed further (C). A replacement of the buildup was required to obtain an acceptable result (D).

When the optimal positions, angulations, and inclinations of the teeth involved are being decided, the anticipated complementary treatments of grinding, buildup with resin composites or veneers, and improvement in shape and color should be the leading factors.[198] When the complementary treatment is carried out by another clinician, preceding consultation is required.

The quality of the result that can be achieved by esthetic dentistry depends largely on the location of the teeth after the orthodontic treatment. In that respect, the distances between the adjacent teeth and the tooth that has to be built up are of great importance, as already indicated. The same applies to the axial orientation of the tooth in the mesiodistal direction (angulation) and the labiopalatal direction (inclination).[172, 241, 243]

Relapses in the location (Fig 15-2) or angulation (Fig 15-3) of the teeth can occur shortly after the appliances have been removed.

It is difficult to determine the best location of the teeth involved without the use of a diagnostic setup. A setup also clarifies which occlusion should be the goal and where and how much grinding of palatal surfaces will be needed. The setup also indicates the necessary adjustments in width and position of the opposing teeth.

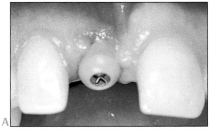
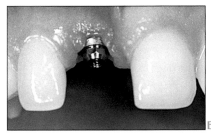
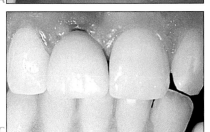
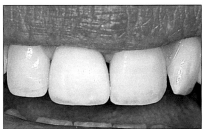

FIGURE 15-4

A woman 20 years of age who had lost her maxillary right central incisor in an accident was treated with a one-stage implant. After an osseointegration phase of 6 months' duration, an abutment with a protective cap was placed (A). After removal of the protective cap (B) an impression was taken, and a crown was made and placed. Because of insufficient bony contour and a shortage in mucosal tissue, the gingival adaptation was not optimal (C). Fortunately, this shortcoming was not visible when the patient was speaking and laughing (D), and generation of alveolar bone and connective tissue was not needed. (Courtesy of Dr B. J. Polder.)

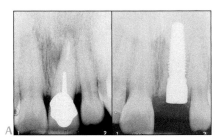
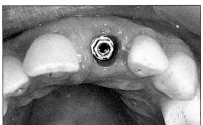
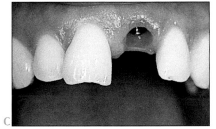
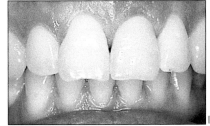

FIGURE 15-5

Fifteen years previously, this 39-year-old man had fractured the crown of his maxillary left central incisor. The tooth was endodontically treated, and a crown with a pinlay was placed. Another trauma, years later, caused a fracture of the root and a periapical infection, and the tooth could not be saved (A: LEFT). Directly after the extraction, an implant with a healing cap was placed (A: RIGHT), by which the gingival contour was preserved (B, C). Six months later, the definitive crown was cemented (D). (Courtesy of Dr B. J. Polder.)

Figures 15-4 and 15-5 show two patients in whom an implant with a crown was used to replace a lost or unsalvageable maxillary central incisor. Both patients were adults and had no need for orthodontic treatment. The application of implants in younger patients, in whom the increase in height of the alveolar processes is not completed yet, will result in an infrapositioning of the implant.[197]

In the Figs 15-6 to 15-15, 10 patients are shown to clarify the possibilities and limitations of orthodontic treatment in patients with missing anterior teeth. In nine of the patients, the defect was located in the maxilla. In one patient, the mandibular right central and lateral incisor could not be preserved (Fig 15-15). Various aspects described earlier are specified and demonstrated by these clinical examples.

FIGURE 15-6

A girl aged 12 years 0 months had large diastemata in the maxillary anterior region because of agenesis of the lateral incisors. She also had diastemata distal to the canines. The mandibular dental arch was normal, but the midlines of the dental arches deviated. The canines and molars were in neutro-occlusion on the left side and in disto-occlusion of half a premolar crown width on the right side (A–D). The maxillary dental arch was moved anteriorly with a Delaire face mask, and on both sides a disto-occlusion of one premolar crown width was reached. With complete fixed appliances, the diastemata were closed and the midlines were aligned. At the age of 14 years 6 months, the intended result was achieved, and the maxillary incisors and canines were retained with a palatally bonded wire (E, F). The radiographs made before (G) and after (H) treatment showed that the maxillary canines were moved more or less bodily to the mesial. However, the apex of the maxillary left central incisor is located too far distally. The maxillary canines were built up with resin composite. Five years later, small diastemata were present distal to the maxillary canines (I, J). These diastemata were closed with resin composite buildups, as shown 5 years later (K, L). This patient had small maxillary canines that differed little in shape and color from the lateral incisors, as is often the case in females. Males have larger and darker canines, which makes it more difficult to reach an acceptable esthetic result in boys. As a rule, agenesis of maxillary lateral incisors is associated with smaller teeth than normal, and spaces in the dental arch are common. Diastemata that have been closed orthodontically tend to open again, so a retention wire is needed; this wire should include the first premolars; otherwise, diastemata can develop distal to the canines, as was the case in this patient.

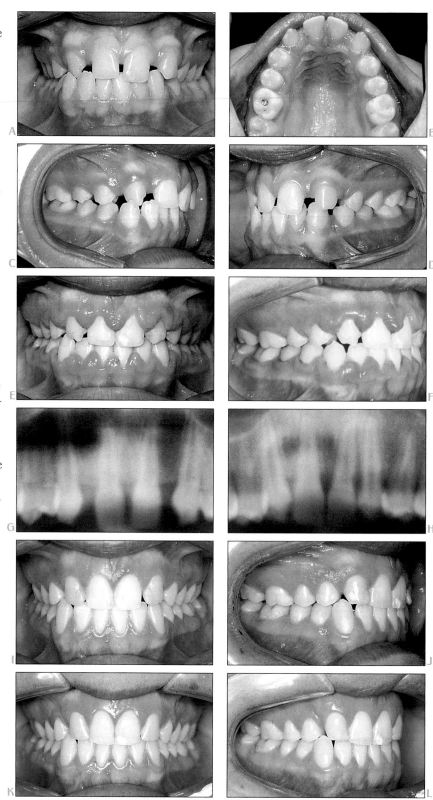

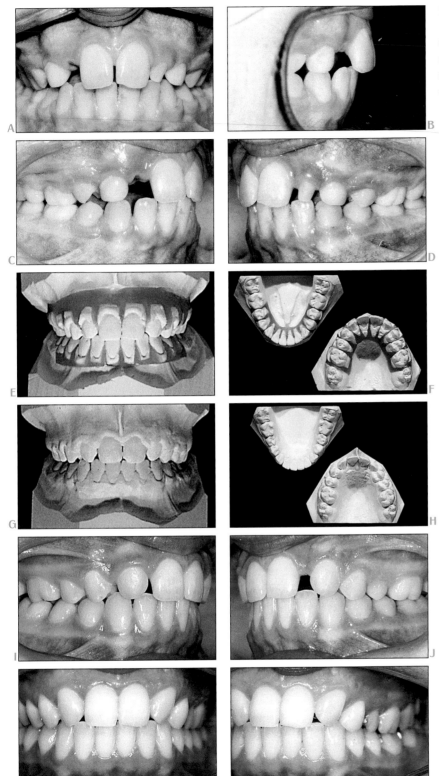

FIGURE 15-7

A girl 10 years 4 months of age had a Class I malocclusion with agenesis of the maxillary left lateral incisor and a peg-shaped right lateral incisor. The mandibular dental arch was normal (A–D). The treatment was started with extraction of the primary maxillary second molars, which resulted in mesial migration of the permanent maxillary first molars and the palatal rotation of their mesiobuccal cusps. This rotation was needed to arrive at a good intercuspation of the first molars in a disto-occlusion. After all premolars and permanent canines had erupted completely, a diagnostic setup was made to assess whether a good occlusion could be obtained by preserving and building up the peg-shaped lateral incisor. Another setup without the peg-shaped lateral incisor seemed to offer the best result, so this tooth was extracted (E, F). At the age of 11 years 4 months, fixed appliances were placed in the maxilla. In 7 months' time a result that matched the setup was obtained (G, H). A positioner was used for detailing of the occlusion and retention purposes. The positioner was worn during the night and 4 hours a day for the first month and only during sleep for the following 5 months. One year after use of the positioner ceased, a small central diastema and a large diastema mesial to the maxillary left canine had developed (I, J). Another year later, a removable plate with a labial arch and a pigtail spring distal to the maxillary left canine was used to close the spaces. Subsequently, the four anterior teeth were connected with a dead-soft braided retention wire. Ten years later, at the age of 25 years, the situation seemed not to have changed. The patient had not accepted the suggestion to build up the mesioincisal corners of the maxillary canines; however, she had agreed to close with resin composite the small diastema that had developed distal to the left canine (K, L).

Figure 15-8

A boy aged 11 years 1 month had a Class I malocclusion. The maxillary central incisors were missing. Both teeth had been lost in a fall on a concrete wall. Subsequently, the lateral incisors had emerged and migrated mesially (A–D). It was decided to use a Delaire face mask to move the entire maxillary dental arch anteriorly. At the age of 11 years 3 months, the permanent maxillary first molars were banded and hooks were inserted in the edgewise tubes to allow attachment of elastics. Brackets were placed on the first premolars for the same purpose. The elastics ran parallel to the occlusal plane to the bar on the mask. During the 14 hours a day that the mask was supposed to be used, the patient had to wear a maxillary plate, which held all teeth firmly in place, so that the forces at the first premolars and molars were distributed over the whole dental arch (E, F). At the age of 11 years 10 months, a disto-occlusion was obtained. Edgewise appliances were placed in the mandible and, 1 month later, in the maxilla. After 12 months of fixed appliance treatment, during which the Delaire mask was worn only during sleep, a retention wire was bonded in the maxilla (G, H). However, the maxillary lateral incisors had not been positioned well. They were too far apart and not uprighted sufficiently (I), which made it difficult to build up the crowns. After loss of the retention wire, a central diastema developed (J). Some years later, the maxillary incisors were built up once more. However, the contact area did not extend to half the crown height, so the central papilla did not fill the interdental space completely. The canines had been ground and built up. However, they were rather large, and their cervical margins were located more superiorly than those of the built up incisors. Nevertheless, the midlines of the dental arches coincided, and both posterior regions were in disto-occlusion with a good intercuspation (K, L).

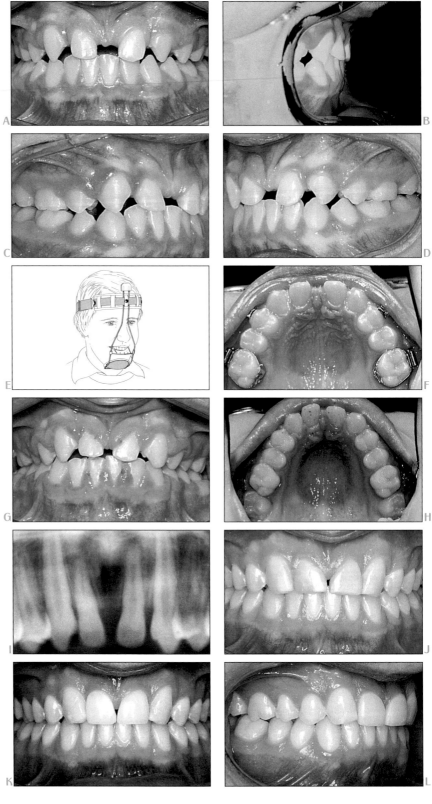

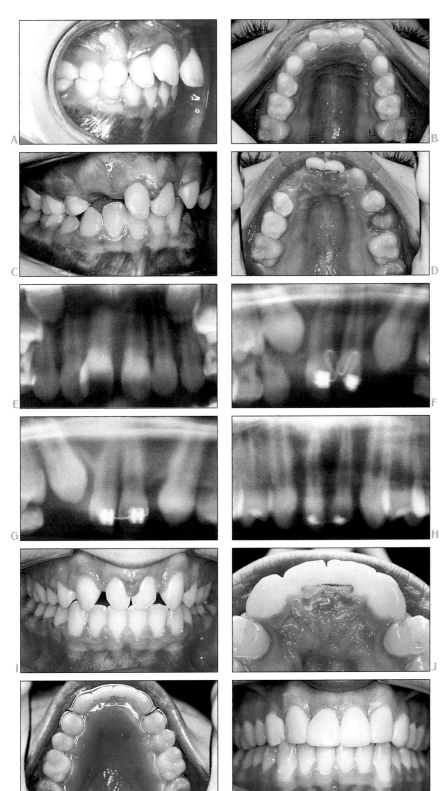

FIGURE 15-9

A boy 9 years 5 months of age, with a Class II division 1 malocclusion, had lost the two maxillary central incisors in a fall at a swimming pool 1 year previously. Reimplantation was not successful, which could have been expected, because the teeth had been out of the mouth considerably longer than 30 minutes. The reimplanted central incisors had to be extracted (A, B). After the extractions, the maxillary lateral incisors were moved to the place of the central incisors, so that the permanent canines could migrate mesially prior to emergence. To that end, 0.022 × 0.028-inch edgewise brackets were placed on the lateral incisors, in which a 0.016 × 0.016-inch stainless steel sectional spring was inserted. The large central diastema was camouflaged by a plate with two artificial teeth, which were gradually reduced in width. After the lateral incisors were in contact with each other, the brackets were removed, and a connecting 0.015-inch dead-soft braided wire was bonded palatally (C, D). The canines erupted in the intended position, as the radiographs from before (E) and after (F) the initial treatment showed. The canines arrived at a more mesial location than otherwise would have been the case. In addition, the lateral incisors were positioned parallel to each other in the middle of the dental arch (G). After all premolars and permanent canines had emerged, complete fixed appliances were placed. In 18 months' time, the goal was reached (H, I). The two incisors were connected with a retention wire that was maintained after the teeth were built up (J). In addition, a retention plate was worn day and night for 6 months and subsequently only during sleep for 2 more years (K). Five years later, the results achieved remained stable (L). The early mesial movement of maxillary lateral incisors is a good example of effective guidance of the development of the dentition. The same applies to the early extraction of primary maxillary second molars to obtain mesial movement and rotation of the permanent maxillary first molars (see Fig 15-7).

FIGURE 15-10

A boy 13 years 1 month of age had lost the maxillary right central and lateral incisors in a fall when he was 10 years of age. Furthermore, the mesial corner of the maxillary left central incisor had fractured. He had a disto-occlusion of one-half premolar crown width on the right side and one-quarter premolar crown width on the left side. The overjet was 5 mm, and the overbite was 4 mm (A–D). It was decided to reduce the diastema to the width of a maxillary central incisor, to replace this tooth with a resin-bonded fixed partial denture, and to establish a neutro-occlusion on the left side and a disto-occlusion of one premolar width on the right side. At the age of 13 years 4 months, the permanent maxillary first molars were banded and an asymmetric headgear was placed. A bracket was bonded on the right canine, to which an uprighting spring was ligated. The end of the spring was attached to the labial bow of the removable plate, which also served to reduce the deep bite. Edgewise appliances were placed 3 months later in the mandible and another 2 months later in the maxilla. With the support of asymmetric elastics, the goal was reached at the age of 15 years 6 months (E–H). Subsequently, a retention plate with an artificial tooth was worn for 6 months, after which the resin-bonded fixed partial denture was made. In the mandible, a canine-to-canine retention wire was bonded. The result was still quite acceptable 5 years (I, J) and 10 years later (K, L). In the maxilla, it is impossible to move a tooth from one half of the arch to the other half. The median suture cannot be passed but only displaced slightly to the other side. When two anterior teeth are lost unilaterally, orthodontic closure of the space is not indicated.

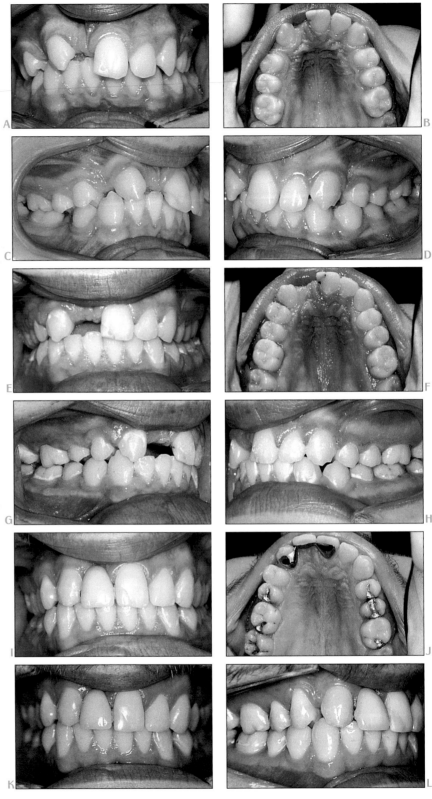

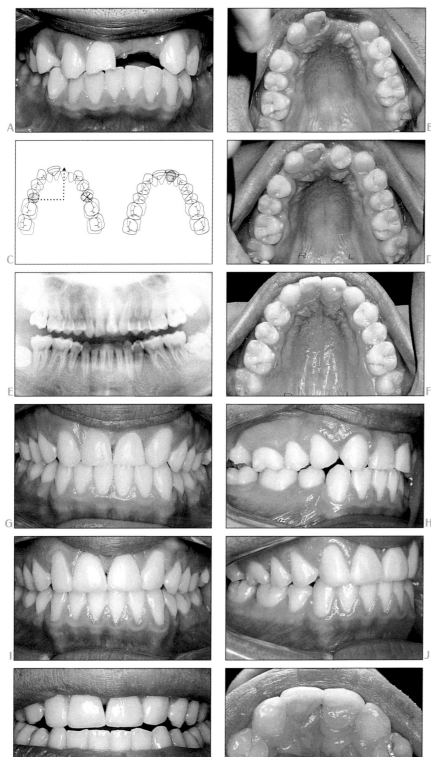

FIGURE 15-11

A boy 14 years 6 months of age had agenesis of the maxillary lateral incisors and had lost his maxillary left central incisor in an accident 2 years previously. A partial denture camouflaged the defect. He had a neutro-occlusion and crowding in the mandibular dental arch (A, B). Although both mandibular second premolars had already emerged, it was decided to transplant one to the location of the missing maxillary left central incisor. Later, the other mandibular second premolar would be extracted (C). At the age of 14 years 8 months, an alveolus was prepared and the mandibular left second premolar was transplanted. However, this tooth developed lateral root resorption, became ankylosed, and had to be removed. During the same session at which the extraction was carried out, the mandibular right second premolar was transplanted in the alveolus, which now had the proper shape and dimensions. The second attempt was successful, and a normal periodontium developed (D). Six months later, the already endodontically treated premolar was ground on the palatal side and complete fixed appliances were placed. After 18 months, the planned result was reached. Subsequently, the transplanted premolar was built up to resemble a central incisor (E–H). The final result met the expectations, and that was still true 5 years later (I–L).

When a single-rooted tooth, with a root formed half to two thirds of its anticipated final length, is removed prior to emergence with no or little damage to the dental follicle and transplanted, the success rate is very high, particularly when a proper alveolus has been prepared at the receiving site.[6, 46, 109, 111] In this patient, the premolars that were transplanted had emerged already, and the alveolar process at the receiving site was extensively resorbed. Consequently, the chance that the transplantation could fail was substantial.

Treatment of Missing Incisors

FIGURE 15-12

A girl with a Class II division 1 malocclusion had damaged her maxillary anterior teeth in an accident, and the left central incisor and the right lateral incisor could not be saved (A, B). It was decided to close the diastemata orthodontically and complement the treatment with esthetic dentistry. After extraction of the two incisors, they were replaced by two artificial teeth on a plate, which were gradually reduced in width. The orthodontic treatment was carried out with edgewise appliances (C). After the appliances were removed, it became clear that the maxillary incisors did not have the proper angulation (D). That had not been obvious when the appliances were in place (E, F). It was an omission not to take a panoramic radiograph during the last phase of the active treatment. Nevertheless, with buildup of the incisors and canines, an attempt was made to arrive at an acceptable-looking anterior region (G). Because the anterior teeth were not retained with a wire at the palatal surfaces, tooth movements occurred, and the situation worsened (H). Two years later, it was decided to treat her for the second time. The mandibular incisors, which had become crowded, were stripped, and again complete fixed appliances were placed (I). This time the angulation of the maxillary teeth was checked radiographically prior to the removal of the fixed appliances. Further uprighting proved necessary (J). After the additional uprighting was carried out (K), the crowns were reshaped (L). In this patient, obtaining a good result was of particular importance because she had a high smile line, so that not only the crowns but also the gingiva superior to them were exposed (a "gummy" smile). With aging the smile line will descend, and the maxillary anterior region will become less visible, so that shortcomings in the maxillary anterior region will be less obvious.

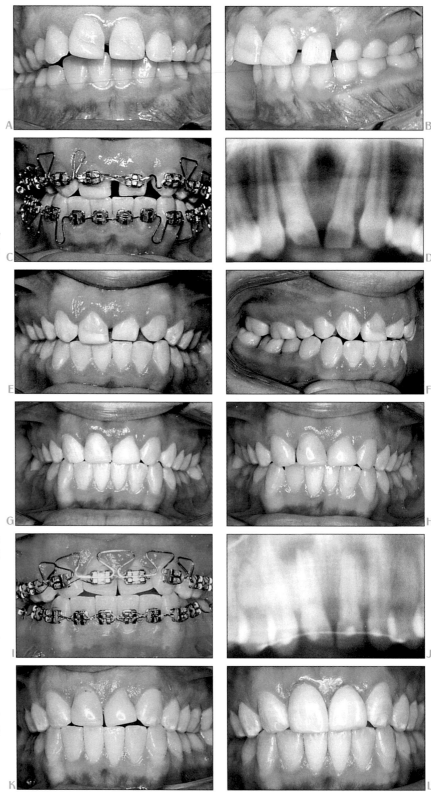

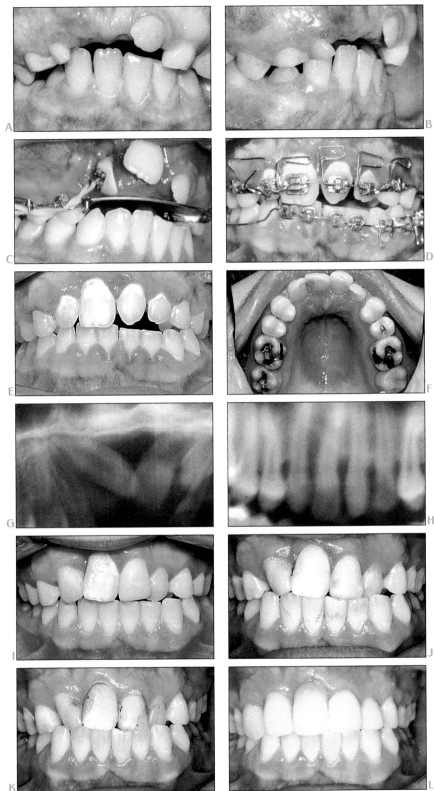

FIGURE 15-13

In a boy 11 years 2 months of age, the permanent maxillary right central and lateral incisors and the left central incisor had not erupted (A, B). The panoramic radiograph revealed that the unerupted incisors were in extremely deviating positions (G). During the surgical exposure of the impacted teeth, a large cyst, which extended from the palate to the nasal floor, was found at the right lateral incisor. The cyst was extirpated, and the right lateral incisor and the left central incisor were removed, because both teeth had severely bent roots. Successively, the remaining maxillary anterior teeth emerged; at the age of 12 years 3 months, the first appliances were placed (C). Gradually the appliances were extended (D) and then removed at 15 years 3 months of age. The anterior teeth were positioned as planned, although the left canine was at the location of the central incisor. An anterior open bite, caused by tongue interpositioning, existed on the left side. The radiographs before (G) and after treatment (H) showed that the teeth had been moved to the intended parallel positions. The teeth were built up, and an adequate result was obtained. However, no retention wire was placed. Six months later, the maxillary anterior teeth were malpositioned (I). The situation deteriorated further, and the left lateral incisors developed a crossbite (J). At the age of 28 years 3 months, the situation was considered to be unacceptable (K), and esthetic dentistry with resin composites was carried out again. A retention wire was not applied, because no further changes were expected. Five years later, the latest improvements appeared stable (L). This case is a good example of the need for adequate retention when teeth are missing in the anterior region; that applies particularly when the teeth have been so abnormally positioned, as in this patient.

FIGURE 15-14

A boy aged 9 years 8 months of age had a Class I malocclusion with crowding in both dental arches. The maxillary left central incisor was excessively wide, and the right central incisor was a double tooth with an unfavorable root morphology (A, B, G). The double tooth was extracted, and the subsequent development of the dentition was awaited. At the age of 12 years 0 months, records were collected again, and based on their analysis it was decided to wait some more before starting orthodontic treatment (C, D). Not until the permanent canines had emerged, at 16 years of age, were various diagnostic setups made to determine the best solution. It became clear that a satisfactory result could not be reached if the very wide maxillary left central incisor were preserved, even if it were reduced excessively in width. Consequently, at the age of 16 years 7 months, the wide central incisor and the mandibular first premolars were extracted for compensatory reasons, and a maxillary plate with two artificial teeth was inserted to camouflage the large anterior gap. One month later, edgewise appliances were placed in the mandible. Another month later, the permanent maxillary first molars were banded, and brackets were placed on the lateral incisors. Four months later, brackets were bonded to the other maxillary teeth, and appropriate archwires were applied. At the age of 18 years 11 months, all appliances were removed, and a dead-soft braided retention wire was placed palatally at the maxillary incisors, canines, and first premolars. In the mandible, a canine bar was bonded. The maxillary lateral incisors were properly positioned with correct angulations and inclinations (E, F, H). Subsequently, the four maxillary anterior teeth and the premolars were built up, and an attractive and functional anterior region was realized (I, J). Two years later, little had changed (K, L).

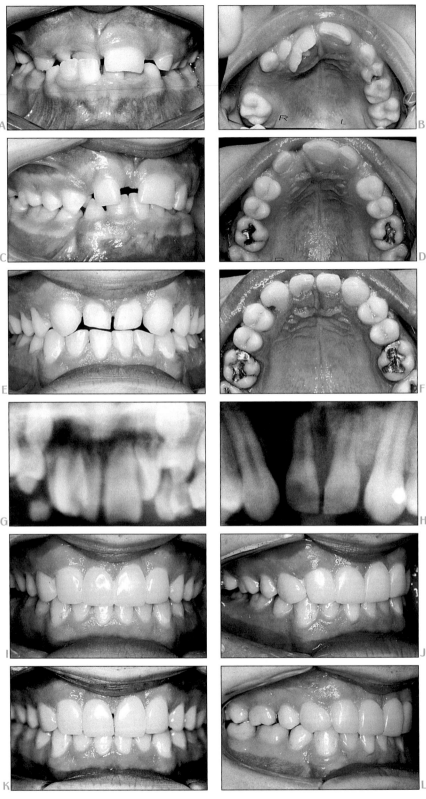

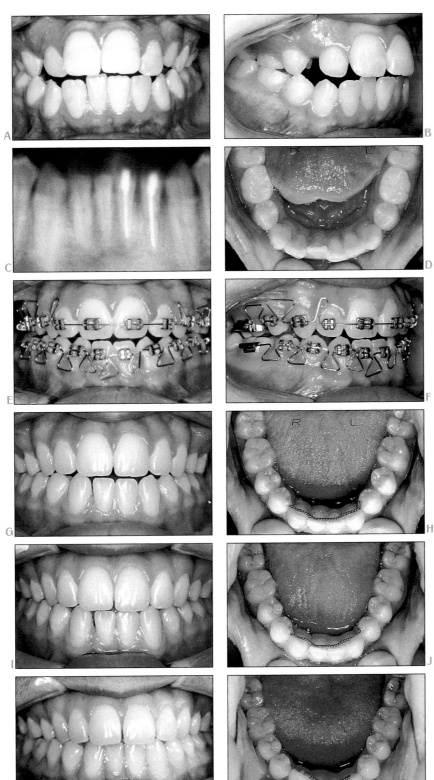

FIGURE 15-15

A boy aged 13 years 5 months had a Class II division 1 malocclusion with an anterior open bite. The two mandibular right incisors were exfoliated when he turned a cartwheel at a swimming pool. These teeth were reimplanted 1.5 hours after the accident. Later, lateral external root resorptions occurred at both reimplanted incisors, and they could not be preserved (A–D). Analysis of various diagnostic setups led to the conclusion that a good result could be obtained if, besides the two mandibular incisors, the maxillary first premolars were removed. Four weeks after the extractions were carried out, a Lehman combined activator-headgear was applied to correct the disto-occlusion. This appliance was replaced later by a cervical headgear and complete edgewise appliances (E, F), and a good result was obtained (G, H). The bonded mandibular retainer became loose during a vacation in a foreign country and was not replaced. Subsequently, a diastema developed (I); it was closed with buttons and elastics and retained again with a dead-soft braided wire (J). Five years later, at the age of 25 years, the result was still satisfactory (K, L). In the mandible, teeth can be moved through the median plane. No structure prevents such movement as the median suture does in the maxilla. As such, the possibilities are more varied in the mandible than in the maxilla. Furthermore, the mandibular central and lateral incisors differ little in size and shape. Mandibular incisors that are moved to another location do not have to be built up. However, proper angulation is essential. Furthermore, with a reduction in the number of anterior teeth, diastemata in the mandible tend to return and permanent retention is indicated.

FIGURE 15-16

The incisal edges of the maxillary lateral incisors have to be situated 0.5 mm higher than those of the adjacent teeth, and their cervical margins should be slightly lower (A). In an asymmetric maxillary anterior region, the incisal edges preferably are placed at the same level (B).

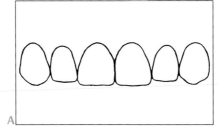

A

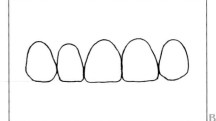

B

FIGURE 15-17

A cervical margin can be positioned more superiorly by gingivectomy; however, the margin of the buildup will become more apically located (A). Intrusion does not have that disadvantage (B).

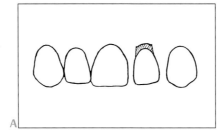

A

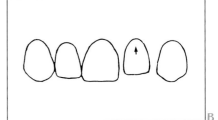

B

FIGURE 15-18

Normal angulation and crown shapes: Papilla fills the interdental space (A1). Abnormal crown shapes and low approximal contact: Papilla is deficient (A2) without reducing crown width (A3). Excess mesial angulation alone (B1) or with deviating crown shapes (B2): Papilla fills in if both are corrected (B3).

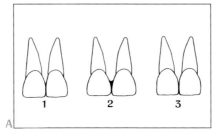

A

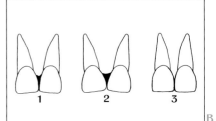

B

As stated already, symmetry in the height of the incisal edges and cervical margins is essential to an attractive dentition. Furthermore, the height of the incisal edges and cervical margins has to meet specific criteria (Fig 15-16).

A correction in the height of cervical margins can be realized by gingivectomy or by intrusion or extrusion of teeth (Fig 15-17).[104]

It is essential that the contact plane between the crowns of the two teeth placed at the center of the maxillary dental arch extend to at least half of the crown height; otherwise, the central papilla will not fill the interdental space (Fig 15-18).

Achieving a functional and esthetically pleasing result in patients with missing maxillary anterior teeth is complex and difficult. Preparation of one or more diagnostic setups can be of great help in determining the treatment goal in detail and comparing alternatives. Indeed, the position, angulation, and inclination of the teeth involved should be specified before treatment is started. It also has to be clear pretreatment which teeth have to be adjusted in size and shape, including the removal of enamel from palatal surfaces.

Role of Occlusion During and After Orthodontic Treatment

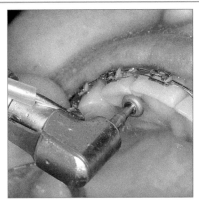

As has been emphasized repeatedly, occlusion plays an essential role in the development of the dentition and in the stability of the permanent dentition. A good intercuspation provides unity to the dentition and maintains the relationship between the dental arches when the dentition displaces in the growing face. The occlusion is of importance not only to the normal and abnormal development of the dentition but also to orthodontic treatment and to subsequent alterations in both the anterior and posterior regions.

The favorable effects of the "cone-funnel" mechanism and the "rail" mechanism in orthodontic treatment are indicated, as are their negative influences. Indeed, both mechanisms play an important role in many aspects.

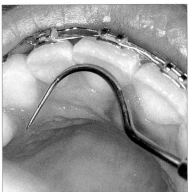

The consequences of space shortage in the maxillary posterior regions for the position of the permanent molars in the developing dentition are demonstrated. After emergence, the roots of the maxillary second molars cannot move distally, because the crowns of the third molars are a barrier. Not before the third molars have emerged can the roots of the second molars upright and become mesially angulated. This limitation is often not realized in clinical orthodontics. The recommendation to end orthodontic treatment with the maxillary second molars in mesial angulation in patients with unerupted third molars, as well as in youngsters whose third molars have erupted but in whom growth is not yet completed, is not realistic.

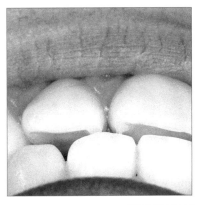

The largest part of this chapter discusses the occlusion in the anterior region, a topic rarely touched. However, the occlusal contacts in the anterior region are of importance for the stability of treatment results and for the maintenance of the arrangement of anterior teeth in nontreated individuals. In that respect, the marginal ridges of the maxillary anterior teeth are essential. When the mandibular incisors start to ride at the maxillary marginal ridges, these teeth will tend to become displaced.

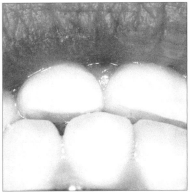

Four treated patients are shown to demonstrate not only the spontaneous improvements but also the undesirable changes caused by occlusal contacts in the anterior region. After the effect of marginal ridges is explained, the benefit of removing them is shown in another four patients. Finally, the role of the occlusion in maintaining approximal contacts is discussed.

Orthodontic Concepts and Strategies

16

FIGURE 16-1

Rarely, opposing posterior teeth will emerge in precisely the correct orientation toward each other. The cone-funnel mechanism guides the posterior teeth into maximal intercuspation.[212] The cone-funnel mechanism plays an important role in the normal development of the dentition as well as in orthodontic treatments. The cone-funnel mechanism acts for the first time when the occlusion becomes established after the emergence of the primary first molars (A, B). Subsequently, this occurs every time emerged opposing teeth in the posterior regions are reaching contact (C, D). In general, maxillary posterior teeth become more displaced than mandibular posterior teeth (E, F). However, when the eruption cannot be completed, as in individuals with a posterior tongue interpositioning, the cone-funnel mechanism will not work. This can occur not only in a naturally developing dentition but also during orthodontic treatment. Furthermore, a tongue interpositioning can displace from the anterior region to a posterior region during treatment, but the reverse can also happen.[227]

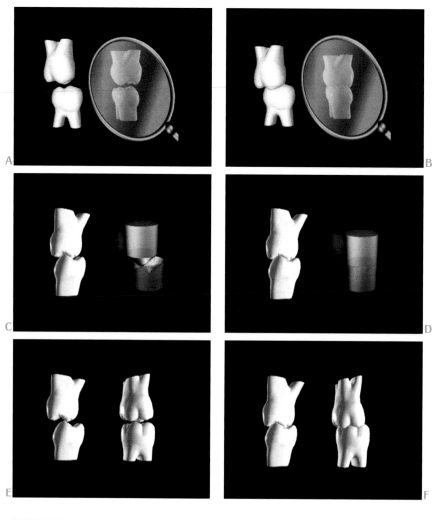

FIGURE 16-2

The positions and inclinations of the permanent first molar deviate because of an abnormal functioning of the cone-funnel mechanism (A). Removal of the too far occlusally placed bracket and an increase in the space for the mandibular first molar, for example, with an open coil spring, will result in spontaneous improvements (B).

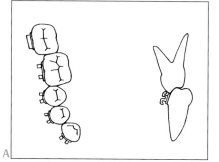 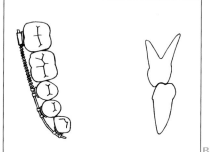

The cone-funnel mechanism not only is important for reaching an optimal intercuspation of the posterior teeth (Fig 16-1) but also plays an essential role in the dentoalveolar compensatory mechanism.[187] Through this mechanism, the inclination of the occluding premolars and molars adapts to compensate for the variation in transverse widths of the opposing apical areas.[214]

Furthermore, orthodontic treatments are facilitated and become more biologic when the cone-funnel mechanism is allowed to function. However, the cone-funnel mechanism can also have a negative effect when it is guided by other structures, as can happen when a bracket on a mandibular molar has been placed too far occlusally and its buccal surface, together with the superior inner side of the bracket, acts as a funnel and a buccal cusp of the opposing tooth acts as a cone (Fig 16-2).

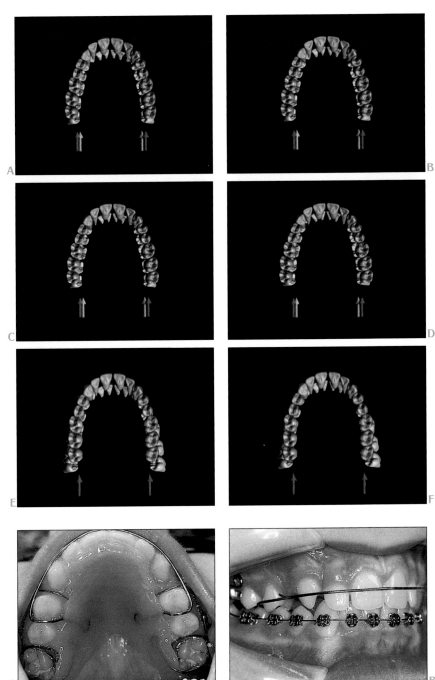

FIGURE 16-3

The occlusion in the posterior regions co-ordinates the width of the maxillary dental arch to the width of the mandibular dental arch. The mandibular dental arch broadens only slightly during growth, because the space within the cortical walls of the mandibular corpus is limited, and the base of the mandible does not widen. Mandibular molars and premolars can move buccally only slightly; however, they can become more upright, particularly when the height of the alveolar processes increases with enlargement of the lower facial height. On the other hand, the maxillary dental arch can increase in width by growth at the midpalatal suture and by apposition of bone at the buccal sides of the alveolar processes. This widening is caused primarily by the gradually mesial movement of the mandibular dental arch in relation to the maxillary dental arch, associated with normal facial growth. In that respect, the mandibular dental arch serves as the rail, or template, on which the maxillary dental arch rides. The rail mechanism only works in the presence of a good transverse and vertical occlusion. That applies to normal development as well as to the correction of Class II malocclusions, in which the posterior teeth can adapt to the occlusion (A–D). However, with open bites and non-occlusions in the posterior regions, the maxillary dental arch will not widen (E, F).[214]

FIGURE 16-4

When a removable plate with an anterior bite plane prevents the posterior teeth from occluding (A), leveling the curve of Spee becomes easier, and obtaining an ideal arrangement of the mandibular teeth is facilitated (B).

The rail mechanism is of importance for the adjustment of the maxillary dental arch width to the mandibular dental arch width, when the sagittal relationship between them alters gradually (Fig 16-3). Like the cone-funnel mechanism, the rail mechanism can be utilized for orthodontic treatment. For example, when the maxillary posterior teeth are not anchored by the appliance during activator treatment, the maxillary dental arch will widen spontaneously in response to the occlusion as the mandibular dental arch advances. The same will happen during treatment with a cervical headgear, if other appliances do not interfere.

On the other hand, keeping the posterior teeth out of occlusion can facilitate the treatment (Fig 16-4). It can also lead to spontaneous improvements, as was demonstrated in chapter 12 for Class II division 2 treatments.

In contrast to the other posterior teeth, permanent maxillary molars attain their final positions not shortly after emergence but only years later, when space for the distal movement of their apices has become available (Fig 16-5 to 16-8).

FIGURE 16-5

The dentition develops in the space available within the jaws (A–D). The space for the developing permanent molars is limited in the maxilla but not in the mandible. In the maxilla, the distal side of the tuberosity is the posterior boundary. In the mandible, there is more space, because the molars can be formed in the anterior area of the ramus, where the apices also can be located later. During their formation, permanent maxillary molars are angulated distally, and permanent mandibular molars are angulated mesially.[223]

FIGURE 16-6

In the maxilla, permanent second and third molars emerge in distal angulation; in the mandible, they erupt in mesial angulation. Occluding permanent maxillary first molars cannot change in angulation as long as the forming second molars are close to their apices. The same applies to permanent second molars, which have the crowns of the third molars close to their roots. Emerged third molars cannot become mesially angulated when the apical areas have not been increased sufficiently in the distal direction by apposition of bone posteriorly at the tuberosity. Indeed, the apices of permanent maxillary first and second molars will not become displaced distally until the bulky crowns of the molars distal to them have descended and are replaced by their narrow tapering roots. In a boy aged 12 years 4 months, the permanent maxillary first molars were not mesially angulated, and the second molars were still distally angulated (A, B). At the end of the orthodontic treatment, at the age of 14 years 7 months, the maxillary third molars were in close proximity to the roots of the second molars, which were still distally angulated (C, D). Not until the third molars had erupted completely, at the age of 18 years 10 months, could the second molars change in angulation (E, F). Three years later, the third molars were also mesially angulated (G, H).

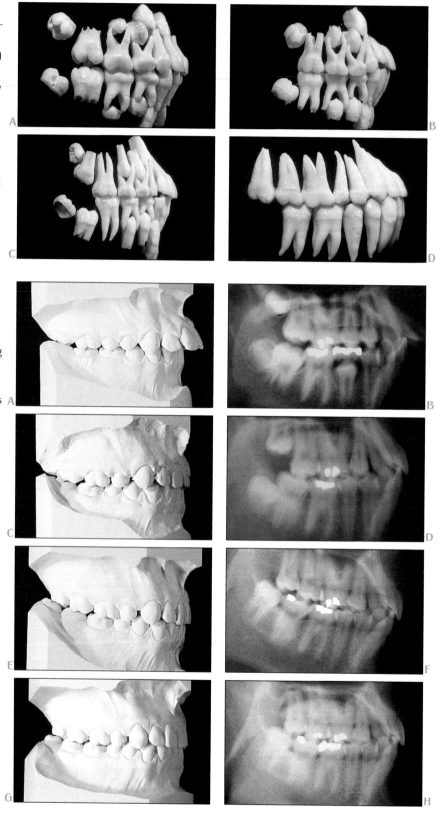

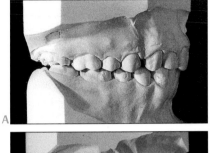

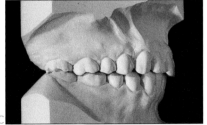

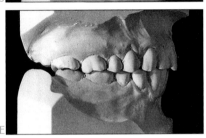

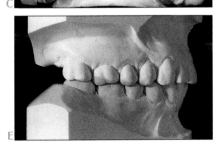

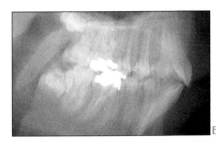

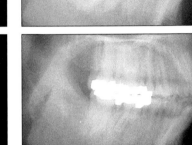

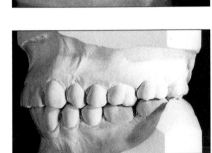

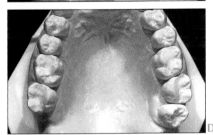

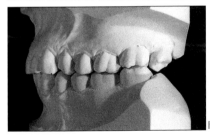

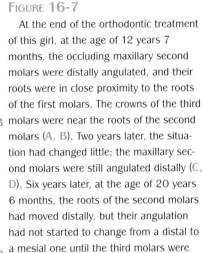

FIGURE 16-7

At the end of the orthodontic treatment of this girl, at the age of 12 years 7 months, the occluding maxillary second molars were distally angulated, and their roots were in close proximity to the roots of the first molars. The crowns of the third molars were near the roots of the second molars (A, B). Two years later, the situation had changed little; the maxillary second molars were still angulated distally (C, D). Six years later, at the age of 20 years 6 months, the roots of the second molars had moved distally, but their angulation had not started to change from a distal to a mesial one until the third molars were removed 2 years previously (E, F).

FIGURE 16-8

In this previously orthodontically treated woman, the maxillary third molars had emerged without sufficient space in the dental arch, particularly on the right side, as revealed by the records collected at the age of 26 years 2 months. The right second molar was angulated distally; the left second molar was oriented almost perpendicular to the occlusal plane (A–C). Shortly after these casts were prepared, the maxillary right third molar was removed. Three years later, both maxillary second molars were angulated mesially (D–F). These illustrations, like the ones presented in Fig 16-7, show that the mesial angulation of the permanent maxillary second molars develops rather late. The early establishment of a mesial angulation through orthodontic means should not be attempted when third molars are present and their crowns are in close proximity to the roots of the second molars. In such cases, give nature a chance.

FIGURE 16-9

A boy 11 years 7 months of age had a Class II division 1 malocclusion with a disto-occlusion of half a premolar crown width on the right side and one-quarter premolar crown width on the left side. There was crowding in the maxilla, where the anterior teeth were displaced to the right side. The maxillary right canine had emerged in a buccal position, and the right lateral incisor was palatally located. The mandibular anterior teeth were malaligned, and the right canine was positioned too far lingually (A–D). In 6 months, a neutro-occlusion was reached on both sides, the midline deviation was corrected, and space was created for the right canine with an asymmetric headgear and a Crefcoeur appliance. Subsequently, edgewise appliances were used only in the maxilla for 9 months. After an active treatment of 1 year 3 months, a Van der Linden retainer was used for 18 months (see Fig 13-10). No appliances were used in the mandible. Nevertheless, at 13 years 1 month of age, when the appliances in the maxilla were removed, the mandibular incisors had arrived at the proper locations and the right canine was almost corrected (E–H). At the age of 20 years 2 months, 5 years after the end of the retention, the mandibular right canine had arrived at the proper location (I–L). These dental casts suggest that the occlusion has an influence on the positions of the anterior teeth. The deviating position of the maxillary incisors initially prevented a good alignment of the mandibular anterior teeth (B, D). These teeth improved spontaneously in position after the disruptive occlusal contacts had been eliminated (F, H). However, it took the right canine longer than it took the incisors to arrive at the proper location (J, L).

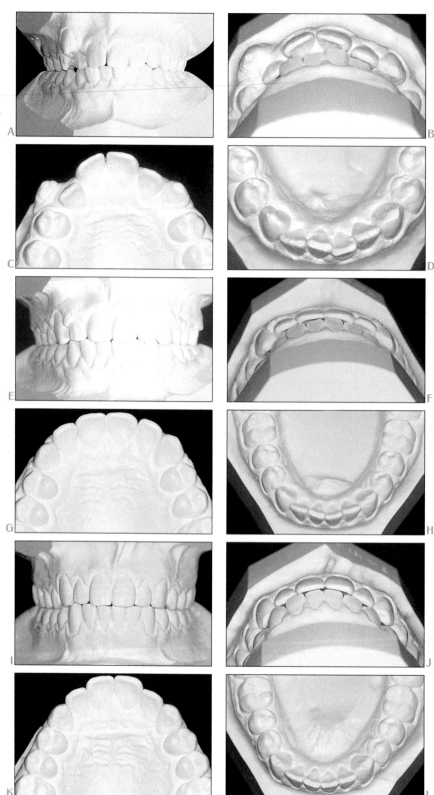

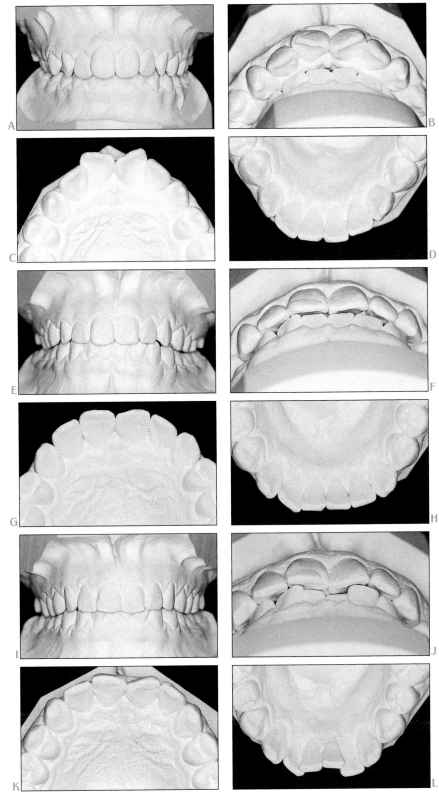

FIGURE 16-10

A boy aged 11 years 2 months had a Class II division 1 malocclusion with a disto-occlusion of one premolar crown width and an overjet of 8 mm. He had crowding in the maxillary dental arch, where the central incisors and canines were rotated. The mandibular anterior teeth were well aligned and not in contact with the maxillary incisors (A–D). He was treated with a cervical headgear and a removable plate in the maxilla. In a later phase, brackets were placed on the canines for rotational purposes, and sectional archwires were inserted, extensions of which were hooked under the labial archwires of the plate. At 13 years 4 months of age, after 2 years of treatment, an acceptable result was reached. The anterior teeth were in maximal occlusal contact, and only the mandibular right lateral incisor was slightly rotated (E–H). A maxillary retention plate was worn day and night for 6 months. For the following year it was worn during sleep, initially 7 nights a week; in the last 4 months, use was gradually reduced to 1 night a week. Two years after the retention ended, the overbite had increased, and the maxillary incisors had rotated slightly. Five years after the end of retention, at the age of 20 years 4 months, the corrected rotation of the maxillary central incisors had relapsed approximately 50%. The maxillary canines had not rotated back to their initial positions. The rotation of the maxillary central incisors was not considered a problem by the patient or his parents, but they were concerned about the severe malalignment of the mandibular incisors, because the central incisors had moved far lingually (I–L). The relapse of the rotation of the maxillary central incisors and the increase in overbite most likely resulted in the malalignment of the mandibular incisors by allowing them to occlude on the marginal ridges of the opposing maxillary teeth.

FIGURE 16-11

A girl 9 years 7 months of age had a Class II division 1 malocclusion with a disto-occlusion of one premolar crown width and sufficient space in both dental arches (A, B, G). After a treatment of 2 years 6 months with a cervical headgear and complete edgewise appliances, a maxillary retention plate was used for 1 year 6 months. In the mandible, a classic canine bar was cemented. It was removed at 15 years 6 months of age (C, D, H). An excellent treatment result was obtained; there were broad occlusal contacts between the well-aligned incisors. However, in later years, the maxillary central incisors rotated slightly, and some irregularities developed in the mandibular incisor region, as was revealed by the records made 13 years postretention (E, F, I, J). In hindsight, detailed inspection of the dental casts collected over many years raised the question of how extensive the late changes in the mandibular incisor positions would have been if the maxillary incisors had not had marginal ridges. The rotation of the maxillary central incisors probably led to the mesiolingual rotation of the mandibular central incisors after these teeth started to ride on the marginal ridges of the maxillary incisors when the overbite increased. The position of the mandibular lateral incisors is obviously also related to the contacts with the marginal ridges of their opposing teeth (I).

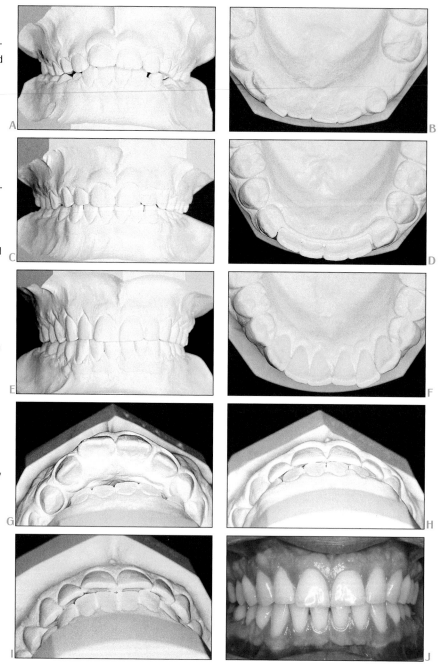

It is generally accepted that a solid intercuspation in the posterior regions secures the position of the premolars and molars. However, little or no attention has been paid to the effect of occlusion on the stability of tooth positions in the anterior region. That applies to natural changes in tooth position with aging as well as to relapses after orthodontic treatment. Although extensive studies have been carried out regarding alterations in anterior tooth positions, particularly of the mandibular anterior teeth, no relationship between such alterations and the occlusion has been suggested. Indeed it has been concluded repeatedly that an orthodontically realized increase in the mandibular intercanine distance is lost after treatment.[116-118] However, a decrease in mandibular intercanine distance has also been observed in untreated individuals with normal occlusions who developed crowding in the mandibular anterior region at a later age.[133]

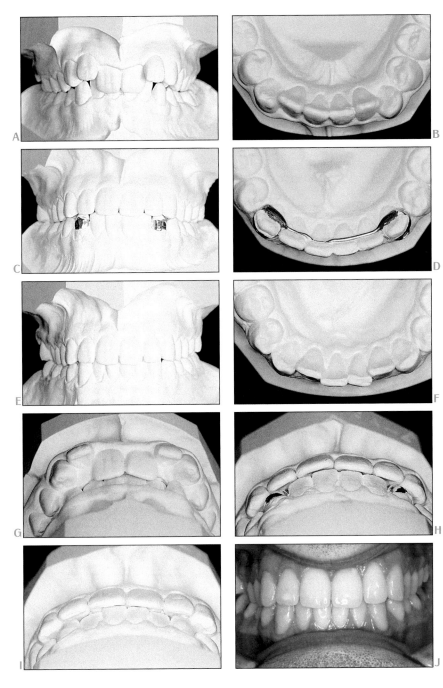

FIGURE 16-12

A boy 13 years 6 months of age had a Class II division 2 malocclusion with a disto-occlusion of three-quarter premolar width (A, B, G). He was treated with a cervical headgear, a maxillary plate, a lingual arch, and standard edgewise appliances. The active treatment lasted 2 years exactly. Subsequently, a retention plate was used in the maxilla for 18 months. In the mandible, a canine bar was placed; it was removed at the age of 18 years 2 months. At that time, the maxillary and mandibular teeth were ideally aligned, and there was only a slight overbite (C, D, H). More than 17 years later, at the age of 35 years 4 months, the position of the maxillary incisors seemed not to have changed. However, the overbite had increased, and the mandibular incisors were positioned irregularly (E, F, I, J). This patient had tight contacts between the mandibular and maxillary anterior teeth, and marginal ridges at the maxillary incisors. These ridges did not extend to the incisal edges but ended a few millimeters more cervically. At the end of the retention, there were broad surface contacts between the labioincisal edges of the mandibular incisors and the palatal surfaces of their opposing teeth (H). However, with the increase in the overbite, the mandibular anterior teeth started to ride on the marginal ridges of the maxillary anterior teeth, leading to a lingual movement of the mandibular lateral incisors (F, I).

Likewise, the cause-effect relationship can be turned around and it can be hypothesized that the occurrence of irregularities in incisor positions causes the reduction in intercanine width. Indeed, irregularities in the mandibular anterior region can be attributed as much, or even better, to riding at the marginal ridges of the maxillary incisors (Figs 16-9 and 16-10).[58, 218]

In many patients at the conclusion of retention, the incisal edges of the mandibular anterior teeth do not have broad contacts with the palatal surfaces of the opposing teeth. Even if they have broad contacts immediately after treatment, they may be changed to point contacts with the marginal ridges when the overbite increases. It is likely that irregularities in the mandibular anterior region that are attributed to relapse, or to late growth changes in untreated individuals, are due to this phenomenon (Figs 16-11 and 16-12).

FIGURE 16-13

Mean nonweighted Peer Assessment Rating (PAR) subscores at the start of treatment (TP), end of active treatment (T00), end of retention (T0), and up to 20 years postretention (T2 –T20) for variables derived from dental casts. (Reprinted with permission from Al Yami et al.[5])

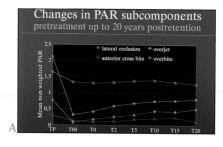

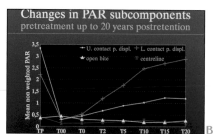

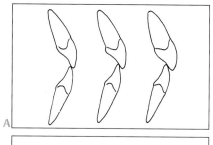

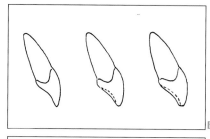

A   B

FIGURE 16-14

Incisors usually are shown in cross section, with their most labial and lingual contours (A). In 50% of white individuals, the palatal surfaces have marginal ridges in a more or less marked form.[167] The labiopalatal dimensions of the crowns can also vary considerably (B). Marginal ridges can extend to the incisal edge (C) or not as far (D). Particularly in Asian individuals, marginal ridges occur often and in a dominant form (shovel-shaped teeth).[91, 157]

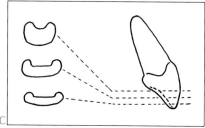

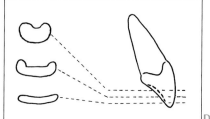

A   B

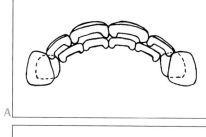

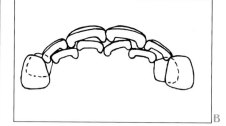

C   D

FIGURE 16-15

Marginal ridges interfere with the establishment of broad, flat occlusal contacts in an ideal arrangement of mandibular and maxillary anterior teeth (A). Irregularly arranged mandibular incisors often have greater occlusal contacts (B). In midline deviations, a mandibular central incisor can fit between the marginal ridges of a maxillary central incisor (C). Occasionally, occlusal contacts can also lead to irregularly positioned maxillary incisors, but less often than and not as markedly as in the mandible (D).

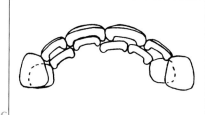

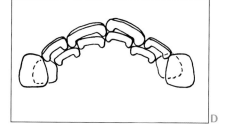

A   B

C   D

A longitudinal study of dental casts to analyze the changes during and after treatment until 20 years postretention in 2,368 patients revealed that the majority of the improvements persist in the long term.[5] On average, the occlusion in the posterior regions does not change. The correction of anterior crossbites also is, by and large, stable. However, the overjet and overbite increase slightly (Fig 16-13, A). Open bites tend to relapse partially, but corrections of midline deviations are quite stable. Improvements in the position of the maxillary anterior teeth get lost for approximately 40% of the measured change, and improvements in the mandibular anterior region dissipate completely and become even worse (Fig 16-13, B).

The morphology of anterior teeth varies considerably (Fig 16-14). The shape of the palatal surfaces of the maxillary anterior teeth determines how extensive the occlusal contacts can be and where these contacts can be located (Fig 16-15).

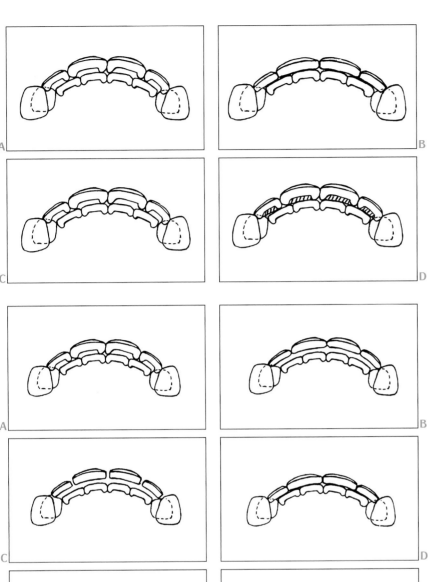

FIGURE 16-16

Pointed occlusal contacts between mandibular and maxillary incisors contribute little to stability. When the marginal ridges are ground away, broad, flat occlusal contacts can be established, increasing the stability. However, without other alterations, the overbite and overjet will increase (A, B). Broad, flat occlusal contacts also can be created by leveling the palatal surfaces with resin composite, which may be indicated when the maxillary incisors should not be positioned more palatally (C, D).

FIGURE 16-17

With the grinding of the marginal ridges, the occlusal contacts disappear (A, B). To avoid an increase in the overbite, the maxillary anterior teeth should be reduced in width and retruded. This will create larger approximal contact areas, which contribute to stability (C, D). When the maxillary incisor crowns have a triangular shape, which is not uncommon if they have marked marginal ridges, reducing the crown widths has the additional advantage of decreasing the risk of papillary recession. Removal of the marginal ridges can solve a tooth size discrepancy, which is usually due to narrow maxillary lateral incisors (E, F).

Malalignments caused by reciprocal influences through the occlusion are more apt to occur in the mandibular than in the maxillary anterior region. Maxillary anterior teeth have a larger root surface than do mandibular anterior teeth. Furthermore, the pressure from the lips on the broad labial surfaces of the maxillary incisors is a stabilizing factor. The mandibular incisors are not as continuously in a comparable contact with the tongue; in addition, their crowns are smaller.

Pointed anterior occlusal contacts can be altered into broad surface contacts in two ways. The simplest, and by far the less time-consuming, method is grinding of the marginal ridges (Figs 16-16, A and B, and 16-17). The other method involves flattening the area between the marginal ridges with resin composite; however, this method is not only more complex but also less secure (Fig 16-16, C and D).

FIGURE 16-18

A girl 12 years 5 months of age had a Class I malocclusion with crowding in both dental arches (A, B). Analysis of the dental casts indicated that the occlusion had played a role in the malalignment of the anterior teeth and that the marginal ridges had been instrumental in that respect (C, D). There was no indication for extraction of teeth, and the treatment was carried out with complete edgewise appliances. At the end of treatment it was obvious that the marginal ridges interfered with the establishment of broad, flat occlusal contacts (E), and they were ground away (F). Various stones can be used to grind marginal ridges. A ball-shaped stone offers a better view at the field of operation than does a wheel-shaped stone, and diamond stones remove enamel faster than do conventional stones (G). The grinding should be done with abundant water cooling, particularly when diamond stones are used. When marginal ridges are ground correctly, the palatal surface becomes smooth and flat (H). When all maxillary incisors are treated, and the mesial marginal ridges of the canines are ground, broad, flat occlusal contacts can be established in the anterior region. Because this patient had small maxillary lateral incisors, which is often the case with tooth size discrepancies, the maxillary anterior teeth did not have to be reduced in width (I, J).

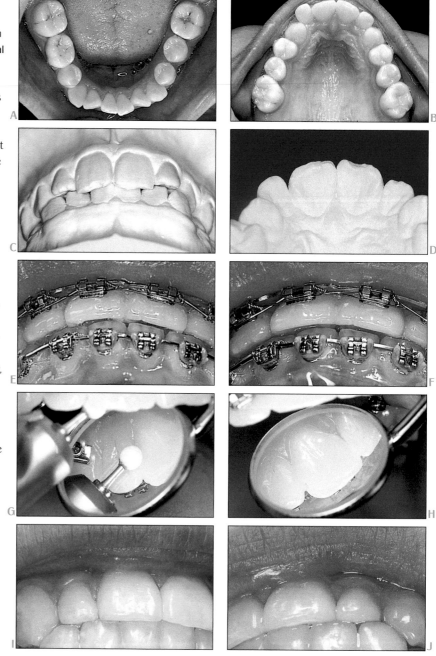

Tooth size discrepancies, like marginal ridges, are commonly encountered.[45, 75, 123, 167, 177] For the combination of both and for other variations in tooth form, Duterloo[58] introduced the term tooth size–shape discrepancy in 1991. Figures 16-18 to 16-20 show three patients who had combinations of tooth size discrepancies and marginal ridges.

As a rule, marginal ridges should not be removed before the last phase of treatment, until the mandibular incisors are aligned and the occlusion in the posterior region is as planned. At this stage, it is clear what adjustments are necessary to arrive at maximal broad, flat occlusal contacts in the anterior region. Furthermore, in that phase, it is much simpler to explain to the patient and the parents why marginal ridges should be removed and to obtain their understanding and consent.

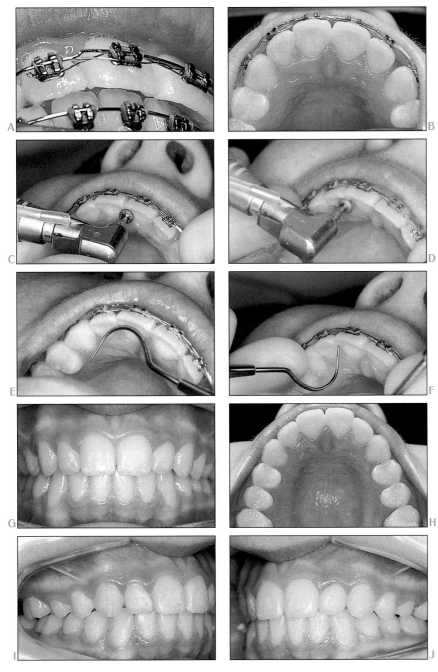

FIGURE 16-19

The girl initially had a Class II division 1 malocclusion. She was treated with a cervical headgear and complete fixed appliances. In the last phase of treatment, she had sagittal contact in the anterior region, but a diastema was still present between the maxillary left lateral incisor and canine (A, B). The marginal ridges were removed to create smooth, flat palatal surfaces, for which a small wheel-shaped diamond stone was used. With such a stone, marginal ridges can be ground through up-and-down movements over the ridges, and two adjacent ridges can easily be brought to a level plane (C, D). The stone can also be turned 90 degrees. This grinding should be done with abundant water cooling. This cooling will prevent pulpal tissues from being damaged, even during removal of a large layer of enamel.[242] The smoothness of the surfaces and their shapes can be ascertained with an explorer during and at the end of the procedure (E, F). In this patient, the removal of the marginal ridges not only resulted in broad, flat occlusal contacts but also eliminated the tooth size discrepancy. Because only the maxillary left lateral incisor was too narrow, the midline of the maxillary dental arch deviated slightly to the left side, but that was not a problem (G–J).

Marginal ridges on the maxillary anterior teeth are always combined with marginal ridges in the mandible. However, the latter do not effect the occlusion. It is not realistic to assume that flat lingual surfaces on the mandibular incisors could contribute to stability by distributing the pressure from the tongue more evenly.

More effective in increasing the stability of the mandibular anterior teeth is a change of the approximal contact points into flat broad contact surfaces. In situations with initial crowding, this method has the additional advantage of creating space, so that the intercanine distance requires no or only a slight increase. Furthermore, it corrects the often encountered tooth size discrepancy resulting from narrow maxillary lateral incisors. However, when there is no tooth size discrepancy, stripping of the mandibular anterior teeth should be combined with stripping of the maxillary anterior teeth, which often leads to better esthetics and causes smaller interproximal areas to be filled by the papillae.

FIGURE 16-20

A girl with a Class II division 1 malocclusion and agenesis of the mandibular right second premolar had been treated with transplantation of the maxillary left second premolar to the location of the agenesis and extraction of the maxillary right first premolar. Subsequently, a cervical headgear, a maxillary removable plate, and complete edgewise appliances were used to realize the corrections (A, B). At the age of 19 years 10 months, 2 years after use of the retention plate in the maxilla ended, there were diastemata in the maxillary anterior region. With the slight increase in the overbite, the mandibular anterior teeth had come in contact with the marginal ridges. The mandibular anterior teeth, still retained with a bonded canine bar, were not displaced (C, D). The marginal ridges were ground away. When the patient was examined again 4 months later, the maxillary incisors had moved palatally because of pressure from the lips at their labial surfaces. However, the diastemata had not been closed completely (E, F). Eighteen months later, at the age of 21 years 8 months, all diastemata were closed and the maxillary incisors were in contact with the labioincisal edges of the mandibular anterior teeth; overall, there were broad, flat occlusal contacts (G–J). Had the marginal ridges not been removed, most likely the mandibular anterior teeth would have become displaced after removal of the mandibular retention wire.

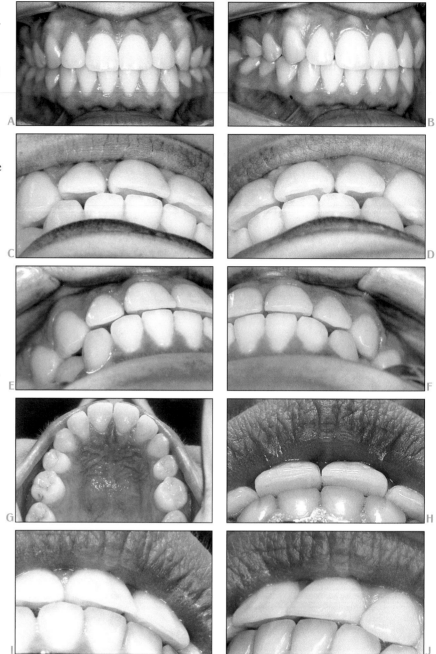

After a successful orthodontic treatment, the ideal arrangement of the anterior teeth can fade when the mandibular incisors start to ride the maxillary marginal ridges. Timely detection of these pointed contacts makes it possible to take measures to improve the stability (Fig 16-20).

Furthermore, attention to the occlusal contacts in the anterior region should not be limited to the situation at the end of treatment. Future changes that may develop when the overbite and overjet increase must also be considered. Hence, marginal ridges should be removed more cervically than the contact level.

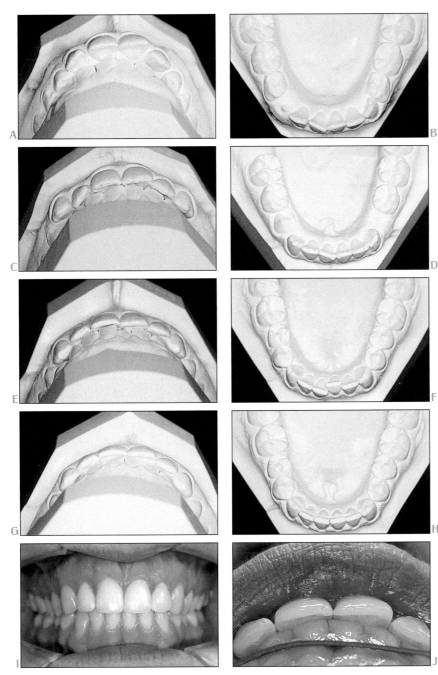

Figure 16-21

A girl with a Class II division 1 malocclusion and irregularly positioned maxillary anterior teeth was treated with an activator that was replaced by a cervical headgear and a maxillary plate later. In the last phase of treatment, brackets were placed on the maxillary incisors (A, B). Prior to the placement of these brackets, the slight irregularities that had existed in the mandibular anterior regions had improved spontaneously (C, D). After the successful completion of the active treatment at the age of 15 years 2 months, a Van der Linden retainer was used for a period of 1 year 6 months. Ten years later, the initial rotation of the maxillary central incisors had returned slightly. Furthermore, the mandibular incisors were riding at the marginal ridges of the maxillary incisors and had become malaligned. It was assumed that these two events were associated (E, F). It was decided to correct the irregularities of the mandibular anterior teeth and to create the space needed for alignment by stripping the approximal surfaces of the incisors and the mesial surfaces of the canines. The stripping was carried out manually with diamond strips. Subsequently, partial fixed appliances were used in the mandible. In addition, the marginal ridges of the maxillary anterior teeth were ground away. Through contact with the well-aligned mandibular anterior teeth, the position of the maxillary incisors improved spontaneously (G–J).

The occlusal reciprocal interaction in the anterior region results in an adjustment of the positions of the mandibular anterior teeth to the positions of the maxillary anterior teeth. The other way around, the effect is limited. However, when the mandibular anterior teeth cannot move, because they are fixed by a retention wire, the maxillary anterior teeth might become malaligned. They can start to rotate, guided by the pointed contacts at their marginal ridges. On the other hand, spontaneous improvements of maxillary teeth can occur when pointed contacts are altered into broad, flat occlusal contacts (Fig 16-21).

FIGURE 16-22

The continuity of the dental arches is maintained when the mesiodistal dimensions of the teeth gradually become reduced by attrition. The approximal contacts are maintained by (1) forces generated by occlusion; (2) forces exerted by the buccal musculature; and (3) forces generated by the supra-alveolar fibers. The occlusal forces (A) can be resolved in vectors along the long axes of teeth and in the mesial and transverse directions (B). Posterior teeth are mesially angulated and have a lingual inclination in the mandible and a buccal inclination in the maxilla (C).[136] The supra-alveolar fibers pull the teeth together (D).

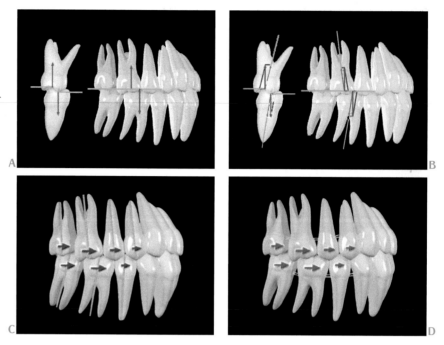

Of course, the grinding of marginal ridges and the removal of approximal enamel should be performed with care. Large, flat contact areas contribute more to stability than do pointed contacts; however, they are more vulnerable to dental caries.

The occlusion is also important for maintaining approximal contacts and the continuity of the dental arch. Even with extensive reduction of mesiodistal crown dimensions through attrition, approximal contacts are preserved. This phenomenon is partly based on the mesial component of forces generated by occlusion (Fig 16-22).[136]

The occlusion in the posterior region plays a special role in the development of the dentition and subsequently in the reinforcement of the transverse and sagittal occlusions. When orthodontic treatment is concluded without the establishment of a solid intercuspation in the posterior regions, the changes in the occlusion realized by treatment will not be stable. Stability can only be expected when premolars and permanent canines are in solid intercuspation.

The occlusion in the anterior region is relevant in the last phase of the development of the dentition and particularly in attaining broad, flat anterior occlusal contacts at the end of treatment. The occlusion in the anterior region also plays an important role in the alterations that occur after retention has been concluded and in the natural changes that occur with aging in individuals who never have been treated orthodontically.

Correction of Incisors in Adults

Because of periodontal breakdown and alterations in the forces generated by the soft tissues, anterior teeth can start to migrate with aging, resulting in an unpleasant appearance.

Migrations can occur in elderly people with an ideal occlusion but occur predominantly in individuals with a Class II division 1 malocclusion. Even with the availability of orthodontic care, patients with Class II division 1 malocclusions are not always treated at a young age, particularly when the teeth are well aligned, the disto-occlusion is not severe, and the lips are competent. Furthermore, Class II division 1 malocclusions are less obvious and less disturbing in adults than in youngsters. With the maturation of the face and subsequent aging, the soft tissues will camouflage the malocclusion. In addition, because of the lengthening of the upper lip, the maxillary incisors become less visible. These patients often have accepted their malocclusion and feel no need to have it corrected.

However, when in later years the maxillary anterior teeth migrate labially, diastemata develop, and vertical malalignments occur, treatment is often desired. A compromise treatment, by which the secondarily developed deviations are corrected in a simple way, can restore a lost feeling of well-being and self-esteem. In the majority of these cases, the patient does not request that the practitioner carry out a comprehensive treatment and correct the primary malocclusion. That usually is not the patient's complaint; rather, he or she only seeks the correction of the secondary deviations.

Indeed, disturbing migrations can have a great psychological impact and affect the patient's behavior. Spontaneous laughter may be suppressed, and a hand may be held in front of the mouth when the patient is speaking. The correction of the disturbing tooth positions is a great service to these patients and does not involve reaching an ideal occlusion.

This chapter explains the use of a removable plate and elastics to correct unattractive tooth positions of maxillary anterior teeth.

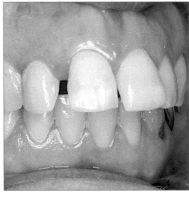
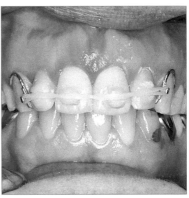
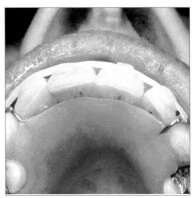
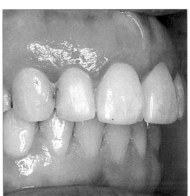

Orthodontic Concepts and Strategies

17

FIGURE 17-1

The mandibular incisors and the lower lips support the maxillary incisors vertically and counteract further eruption. In addition, the lower lip resists the labial movement of the maxillary incisors by partially covering their labial surfaces (2 to 3 mm). The upper lip, which covers the greater part of the maxillary incisors, also prevents their labial movement (A). In Class II division 1 malocclusions with a disto-occlusion of half a premolar crown width, the overbite and overjet are increased, but the lower lip still supports the maxillary incisors vertically. However, the lower lip will be positioned also partly lingual to the maxillary incisors (B). In Class II division 1 malocclusions with a disto-occlusion of one premolar width, the overjet is so great that the lower lip will be positioned mostly lingual to the maxillary incisors (C) or will be "trapped" behind the maxillary incisors (D). Particularly in the latter situation, maxillary incisors can be displaced labially by the lower lip and overerupt.

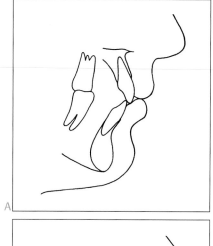
A
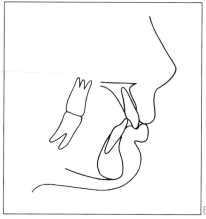
B
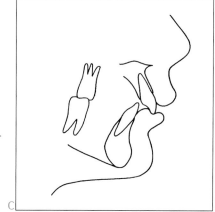
C
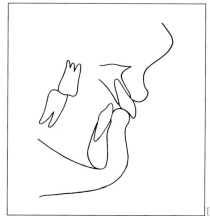
D

FIGURE 17-2

The pressure from the tongue on the anterior teeth is greater than the pressure from the lips. Normally, the alveolar bone and the periodontium provide sufficient resistance to prevent a labial movement of the maxillary incisors (A).[165] With resorption of the marginal alveolar bone and the associated loss of periodontal attachment, the equilibrium becomes disturbed, and the maxillary incisors will move labially and erupt further (B).

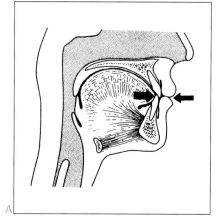
A
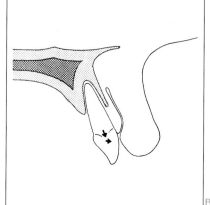
B

The position of the mandibular and maxillary incisors depends on the maxillomandibular relationship, the occlusion, and the position of the tongue and lips at rest. Normally, the tongue is positioned within the dental arches and in contact with the lingual surfaces of the mandibular and maxillary anterior teeth. The lower lip rests against the labial surfaces of the mandibular incisors and the incisal edges of the maxillary incisors (Fig 17-1).

With aging, the upper lip lengthens, and the level at which the lips are in contact (stomion) descends. In addition, the muscle tone alters, and the lips become thinner.[232] These changes can contribute to a disturbance in the equilibrium of the forces on the maxillary incisors and result in tooth migrations (Fig 17-2).

Root resorptions arising from orthodontic treatment occur more frequently in adults than in children. In addition, some marginal bone is often lost in adults, particularly with the intrusion of teeth that are not free of plaque (Fig 17-3).[55, 81, 121, 145]

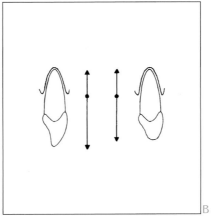

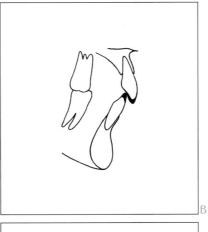

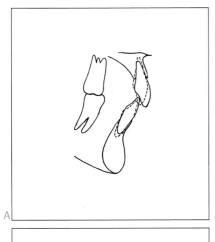

FIGURE 17-3

With intrusion of teeth, the amount of the root that is periodontally attached is reduced by apical root resorption at one side and by loss of marginal bone at the other side. Consequently, the ratio between the attached part of the root and the unattached part worsens (A). With incisal grinding, the unattached part of the root is reduced, rather than the attached part, so the ratio improves (B).

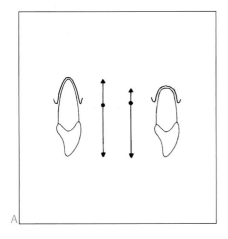

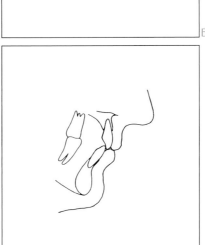

FIGURE 17-4

Labial migration of maxillary incisors is associated not only with their overeruption but also with overeruption of mandibular incisors, so that the overjet and overbite increase (A). Orthodontic movement of the displaced teeth to their previous positions has disadvantages and involves risks.[66, 115, 135] Often the best approach is to shorten the mandibular anterior teeth and to grind the maxillary incisors palatally and incisally (B). Through this removal of tooth material, space is created to retract the maxillary anterior teeth. Subsequently, the overeruption of the mandibular anterior teeth should be prevented (C). The maxillary incisor will tip palatally and become more upright, with slightly more inferiorly positioned incisal edges. After treatment, the lips will be positioned correctly, which contributes to the stability of the improved tooth positions (D).

Especially in periodontally compromised patients—and these are often the ones who have disturbing tooth migrations—comprehensive and lengthy orthodontic treatments should be avoided. Intrusion of mandibular incisors is impossible without the use of fixed appliances, and such treatments are protracted. The same holds true for the intrusion of maxillary incisors. However, when the crowns of the mandibular incisors are shortened and the maxillary incisors are ground incisally, tooth corrections can be limited to the maxillary anterior teeth and carried out through simple means in a short period of time. In addition, grinding can eliminate irregular incisal edges (Fig 17-4). Such treatment can be carried out not only in a short period of time but also with limited discomfort and minimal visibility of orthodontic appliances. The goal can be reached through the use of a maxillary removable plate and elastics, which deliver the appropriate forces. The limitation of this approach is that only tipping movements can be realized; however, in most patients, that suffices (Fig 17-5).

FIGURE 17-5

The shortening of the mandibular anterior teeth and the grinding of the maxillary incisors should not be carried out before the plate, which should be thin in the anterior region, is available (A). When the plate is inserted, occlusion of the mandibular anterior teeth at the acrylic resin will prevent the posterior teeth from reaching occlusion (B). The labial surfaces of the mandibular anterior teeth are scratched with a sharp instrument (scaler B) to mark the region where the teeth touch the plate. Subsequently, the acrylic resin is trimmed away posterior to that line to allow the mandibular incisors to occlude further superiorly. After these preliminary steps have been taken, the mandibular anterior teeth are shortened to the desired length. If the posterior teeth do not make occlusal contact yet, the groove for the mandibular teeth should be deepened or widened. Subsequently, the maxillary incisors are ground (C). The groove for the mandibular anterior teeth and the area behind the maxillary incisors, where their labial surfaces have been ground, are filled with quick-curing acrylic resin. After the acrylic resin has hardened, excess is removed, and the surface where the mandibular incisors occlude is trimmed to a smooth plateau (D). Subsequently, the maxillary incisors are built up with resin composite slots to guide the elastics. The acrylic resin behind the maxillary incisors is trimmed away where they have to move palatally (E). After all corrections have been realized, a retention plate is provided. It is to be worn day and night for 6 months and subsequently only during sleep to prevent relapse (F).

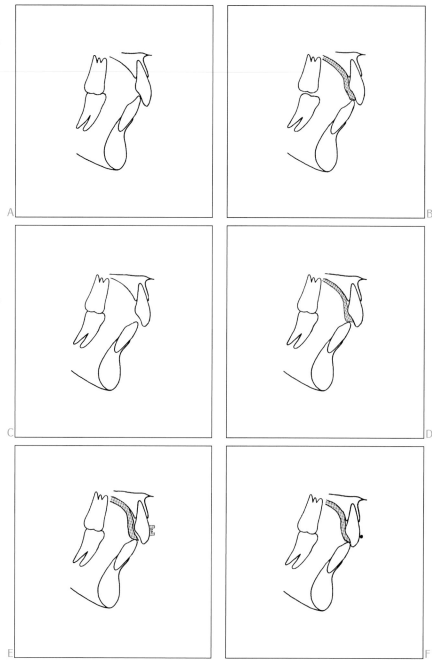

The orthodontic treatment of periodontally compromised patients has to be preceded by initial periodontal therapy, followed by a healthy period of 6 months. During orthodontic treatment, regular bimonthly professional cleaning should be arranged.

Dental casts can be examined to estimate how much of the mandibular and maxillary incisors should be ground away. In a dentition with an anterior open bite or non-occlusion, shortening of the mandibular incisors is usually not needed. The maxillary anterior teeth can be retruded even further than their initial positions when the mesiodistal crown dimensions are reduced. This reduction in tooth material can substantially improve the result, particularly in Class II division 1 malocclusions. The same also applies to arriving at well-aligned anterior teeth in situations with initial crowding.

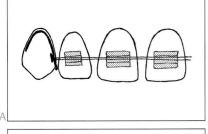

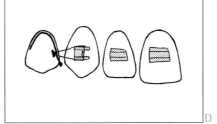

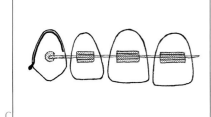

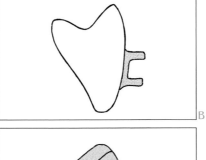

FIGURE 17-6

A three-quarter clasp that encompasses the canine from the mesial direction works well (A). Less desirable is a clasp coming from the distal direction; such a clasp should have a firm grip on the canine and not become displaced when the elastic is attached (B). When visibility is to be avoided, a small resin composite ball with an undercut at the distal side can serve as a hook at a tooth firmly anchored with a clasp (C). When a canine has to be moved distally, the clasp with a hook for the elastic can be placed at the first premolar (D).

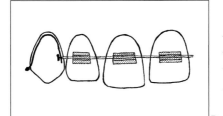

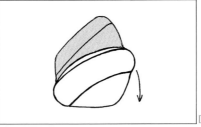

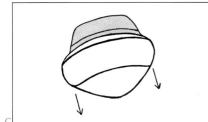

FIGURE 17-7

To guide the elastics, resin composite slots are bonded at the labial surfaces of the incisors (A, B). The proper places for the guiding slots should have been determined beforehand by attachment of the elastic. When the tooth has to be retracted without rotation, the slot should be parallel to the labial surface (C). When a tooth has to be rotated, the slot should extend at the side that should receive the greater force (D).

The elastic should extend in a straight line and not be used to correct vertical malalignments. Differentiated selective grinding is more effective and does not involve unwanted vertical movements of adjacent teeth by reaction forces, as would elastics. However, elastics are well-suited for moving teeth in a mesiodistal direction.

Preference should be given to placing the hooks for the elastics on three-quarter clasps, which encompass the canines from the mesial direction with a firm grip. The shorter the piece of wire between the hook and the site where it is embedded in the acrylic resin, the less likely the clasp will deform. In addition, the clasp will block the mesial movement of the canine (Fig 17-6).

An important advantage of the use of tooth-colored elastics and of resin composite for guidance purposes is that both materials are barely visible. Most patients accept the appliance readily, because it does not cause much discomfort and does not interfere with the occlusion.

Without the use of guiding slots, elastics tend to move cervically. In addition, without guiding slots, tooth movements are difficult to control, and mesiodistal movements cannot be carried out (Fig 17-7).

FIGURE 17-8

The elastics should exert small forces, especially when roots are attached only for a small part of their length. For a very light force, two long, thin elastics (Ormco, Eagle, 7B (five-eighths inch) 2 oz) can be connected (A). For rotations, the margin of the plate should be in a pointwise contact at the one side of the crown, and the resin composite slot should extend at the other side (B). Lateral incisors are particularly difficult to rotate without these one-sided extended buildups (C). With an additional elastic, a tooth can be moved in the mesiodistal direction (D).

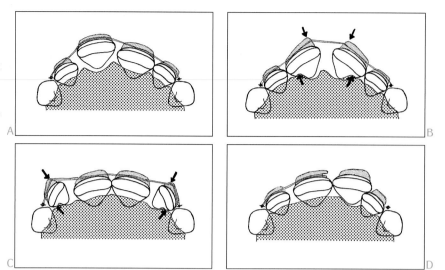

FIGURE 17-9

In this patient, the maxillary anterior teeth were reduced in width to retrude them further. Hooks for elastics have been welded at three-quarter clasps coming from the mesial side. Even without guiding slots, the elastics extended across a broad area of the crowns and stayed in place, because the hooks were positioned correctly for that purpose (A, B). In addition, the resin composite hook placed at the right central incisor to move that tooth distally held the long elastic in place (C). The incisal edges have not yet been ground to improve the vertical alignment (D).

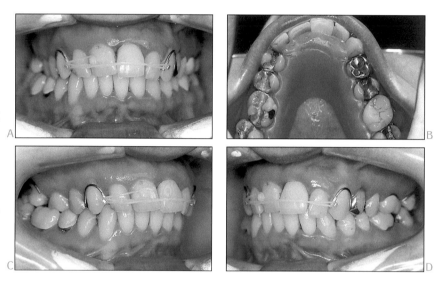

For a controlled movement of teeth, the forces from the elastic on the one side and the contact between the margin of the plate and the palatal surfaces of the maxillary incisors on the other side should be coordinated (Fig 17-8). Where teeth have to move palatally, the acrylic resin has to be trimmed not only at the crowns but also at the area where the alveolar process had to be rebuilt (Fig 17-5, E).

Rotational movements require contact between the plate and the tooth at the corner that should not move palatally as well as an extra thickness of the slot on the side of the tooth that should move palatally. Without these modifications, rotations are difficult to realize (Fig 17-7, D).

Where teeth have to be moved in the mesiodistal direction, the margin of the plate should be smooth and provide guidance (Fig 17-9).

The correct trimming of the margin of the plate is essential for successful treatment. It is often difficult to detect where the plate is touching and whether it is free at the right spots. For a good assessment, observation from different angles, with and without a mouth mirror, is helpful. Lifting the plate slightly also helps. In addition, careful pushing against a tooth will reveal if the tooth is in contact with the plate, because the tooth will move when there is space. These aspects should also be checked while the patient is biting on the plate.

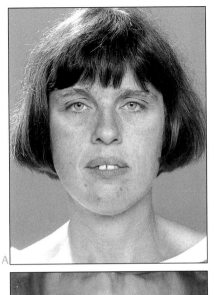

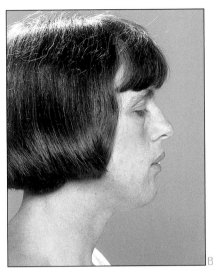

Figure **17-10**

This 40-year-old woman with a Class II division 1 malocclusion had an open mouth posture (A, B). She held her lower lip at rest behind the maxillary anterior teeth, which were labially displaced and had diastemata between them. However, the large overjet was not combined with a deep bite (C–F). Tongue interpositioning had interfered with the eruption of the mandibular anterior teeth.

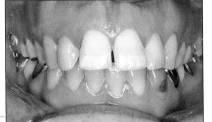

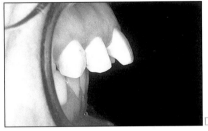

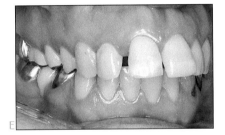

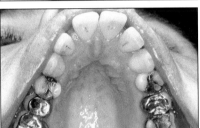

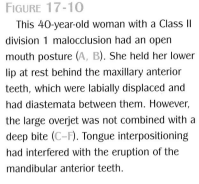

When a large overjet is combined with an anterior open bite or non-occlusion, the mandibular incisors do not have to be shortened, because enough space is available to retract the maxillary incisors. When the maxillary incisors have overerupted, and particularly when they have long clinical crowns, the grinding of their incisal edges will facilitate the treatment and improve the result (Figs 17-10 and 17-11).

In Class II division 1 malocclusions, further retraction of the maxillary incisors after the diastemata have been closed is often desirable. The extra space needed can be obtained by removing enamel from the approximal surfaces of the incisors and the mesial sides of the canines. Diamond strips (Horico strips, Pfingst, South Plainfield, New Jersey) can be used for this stripping of anterior teeth. These strips provide good control of the amount of enamel that is removed and of the remaining contour of the tooth. Additional interproximal stripping is usually needed at the end of treatment to obtain satisfactory approximal contact areas.

The esthetics of the anterior teeth can be improved not only by grinding but also by buildup with resin composite. With a combination of both techniques, satisfying results can be obtained. However, in periodontally compromised patients, resin composite must be applied with care at the cervical regions.

FIGURE 17-11

After a treatment of 7 months, an adequate result was obtained. Although the maxillary incisors were retracted extensively, no competent lip seal had developed (A, B). When that is the case, retention is of particular importance. The crowns of the maxillary incisors had been shortened. The incisal edges of the lateral incisors purposely were located slightly more cervically than the incisal edges of the central incisors (C–F).

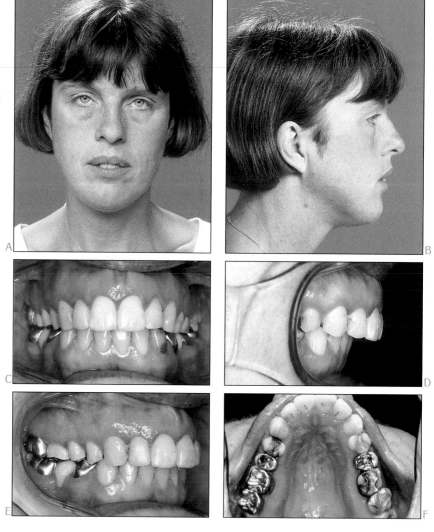

More than 10 years have passed since the patient shown in Figs 17-10 to 17-14 has been treated. She returns for reexamination once a year. The position of the teeth has not changed noticeably over these 10 years.

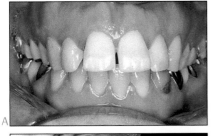

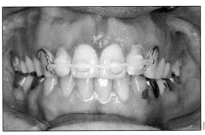

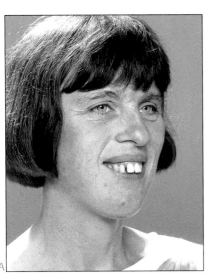

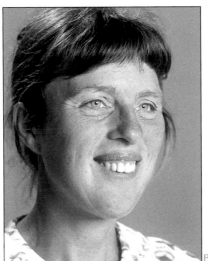

FIGURE 17-12

The maxillary central incisors were positioned far labially (A). The appliance used consisted of a maxillary acrylic resin plate with 0.8-mm-thick three-quarter clasps (C-clasps) at the last molars. The 0.7-mm three-quarter clasps around the canines came from the mesial side and secured a good fixation anteriorly (B). Hooks had been welded at the canine clasps for the elastic, which was guided by resin composite slots (C). At the end of the treatment, the plate was in contact with the anterior teeth, and only kept free from the mesial sides of the lateral incisors, which still had to be rotated (D).

FIGURE 17-13

Photographs of the smiling patient before treatment (A) and 5 years after the conclusion of active treatment (B). The result was stabilized by retention.

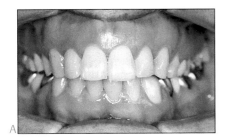

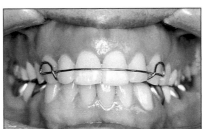

FIGURE 17-14

Intraoral photograph 5 years after the conclusion of active treatment (A). A Van der Linden retainer was still worn during sleep (B).

When the mouth is not closed at rest, retracted maxillary incisors will tend to move labially again. This relapse can only be prevented when the active treatment is followed by continuing retention.

Correction of Incisors in Adults

FIGURE 17-15

In this 38-year-old woman with a Class II division 1 malocclusion, the maxillary incisors had migrated labially, and the overbite and overjet had increased (A, B). There were diastemata between the maxillary incisors as well as distal to the right canine (C–E). Prior to orthodontic treatment, space was created distal to the left canine by grinding the restoration in the first premolar and stripping the distal surface of the canine (F).

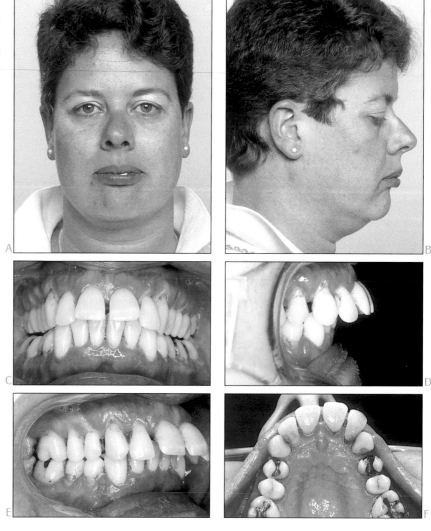

In patients with a deep bite and anterior contact, retraction of the maxillary incisors has to be preceded by creation of space in the vertical direction (Figs 17-15 and 17-16). When no other orthodontic treatment is needed, shortening of the mandibular anterior teeth is the best solution. The grinding of these teeth should be done strategically and according to the specific needs. Grinding of the labioincisal edges is most effective. The removal of extending corners can contribute substantially. The grinding should be done with abundant water cooling and is usually painless, because pulpal chambers become smaller with increasing age. Sometimes it is better to carry out the grinding over more than one visit. Limited additional grinding is often needed at the end of treatment to obtain good contacts.

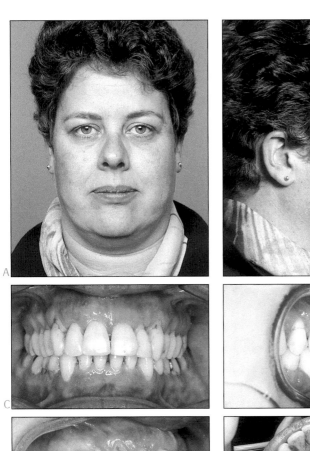

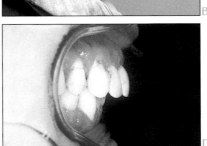

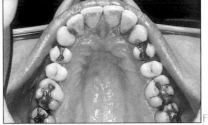

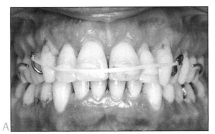

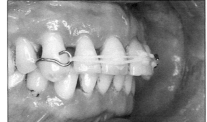

FIGURE 17-16

After 11 months' treatment, a good result was obtained. At rest, the lower lip was in contact with the labioincisal region of the maxillary incisors, and a competent lip seal had been established (A, B). All diastemata had been closed, including those distal to the canines. The inclination of the maxillary incisors was improved, and the overjet was reduced substantially (C–F).

FIGURE 17-17

In this patient, the heavy (0.8-mm) wire hooks were placed in contact with the first premolars to allow distal movement of the canines (A). In another patient, this type of hook also fulfilled a clasp function (B).

When the treatment starts with distal movement of the canines, they must be anchored firmly after arriving at the proper location. This fixation can be realized by adding acrylic resin to the margin of the plate at the palatal and mesial surfaces of the canines and by the elastic at the labial side (Fig 17-17, A). Hooks attached to the labial surfaces of the canines also can serve to secure the canines in the new position (Fig 17-17, B).

FIGURE 17-18

One of the basic rules in the use of removable appliances is that occluding on metal parts should be avoided, and the occlusion should not be disturbed (A). Furthermore, the palatal side of the cervical regions should be kept free of acrylic resin, which can easily be achieved by applying wax at the cervical borders of the dental cast prior to application of the acrylic resin. In addition, the clasps should not endanger the gingival and periodontal tissues and should not be too close to the cervical border (B). When maxillary incisors are retracted, the bite plane should prevent the mandibular anterior teeth from erupting. When the acrylic resin is trimmed from the palatal side of the maxillary incisors to create space for their palatal movement, the incisors will make a tipping movement. The rotation point will be located at approximately the midpoint of the attached part of the root (C). After a maxillary incisor has arrived at the correct position, the plate should be built up with quick-curing acrylic resin to support this tooth at the palatal side (D).

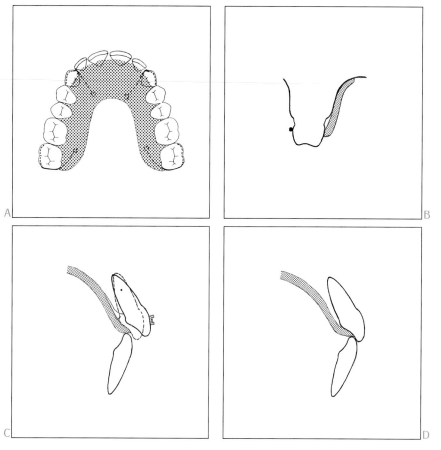

At every recall examination, the patient first should be asked about his or her experience with the appliance, before it is carefully checked. The clasps at the molars should offer sufficient retention and be positioned at the proper height of the crowns. That also applies to clasps around the canines (Fig 17-18).

The dentition and the periodontium should be inspected, and irritations caused by the plate should be noted.

In addition, the appliance and the position of the elastic should be checked while the patient is in habitual occlusion. The opposing posterior teeth should be in contact, and the plate should not move when the mandibular anterior teeth contact the bite plane. If the plate starts to tip, insufficient support is provided at the palatal and mesial surfaces of the canines and at the palatal sides of the incisors that do not have to be moved.

Furthermore, the incisors that have to be moved should not shift when the patient occludes on the plate. If they do, not enough acrylic resin has been trimmed away. There should be sufficient space between the tooth and the margin of the plate that the associated excessive tooth mobility will not develop between appointments.

The proper location of the elastic should be confirmed. The examiner must verify that appropriate forces are applied to the correct points. The elastic should not shift during speech or when the lips are moved; this shifting can occur when the resin composite slots are too shallow.

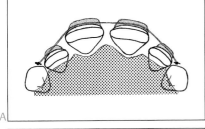
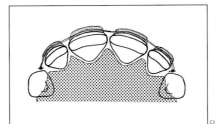

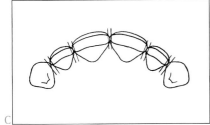
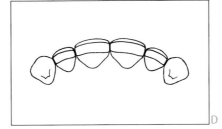

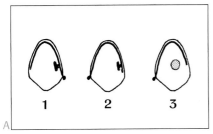
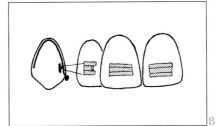

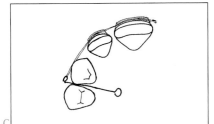
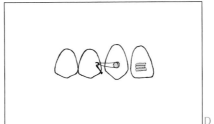

FIGURE 17-19

Incisors that are inclined labially should be retracted first, and the acrylic resin should be left in contact with the other teeth. That contact should always be maintained for teeth that are not supposed to move palatally (A). After a well-shaped arch has been established, the four incisors can be retracted at the same time (B). More space can be created in the dental arch by mesial and distal grinding of the anterior teeth (stripping) (C). In the maxilla, broad, flat contact areas contribute to stability (D).

FIGURE 17-20

A clasp that encompasses the canine from the mesial side is preferred (A1). When space between the lateral incisor and the canine is insufficient, the clasp can come from the distal direction, usually without interfering with the occlusion (A2). When visibility is a concern, a resin composite hook can be applied, provided that a clasp fixes the canine rigidly (A3). A lateral incisor is distalized (B). A hook is attached to a wire extension (C); the same method is used for retracting a canine (D).

Control over the movement of the incisors depends on the margin of the plate; the shape, size, and location of the resin composite slots; the location of the hooks; and the elastic used. The forces exerted by the elastics will vary with the degree that teeth are labially positioned. If the thickness of a guiding slot is increased, the built-up tooth will extend farther and be exposed to a substantial force. When such a tooth starts to move, the applied force will decrease, while the forces exerted on the adjacent teeth will increase (Fig 17-19). The hooks for the elastics can be placed at different locations (Fig 17-20).

Maxillary lateral incisors are smaller labiopalatally than are central incisors. Normally, the labial surfaces of the lateral incisors are located more palatally than are the labial surfaces of the central incisors. For the elastic to exert an effective force on the lateral incisors, they have to be provided with thicker resin composite slots than the central incisors.

However, resin composite guiding slots are not always needed. When teeth do not have to be rotated, and the needed correction is limited to one or two teeth, one small resin composite addition can suffice to hold the elastic in place (Fig 17-9); occasionally, none at all is necessary (Fig 17-21).

In addition to the space generated by removal of enamel from the approximal surfaces of the maxillary anterior teeth, extra space for further retraction will be gained in the sagittal direction through palatal grinding. That applies particularly to excessively thick central incisors and to incisors with artificial crowns that extend too far palatally (Fig 17-22).

FIGURE 17-21

The maxillary left central incisor was too far labially positioned in a 25-year-old woman with a neutro-occlusion (A, B). The space needed to align that tooth was created by stripping all four incisors and the mesial sides of the canines. With a removable plate combined with elastics, and without the placement of resin composite slots for guidance, an ideal arrangement was reached in a period of 6 months (C, D).

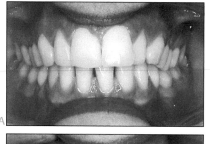
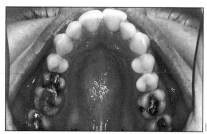
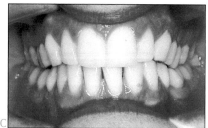
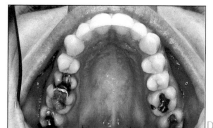

FIGURE 17-22

The maxillary incisors were too far labially positioned and inclined in a 40-year-old woman with a severe Class II division 1 malocclusion. The maxillary dental arch had a tapered shape, and the central incisors were restored with excessively thick crowns (A, B). The mesiodistal crown dimensions of the anterior teeth were reduced to create space for palatal movement of the maxillary incisors. The palatal surfaces of the crowns on the central incisors were ground to gain more space in the sagittal direction to retract these teeth further and to arrive at a better arch form (C, D).

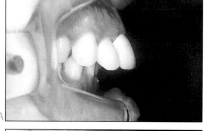
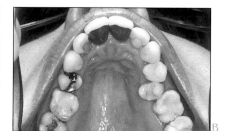
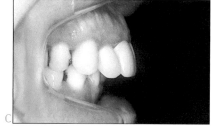
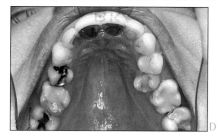

Irregularities in the positions of maxillary anterior teeth are perceived as the most disturbing orthodontic deviations. In that perception, the size of the overjet plays a limited role, as long as the teeth do not protrude too much. Particularly disturbing are diastemata, an irregular incisal line, and malalignment associated with crowding. Sometimes only one tooth is in an abnormal position, but usually more teeth are involved. Rotations can be very disturbing, especially when the arrangement allows the observer to look between the teeth.

All the aforementioned deviations can be corrected with the method presented in this chapter. Although the result might not be perfect, the complaint of the patient is solved.

In patients with these conditions, treatment usually goes smoothly, because their appearance is of great importance to them. Their compliance and cooperation are excellent, and oral hygiene is good. These patients are careful with the appliance and follow the progress with great interest.

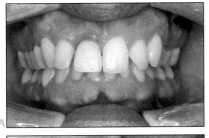

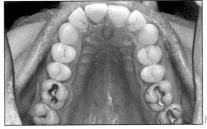

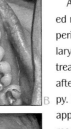

FIGURE 17-23

A 39-year-old man did not like his rotated maxillary lateral incisors. In addition, a periodontal problem existed at the maxillary right central incisor (A, B). Orthodontic treatment was not started until 6 months after the end of the initial periodontal therapy. In a period of 5 months, and with four appointments, an acceptable result was reached (C, D).

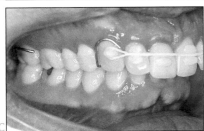

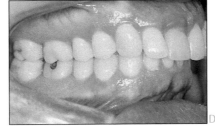

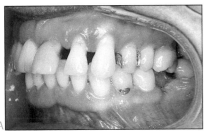

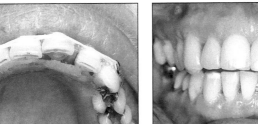

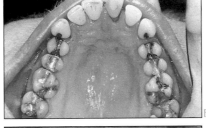

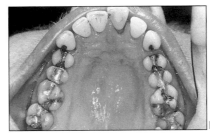

FIGURE 17-24

In a 48-year-old woman, the initially well-aligned maxillary incisors had migrated. The labially displaced left central incisor and the large diastemata were perceived as particularly disturbing (A, B). With an elastic attached to hooks welded to clasps, which did not extend to the cervical region around the canines, the anticipated result was reached (C). Subsequently, the situation was improved by building up the cervical regions with resin composite (D).

In addition to patients in whom an unacceptable situation has developed at a later age, patients with deviations that should have been treated at an early age can also benefit from the method presented (Figs 17-21 to 17-23).

Often the gingiva is receding, and open spaces are present cervically between the anterior teeth, because the papillae do not fill the interdental areas anymore. At the conclusion of orthodontic treatment, the teeth might be well aligned, but dark triangular areas may be present cervically.

This shortcoming can be perceived as disturbing when it is visible during laughter and speech. Buildup of the cervical regions with resin composite can solve this problem (Fig 17-24). As has been explained in an earlier chapter, the risk for the occurrence of receding papillae can be decreased by reduction of the mesiodistal crown dimensions and subsequent closure of the resulting interdental spaces. However, this approach is not indicated in dental arches with an excess of space.

FIGURE 17-25

In the transition to the retention phase, limited improvements can be realized directly. The wide periodontal spaces around the teeth that have been moved offer the opportunity for instant corrections. Through modifications of the plaster cast on which the retainer is made, an appliance that had the instant corrections included was fabricated (A, B). After insertion of the retention plate, the teeth involved were instantaneously forced into the desired positions (C, D).

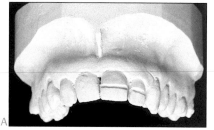
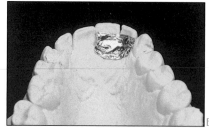
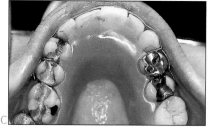
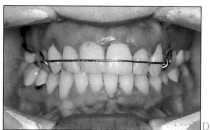

FIGURE 17-26

The instant correction procedure at the transition from the active treatment to the retention phase is shown. On the plaster cast, the teeth were slightly rotated and some space existed between the crowns and the margin of the plate (A). After insertion in the mouth, the teeth attained the proper positions instantaneously (B).

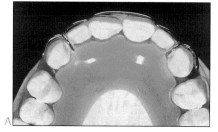
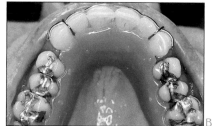

At the end of every orthodontic treatment, the periodontal spaces around the teeth that have been moved are extra wide. Consequently, these teeth exhibit increased mobility, which allows the implementation of instantaneous corrections when retention is applied (see chapter 18). Particularly in patients with extremely mobile teeth, this approach can facilitate attainment of the goal and shorten the active treatment time (Figs 17-25 and 17-26).

The type of patients presented in this chapter are the most grateful ones in a practice. Their appearance is improved considerably and the disturbing deviations are eliminated.

When the irregularities in tooth positions are caused by secondary migrations at a later age, securing the obtained result is essential and requires retention of one type or another. For this purpose, a removable plate is well suited. Such a retention plate should be worn day and night for the first 4 to 6 months and only during sleep subsequently.

A well-designed, well-fabricated, and well-applied retention plate can function effectively for many years, without allowing any loss of the obtained improvements. An examination once a year suffices to confirm stability. The theoretical and practical aspects of retention, and particularly those of a maxillary retention plate, are discussed in the next chapter.

Effective Retention

After orthodontic treatment, the periodontal structures have to adapt to the new situation and altered circumstances.[166] That applies particularly to the teeth that could not fully respond to the forces exerted by the occlusion, tongue, cheeks, and lips because they were held by the appliances. After removal of the appliances, functional influences should have the freedom to affect the position of the posterior teeth, which will lead to adjustments in the occlusion. Consequently, retention appliances should, on the one hand, leave the posterior teeth free and, on the other hand, anchor the anterior teeth, which can attain undesirable positions. Indeed, posterior teeth are three-dimensionally consolidated by the occlusion and intercuspation, and that is not the case for incisors and canines.

As explained in chapter 17, at the end of active treatment the mobility of the teeth is increased, because the periodontal spaces are wider. This phenomenon offers the opportunity to move teeth instantaneously to better positions after the removal of the appliances, through the insertion of the retainer. With the introduction of bonding, closure of remaining spaces after band removal is no longer needed. Bonding not only has facilitated the use of fixed appliances but also has opened the way for more detailed finishing and arrival at an ideal arrangement of teeth. Consequently, retention appliances are no longer required to move teeth to their final positions; they should now be used only to anchor the teeth.

The fact that it takes 4 to 6 months for periodontal structures to adapt to the new situation determines the retention protocol to a large extent. Consequently, active treatment should be followed by 24-hour daily retention for 6 months. Subsequently, the use of a removable appliance during sleep suffices. How long retention should be maintained depends on the initial malocclusion, the treatment performed, the functional conditions, the periodontal situation, the anticipated facial growth, and the wishes of the patient.

Rarely will it be indicated that the patient will have to wear a retainer for the rest of his or her life. In most instances, it is better to accept a slight relapse than to attempt permanent retention without an end in view. If needed, grinding and buildup with resin composite can camouflage subsequent changes in tooth positions.

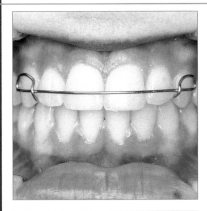

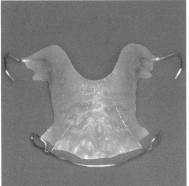

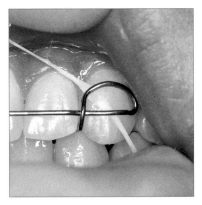

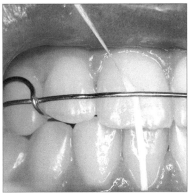

Orthodontic Concepts and Strategies

18

Effective Retention

FIGURE 18-1

In normal functional conditions, the tongue is situated at rest within the dental arches. The position of the posterior teeth depends on the width of the mandible, the occlusion, and the forces from the tongue and cheeks. The width of the maxillary dental arch adapts to the width of the mandibular dental arch, as does the maxilla itself, but to a smaller degree (A). In the anterior region, the tongue and lips lie against the teeth (B).

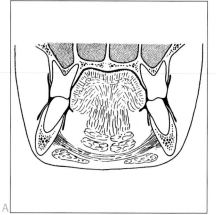
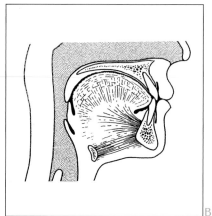

FIGURE 18-2

Opposing teeth do not overlap in an open bite (A3). In a non-occlusion, the anterior teeth do not make contact but overlap in habitual occlusion (A1, A2, B1–B3). The sizes of open bites and non-occlusions can vary considerably.

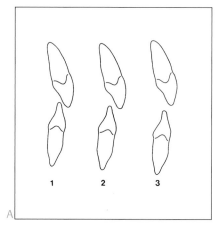
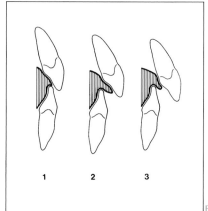

FIGURE 18-3

Open bites and non-occlusions also occur in posterior regions. In a local open bite, some teeth do not overlap, but others are in contact or in non-occlusion (A). An open bite and a non-occlusion can occur in an entire quadrant. In a total non-occlusion, whether or not combined with an open bite, there is no solid contact anywhere. Open bites and non-occlusions are mostly caused by tongue interpositioning (B).

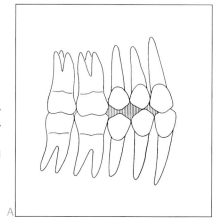
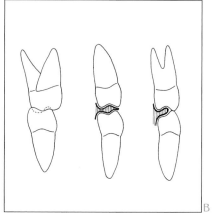

Functional aspects also play an essential role in retention, as is emphasized with illustrations shown previously in another context (Figs 18-1 to 18-3). In patients with an anterior open bite or non-occlusion, in whom irregularities in the anterior region have been corrected, retention with a thin dead-soft braided wire is the best method. Such a wire compensates for the lack of support normally provided by the occlusal contacts in the anterior region. When teeth are missing or large diastemata have been present, a bonded retention wire is the best choice. In open bites and non-occlusions, the intraoral space is relatively restricted, and a retention plate should mean an additional limitation.

As has been stated previously, the size of an open bite and a non-occlusion often reduces with aging. In one third of adolescents, spontaneous closure occurs later. The same applies to both the anterior region and the posterior regions. When an open bite or non-occlusion does not dissolve, the retention wire should be maintained for a long time (Figs 18-4 and 18-5).

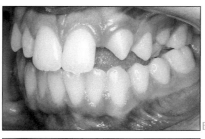

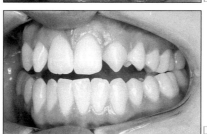

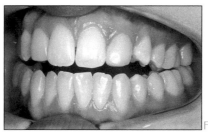

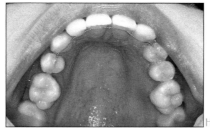

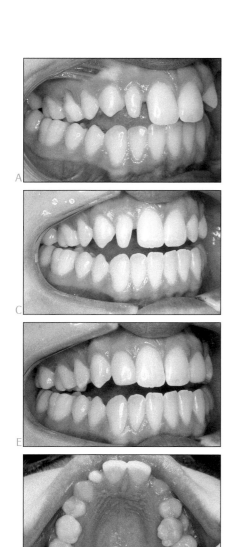

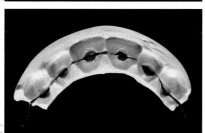

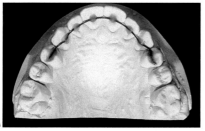

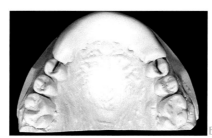

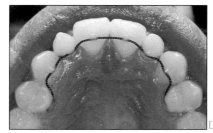

Figure 18-4

In a total non-occlusion, there is no solid intercuspation anywhere, as in this patient, shown previously (see Fig 14-15). At rest and during swallowing, the tongue is kept between the teeth, and the "cone-funnel" mechanism does not work. When the patient is asked to occlude, only some teeth make a pointwise contact (A, B). The maxillary dental arch is too narrow (G). The mandibular dental arch is broad and usually well shaped. These characteristics are caused by the position of the tongue at rest. The tongue lies against the lingual and occlusal surfaces of the mandibular teeth and is not in contact with the palate; this factor, together with the absence of intercuspation, leads to the narrow maxillary dental arch. In this patient, during treatment with fixed appliances in only the maxillary dental arch, the open bite increased (C, D). Later, the teeth were built up with resin composite (E, F). The maxillary dental arch was widened in the premolar region. The bonded 0.0175-inch dead-soft braided wire used for retention also stabilized the first premolars (H).

Figure 18-5

The thin, flexible wire is bent at the plaster cast and attached with wax where the resin composite has been placed (A). After the open areas in the silicone mold are filled with resin composite, the wire can be bonded at all teeth at the same time (B, C). The ends can also be bonded first with light-curing resin composite and can subsequently be bonded at the intervening teeth. Depending on the occlusion, the wire at the premolars has to be placed at the palatal surfaces (D) or can be located in the occlusal fissure (A).

FIGURE 18-6

The position of the molars and premolars is solidified by the occlusion. The opposing teeth stabilize each other reciprocally in the vertical, mesiodistal, and transverse directions (A). Even when the periodontal structures are severely broken down, and the teeth are extremely mobile, their position is maintained by the intercuspation. In normal circumstances, the occlusion, tongue, and cheeks should be allowed to influence the position of the teeth after removal of the orthodontic appliances, so that a solid intercuspation and a balanced position of the posterior teeth can be established. Incisors and canines are not three-dimensionally stabilized by a supporting and anchoring occlusion and can become displaced in all directions (B). If there is a good intercuspation of the posterior teeth, retention can be limited to the incisors and canines (C, D).

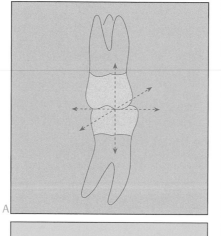
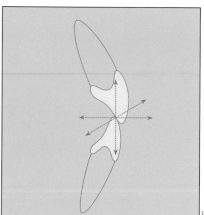
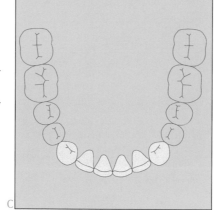
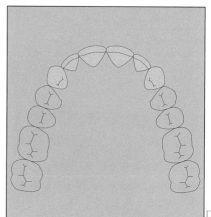

FIGURE 18-7

Maxillary incisors and canines have to be fixed with a retention device in three directions (A). They have to be supported vertically to prevent eruption, for which a removable plate that fits well and is in contact with the palatal surfaces is particularly suited. The oblique orientation of the palatal surfaces will load the teeth in the labial direction, but that can be counteracted by a stiff labial wire (B). The margin of the plate and the labial arch also prevent labiolingual movements (C). A good adaptation of the labial arch to the contours of the incisors and canines hinders mesiodistal movements and prevents the reoccurrence of rotations. The sections of the wire that pass between the lateral incisors and the canines also contribute to the stability in the mesiodistal direction (D).

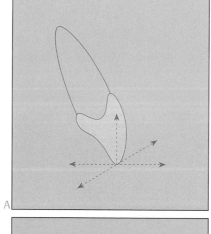
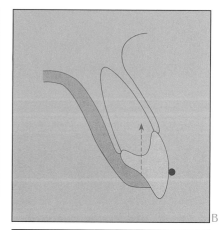
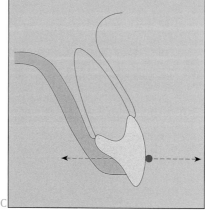
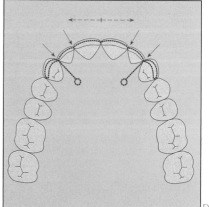

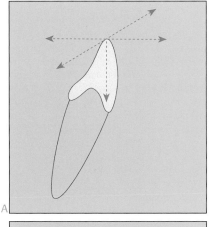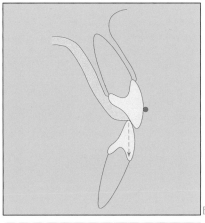

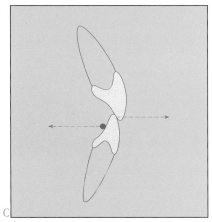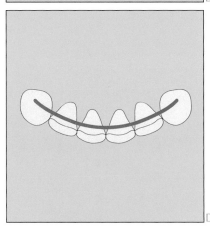

FIGURE 18-8

Mandibular incisors and canines have to be stabilized in three directions (A). Eruption can be hindered by the contact with the bite plane of the retention plate while the posterior teeth occlude (B). To that end, the plate has to be trimmed or built up with quick-curing acrylic resin and subsequently flattened. The surface should be smooth, so that transverse and sagittal excursions can be made without interferences. The labial movement is prevented through contact with the maxillary anterior teeth. A canine bar in contact with the incisors can hinder their lingual movement (C). The canine bar also hinders the mesiodistal movement (D). Depending on the initial situation, and the risk of local movements, bonding of the bar to all six anterior teeth may be required.[244]

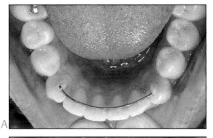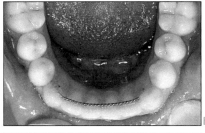

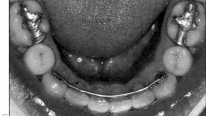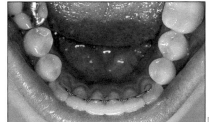

FIGURE 18-9

Retention can be provided by a canine bar of rectangular wire (0.016 × 0.022-inch), only bonded at the canines (A). A multistranded round wire (0.032-inch) is easier to adapt to the lingual surfaces than a rectangular wire (B). Preformed bars are commercially available in various lengths and usually have to be adapted slightly, but stay in place well (C). For the individual fixation of all mandibular anterior teeth, a thin dead-soft braided wire (0.015-inch) works well (D).

Molars and premolars are solidified in their position by the contacts in intercuspation, mainly during swallowing.

Under normal functional conditions, only the anterior teeth have to be retained (Fig 18-6). For that purpose, a retention plate is the best solution in the maxilla (Fig 18-7). A canine bar is preferred in the mandible (Fig 18-8). For fixed retention in the mandibular anterior region, various materials and designs have been introduced (Fig 18-9).

Figure 18-10

The wire has to be well adapted at the contours of the labial surfaces of the six anterior teeth (A). The labial arch is made of 0.7-mm-thick, round, stainless steel spring hard wire. A firm grip of the labial arch and the plate is essential for good retention, so clasps are needed. The last molars are well suited for anchorage at the posterior side. However, most important is adequate retention anteriorly, for which the canines can serve best (B). Connection of the three wire sections results in a continuous construction, which is stiff because it contains closed loops and not open loops (C). Two sections of wire cross over the canines. The cervical section has the clasp function. The more occlusally located section stabilizes the canine firmly against rotations as well as other movements (D).

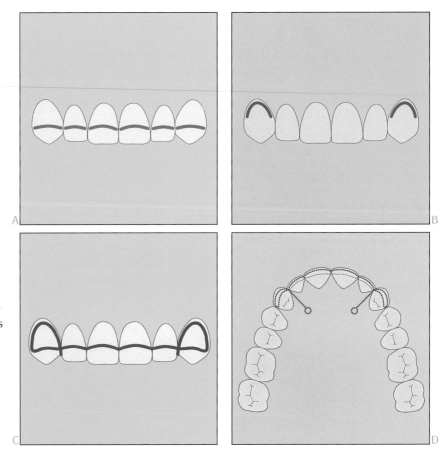

Figure 18-11

A cervically located labial arch offers insufficient resistance against rotations. At the incisal region, the retainer is too visible. At the center of the tooth, the grip is still adequate (A). When located at the center of the teeth, the archwire is at the proper height in relation to the acrylic resin at the palatal surfaces (B).

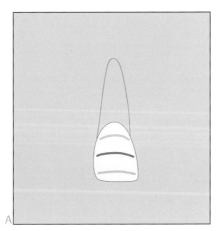 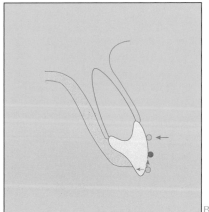

A retention plate has the advantage over a bonded wire that, with proper use, tooth movements rarely occur. When a retention wire is bonded to two teeth only, the patient will notice immediately when one end is loose. However, when a retention wire is bonded to more teeth, a loose spot that is not located at the end of the wire usually is not noticed before a disturbing movement has become obvious. The patient will not call for repair before that has happened.

A retention plate fabricated according to the design advocated in this chapter offers considerable security (Figs 18-10 and 18-11). In addition, oral hygiene is not restricted. A retention plate has the additional advantage that its use can be reduced gradually.

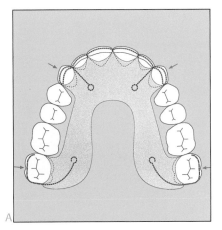
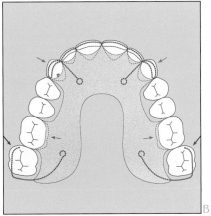

Figure 18-12

The acrylic resin should not be removed palatal to the most posteriorly located molars, which are encompassed by the three-quarter clasps. The other posterior teeth should be free of the acrylic resin (A). Second molars that have erupted too far mesially and buccally can be moved distally and palatally with the three-quarter clasps when the acrylic resin has been removed from their palatal sides but has been maintained at the first molars (B).

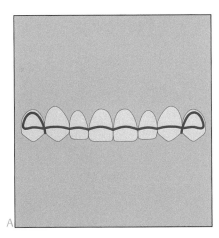
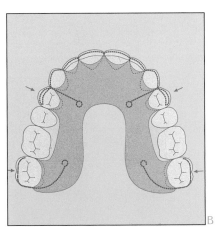

Figure 18-13

Sometimes insufficient space is available for the 0.7-mm wire to pass distal to the lateral incisors. Furthermore, to avoid occlusion at that section, the wire has to cross more distally (A). The clasp function also moves distally, but premolars are less suited for that purpose than are canines, because premolars have shorter crowns and smaller buccal undercuts. The acrylic resin now has to be maintained at the palatal side of the first premolars (B).

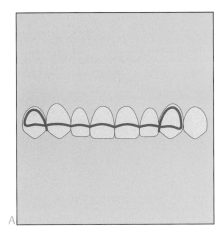
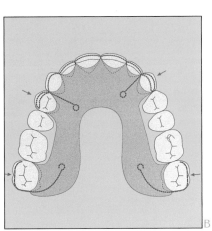

Figure 18-14

Sometimes the wire can pass between the lateral incisor and canine on one side, and not on the other side, so only one clasp function has to move distally (A). Only when necessary should the labial arch be lengthened and premolars be used for the clasp function (B).

The acrylic resin has to be trimmed away at the palatal sides of the posterior teeth (Fig 18-12). The plate should not interfere with the occlusion. Hence, whether a 0.7-mm wire can pass between the lateral incisor and the canine without disturbing the occlusion should be confirmed in the patient's mouth. If not, sufficient space is usually available distal to the canine (Figs 18-13 and 18-14).

The trimming away of the acrylic resin in the region of the posterior teeth provides freedom to the occlusion, the tongue, and the cheeks, so that a functionally adapted position of the premolars and molars can be established and maintained.

FIGURE 18-15

The Van der Linden retainer does not disturb the occlusion. Most lateral incisors have rounded distal corners, which allow palatal passage of the wire at a sufficiently high level. In this patient, the occlusion in the posterior regions was excellent. The maxillary first molars were mesially angulated and in solid intercuspation with their opposing teeth. Clasps that passed distal to the first molars would have disturbed the occlusion (A, B). The plate has to be kept thin, and the palate should be covered only partially (C, D). The acrylic resin in the posterior regions should be removed, except where it has to withstand the force of the clasps. The free area should be rather wide, and the margins rounded, to avoid food collection and to facilitate cleaning by the tongue (E, F).

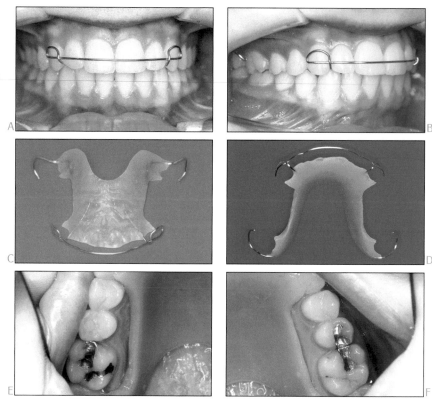

FIGURE 18-16

The morphology of the lateral incisors and canines did not allow passage of the wire between these teeth without a disruption of the occlusion (A). There was sufficient space distal to the canines (B). However, this resulted in a longer labial arch (C). In addition, first premolars and especially second premolars have shorter crowns and smaller buccal undercuts than canines. As already indicated, if clasp functions are located at the premolars, the acrylic resin should be maintained at their palatal sides (D).

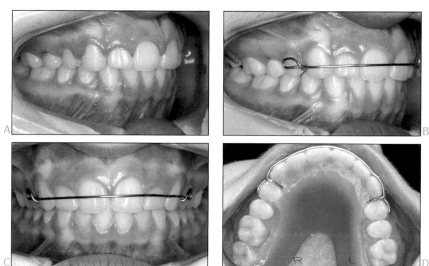

When the acrylic resin is not removed from the palatal sides of the posterior teeth, a plate that is worn only during sleep will force the premolars and molars in unnatural positions when it is inserted at night (Figs 18-15 and 18-16).

The patient's compliance in wearing a retention plate depends largely on the associated discomfort. Hence, it is essential to aim for an appliance that causes as few inconveniences as possible. To that end, the plate should be thin, except behind the incisors, where the mandibular anterior teeth have to be supported vertically. The more the palate is uncovered, the better. Occluding on acrylic resin and particularly on metal parts of appliances is annoying to the patient.

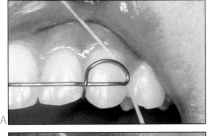

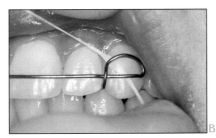

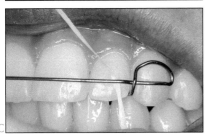

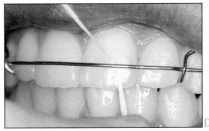

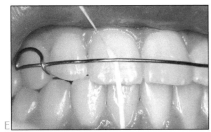

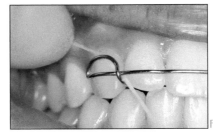

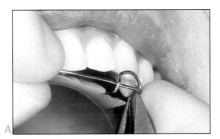

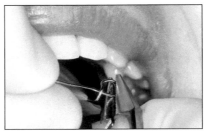

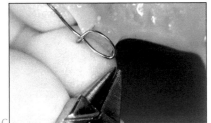

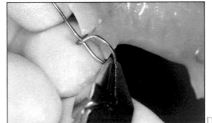

FIGURE 18-17

The clasp function at the canines and the adaptation to the contours of the labial surfaces can be controlled with silk dental floss. The most suitable method for right-handed practitioners is to start at the left canine. Silk floss can be used to feel if the wire is properly located and how much pressure is exerted (A, B). This is also revealed by the degree the floss becomes flattened and by the angle in the course of the silk floss when it is shifted between the teeth and the wire. After the wire at the canine has been examined, the floss is placed under the labial arch, and the adaptation at the incisors is controlled (C–E). Finally, the situation at the right canine is examined (F).

FIGURE 18-18

When needed, the clasp function at the canines can be tightened with a No. 139 (bird-beak) pliers. The round beak is placed at the inner side of the wire sections at the canine and subsequently the top is turned slightly inward (A, B). If the corner of the wire at the canine is moved slightly more distally, the tension at the incisors can be somewhat increased (C, D). However, this adjustment is rarely needed and is not easy to accomplish without losing control.

Retention plates should not be used to move anterior teeth, because the technique involves loss of control over adjacent teeth. A retention plate should have a rigid labial arch that does not deform in normal use. The recommended design and construction fulfill these requirements (Fig 18-17). A patient who handles such a retention plate with care does not have to return for reexamination more than once a year, and even then adjustment of the labial arch is rarely needed. However, sometimes the clasp function has to be increased (Fig 18-18). A retention plate that is worn only during sleep can function well for many years (Fig 18-19).

FIGURE 18-19

A 39-year-old woman had a Class I malocclusion, periodontal destruction, and secondary tooth migrations (A, B). Six months after the end of the initial periodontal therapy, fixed appliances were placed in a healthy environment. In a period of 18 months, an excellent result was reached. Subsequently, a maxillary plate and a mandibular canine bar were placed for retention (C, D). After 6 months, the plate was worn only during sleep. Ten years after the conclusion of active treatment, the position of the teeth seemed not to have changed (E, F). The retention plate still fitted well. In adult patients, and particularly in periodontally compromised patients, the clasps on the molars should not be in close proximity to the gingiva (G). The labial arch stayed in contact with the contours of the teeth, and the clasp functions at the canines worked well (H). The same Van der Linden retainer had been used for more than 10 years (I).

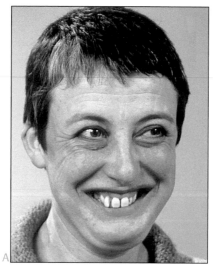

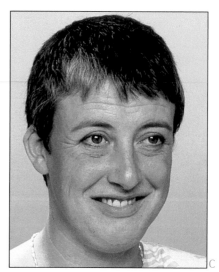

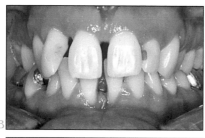

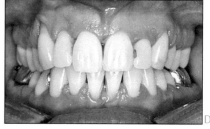

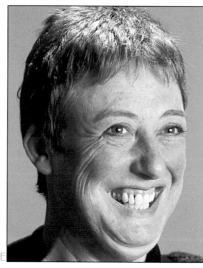

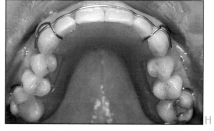

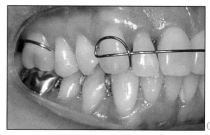

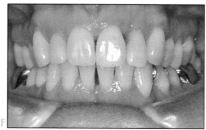

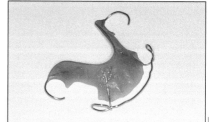

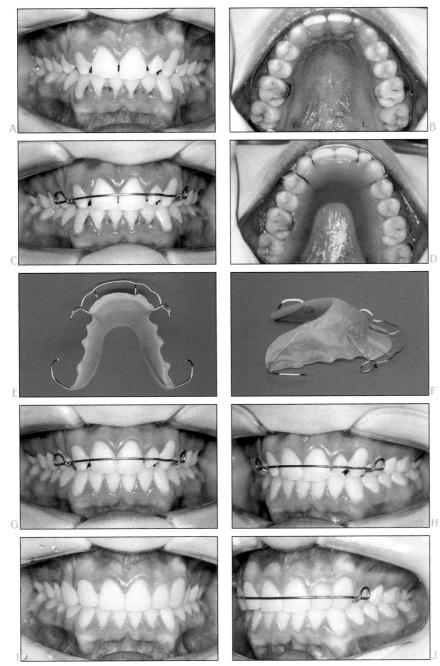

FIGURE 18-20

A girl aged 13 years 11 months is shown on the day that the fixed appliances were removed. The right lateral incisor was absent and the left lateral incisor was small and peg shaped. During fixed appliance therapy, oral hygiene had not been ideal, and the gingiva was irritated and slightly inflamed (A, B). The clasp function was located at the first premolars, because it was impossible to arrange for a new retainer to be made directly after buildup of the incisors (C). Because of the loss of a bracket in the period preceding the day of appliance removal, a central diastema had developed. To close that space, two straight pieces of 0.6-mm stainless steel wire were placed distal to the central incisors, with some tension built in. After the insertion of the plate, the diastema closed almost completely (C, D). Even if the central diastema had not developed, these pieces of wire should have been included to keep the central incisors together (E, F). This preliminary retention plate was used for a 4-month period (G, H). After the right lateral incisor and the canines were built up with resin composite, a new retention plate was made. Because it was impossible to have the wire pass mesial to the canines, the first premolars were used for the clasp function (I, J).

It is usually not feasible to carry out the esthetic dental treatment the same day the orthodontic appliances are removed or shortly thereafter. Consequently, the first retention plate can be used only for a limited period of time. Immediately after the teeth have been built up, a new retention plate has to be fabricated, because it is impossible to readjust the existing rigid labial arch so that it will provide the required control (Fig 18-20).

FIGURE 18-21

Prior to the introduction of bonding, ideal occlusions and tooth positions could not be reached with fixed appliances. Bands interfered with the placement of adjacent teeth in contact with each other. Sometimes incisal contacts could not be established, because the palatal surfaces of the maxillary incisors were covered with band material (A–D). In addition, with bands it was difficult to assess if the teeth were properly positioned. That applied particularly to contact points. Consequently, interproximal spaces had to be closed, and the positions of the anterior teeth refined (E, F). These minor tooth movements were carried out with removable appliances, which were subsequently utilized as retention devices. Occasionally, a positioner was used for that purpose, especially when extensive adjustments had to be made. Therefore, not directly after removal of the bands, but at a later stage, an ideal occlusion and correct tooth positions were obtained (G, H).

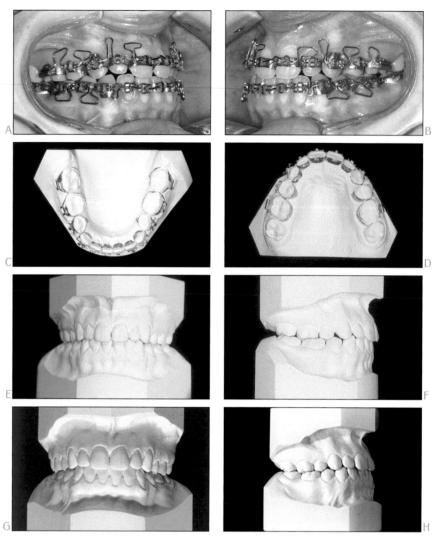

FIGURE 18-22

Bands and interdental spaces after treatment can be avoided when tubes and brackets are bonded to the enamel (A, B) and an ideal occlusion and arrangements of teeth can be achieved before the fixed appliances are removed (C, D). Consequently, the need to use retention appliances to close spaces and refine tooth positions has largely disappeared.

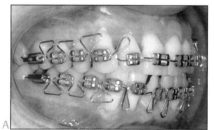
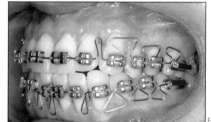
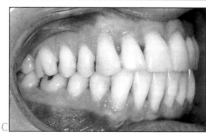
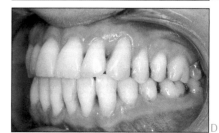

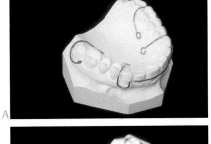

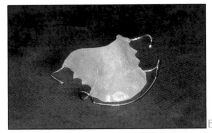

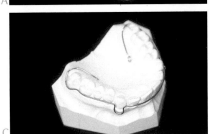

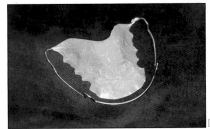

FIGURE 18-23

These retention plates were designed before bonding was available, when the use of fixed appliances involved the cementation of bands. The Hawley retainer has U-loops at the canine regions (A, B). The wraparound retainer has a continuous wire at the labial and buccal surfaces of all teeth (C, D). At the beginning at the 21st century, both of these retainers are still the most frequently used types, worldwide. It is astonishing that, more than 35 years after the introduction of bonding, the advantages of this technique have not affected the standard concepts of retention, introduced a century ago and to which many clinicians still adhere. It is difficult to understand why so many practitioners still use U-loops, which are flexible, cannot provide rigid control, and are no longer necessary to close spaces.

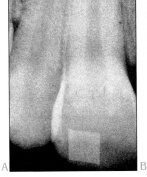

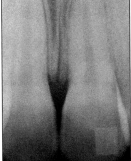

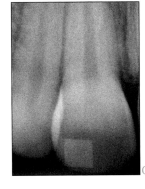

FIGURE 18-24

Radiographs of the maxillary incisors before the start of treatment (A), at the day of fixed appliance removal, when the periodontal spaces were extra wide (B), and 2 years later (C).

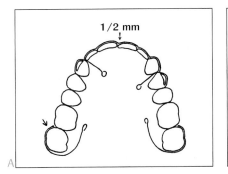

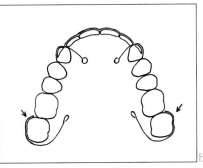

FIGURE 18-25

Two examples of a design for a Van der Linden retainer. If the movements to be carried out (arrows) are indicated on the plan, the plate can be adjusted accordingly (A). The need for movement of second molars should be indicated as well as the required space between their palatal and distal sides and the clasps (B).

Because of the introduction of bonding, orthodontic treatment can be finished so well that teeth no longer have to be moved during the retention phase or have to be moved very little (Figs 18-21 to 18-23). Indeed, minor corrections are often still needed. Fortunately, the wide periodontal spaces at the end of active treatment allow teeth to be brought directly to slightly better positions (Fig 18-24). Consequently, instant corrections of minor dimensions can be performed when retention is implemented (Fig 18-25).

When that is necessary, the required improvements are included in the retention plate (Fig 18-26). After the retention plate is inserted, the teeth are forced instantaneously to the desired positions. When teeth have to be moved labially, plaster should be removed from that palatal side so that the plate will exert pressure there, and the labial arch should be at the desired distance from the labial surface on the plaster cast.

Figure 18-26

A good plaster cast is needed to fabricate a retention plate (A). The desired instant corrections should have been indicated by the clinician in the design (B). Plaster has to be scraped away where the labial arch has to be placed more palatally (C). The 0.7-mm spring hard stainless steel wire is bent so that it fits into the grooves (D). The wire is bent around to create the clasp function at the canine (E–G). Layers of tin foil are adapted closely to the surfaces where the teeth have to move palatally. The thickness of the tin foil layers should be matched to the distance the tooth has to move palatally, so that the acrylic resin will support the tooth when it has reached its destination (H). The 0.8-mm clasp around the last molar should lie against the buccal surface at the undercut. Banding around the end of the clasp increases the retention, which is of special importance when the molar has to be moved (I, J). The plate is shown on the plaster cast (K) and before fitting in the mouth (L).

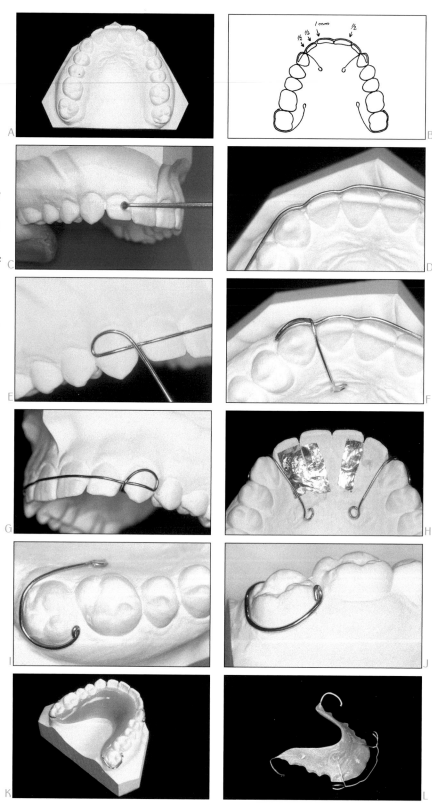

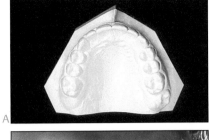

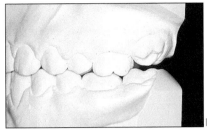

FIGURE 18-27

At the end of orthodontic treatment, the permanent maxillary left second molar had emerged and erupted too far mesially and buccally (A, B). With the three-quarter clasp around this tooth, it could be moved in the distal and palatal directions (C, D).

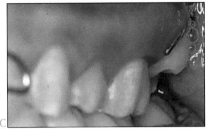

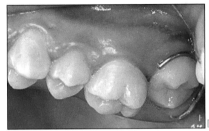

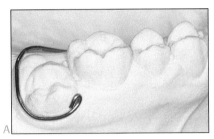

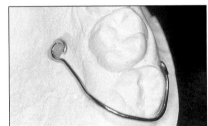

FIGURE 18-28

To move the second molar, the wire should be placed some distance from the tooth, distally as well as palatally (A, B).

Second molars that emerge during orthodontic treatment quite often erupt too far mesially and buccally, at the risk of ending up in crossbite (Fig 18-27, A and B). These teeth can be moved to the proper positions by the clasps on the retention plate (Figs 18-27, C and D, and 18-28). In that case, the acrylic resin has to be trimmed palatal to the second molar and maintained at the first molar; otherwise the plate will be pulled buccally by the clasp. After the second molar has arrived at the proper location, the acrylic resin is built up again on its palatal side and removed at the location of the first molar.

The plate shown here is known as the Van der Linden retainer.[220] It has, like all maxillary retention plates, two shortcomings. First, corrections in angulation are not stabilized; if necessary, a bonded dead-soft braided wire should be applied. Such a bonded retainer can be combined with a retention plate (Fig 18-29).

Second, the movement of an incisor in the apical direction, that is, the return to infraposition, is not prevented. A lateral incisor that has been extruded can move in the apical direction between the labial arch and the margin of the plate. In these situations a bonded retention wire will provide the needed fixation, applied in combination with or applied without a retention plate. However, such an intrusion can also be prevented by the placement of a little resin composite at the involved tooth incisal to the labial arch of the retention plate.

Bonded retainers that span a large distance and are not bonded to the intervening teeth, such as mandibular canine bars, should be rather thick (0.016 × 0.022-inch or 0.032-inch multistranded). When a bar is bonded to all teeth it passes, a thin dead-soft braided wire should be used, because the fixed teeth should maintain their individual mobility. When the distances between them are small, as in the mandibular anterior region, a 0.015-inch diameter archwire will meet that criterion. In the maxillary anterior region, where the distances between teeth are larger, a 0.0175-inch dead-soft braided wire should be used.

Bonded retention wires complicate the maintenance of adequate oral hygiene, because plaque and calculus tend to collect around them. However, the occurrence of dental caries in mandibular teeth anchored with a bonded retainer is very rare.

FIGURE 18-29

The maxillary lateral incisors were moved to the sites of the central incisors, which had been lost in an accident (A). At the end of active treatment, a 0.015-inch dead-soft braided wire was bonded at the palatal surfaces of the two incisors. After these teeth were built up, a new retention plate was made (B). The retention plate was combined with the small bonded dead-soft braided wire (C, D).

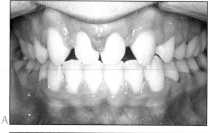
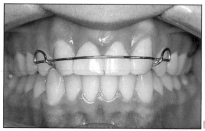
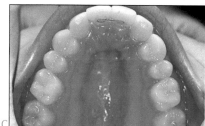
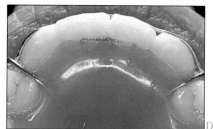

FIGURE 18-30

When the labial arch cannot be bent to deliver the required support to the maxillary incisors, application of a strip of clear acrylic resin at the labial arch can provide adequate coverage of the labial contours (A, B).

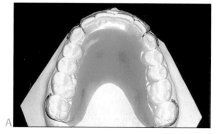
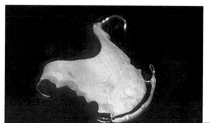

FIGURE 18-31

The Van der Linden retainer should be removed carefully; the fingernails are placed on top of the wire at the cervical area of the canines, so deformation of the labial arch will be avoided (A, B).

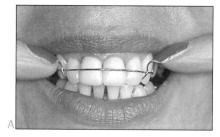
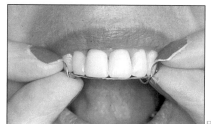

When the adaptation of a labial arch to the contours of the maxillary incisors causes problems, an acceptable compromise is application of a strip of clear acrylic resin at the labial arch (Fig 18-30).

The effect of a retention appliance depends on the way it is handled. The patient should be careful with a removable retainer and insert and remove it gently. Instruction in this matter is essential (Fig 18-31).

References

Orthodontic Concepts and Strategies

References

1. AAO issues special bulletin on extraoral appliance care [editorial]. Am J Orthod 1975;68:457.
2. Ackerman JL, Ackerman MB, Brensinger CM, Landis JR. A morphometric analysis of the posed smile. Clin Orth Res 1998;1:2-11.
3. Ackerman JL, Proffit WR. Soft tissue limitations in orthodontics: Treatment planning guidelines. Angle Orthod 1997;67:327-336.
4. Altenburger E, Ingervall B. The initial effects of the treatment of Class II, division 1 malocclusions with the Van Beek activator compared with the effects of the Herren activator and an activator-headgear combination. Eur J Orthod 1998;20:389-397.
5. Al Yami EA, Kuijpers-Jagtman AM, Van 't Hof MA. Stability of orthodontic treatment outcome: Follow-up until 20 years postretention. Am J Orthod Dentofacial Orthoped 1999;115:300-304.
6. Andreasen JO, Paulsen HU, Yu Z, Bayer T. A long-term study of 370 autotransplanted premolars. Part IV: Root development subsequent to transplantation. Eur J Orthod 1990;12:38-50.
7. Andresen V. Über das sogenannte "norwegische System der Funktions-Kiefer-Orthopädie." Dtsch Zahnärztl Wochenschr 1936;39:235-283.
8. Andresen V, Häupl K, Petrik L. Funktionskieferorthopädie. 6. Aufl. München: Johann Ambrosius Barth, 1957.
9. Balters W. Eine Einführung in die Bionatorheilmethode. Hrsg. C. Hermann. Hölzer, Heidelberg, 1973.
10. Barrer HG. Protecting the integrity of mandibular incisor position through keystoning procedure and spring retainer appliance. J Clin Orthod 1975;9:486-494.
11. Bass NM. Innovation in skeletal II treatment including effective incisor root torque in a preliminary removable appliance phase. Br J Orthod 1976;3:223-230.
12. Bass NM. Dento-facial orthopaedics in the correction of class II malocclusion. Br J Orthod 1982;9:3-31.
13. Baume LJ. Physiological tooth migration and its significance for the development of occlusion. I. The biogenetic course of the deciduous dentition. J Dent Res 1950;29:123-132.
14. Baume LJ. Physiological tooth migration and its significance for the development of occlusion. II. The biogenesis of the accessional dentition. J Dent Res 1950;29:33-337.
15. Baume LJ. Physiological tooth migration and its significance for the development of occlusion. III. The biogenesis of the successional dentition. J Dent Res 1950;29:338-348.
16. Baumrind S, Korn EL, Molthen R, West EW. Changes in facial dimensions associated with the use of forces to retract the maxilla. Am J Orthod 1981;80:17-30.
17. Becker A. The Orthodontic Treatment of Impacted Teeth. London: Martin Dunitz, 1998.
18. Behrents RG. Personal communication, 2004.
19. Berger H. Idiopathic root resorption. Am J Orthod Oral Surg. 1943;29:548-549.
20. Beyer JW, Lindauer SJ. Evaluation of dental midline position. Semin Orthod 1998;4:146-152.
21. Bimler HP. The Bimler Appliance: Construction and Adjustment. Great Falls, MT: V.A. Nord, 1966.
22. Bishara SE, Burkey PS, Kharouf JG. Dental and facial asymmetries: A review. Angle Orthod 1994;64:89-98.
23. Björk A. The face in profile. Svensk Tandläkare-Tidskrift 1947;40(suppl 5B).
24. Björk A. Facial growth in man, studied with the aid of metallic implants. Acta Odontol Scand 1955;13:9-34.
25. Björk A. Variations in the growth pattern of the human mandible: Longitudinal radiographic study by the implant method. J Dent Res 1963;42(pt 2):400-411.
26. Björk A. Sutural growth of the upper face studied by the implant method. Rep Congr Eur Orthod Soc 1964;40:49-64.
27. Björk A. Kaevernes relation til det øvrige kranium. In: Lundstrom A (ed). Nordisk Lärobok i Orthodonti, ed 4. Stockholm: Sveriges Tandläkarforbunds Förlagsförening, 1975:69-110.
28. Björk A, Skieller V. Facial development and tooth eruption. An implant study at the age of puberty. Am J Orthod 1972;62:339-383.
29. Boersma H. Eenvoudige Orthodontische Therapie. 4e druk. Alphen aan den Rijn: Samsom Stafleu, 1989.
30. Boersma H, Van der Linden FPGM, Prahl-Andersen B. Craniofacial development. In: Prahl-Andersen B, Kowalski CJ, Heydendael PHJ (eds). A Mixed-Longitudinal Interdisciplinary Study of Growth and Development. New York: Academic Press, 1979:537-571.
31. Booy C. Over het distaalwaarts verplaatsen van hoektanden na extractie van de eerste premolaren. Ned Tijdschr Tandheelkd 1960;67:353-368.
32. Booy C. Over het roteren van frontelementen. Ned Tijdschr Tandheelkd 1967;74:302-313.
33. Booy C. Orthodontie in de algemene praktijk. In: Sociale Tandheelkdunde, nu en in de toekomst. Utrecht: Bohn, Scheltema & Holkema, 1981:95-107.
34. Brattström V, Ingelsson M, Aberg E. Treatment co-operation in orthodontic patients. Br J Orthod 1991;18:37-42.

35. Brauer JE. A report of 113 early or premature extractions of primary molars and the incidence of closure of space. J Dent Child 1941;8:222-223.

36. Breakspear EK. Further observations on early loss of deciduous molars. Dent Pract Dent Rec (Bristol) 1961;11:233-252.

37. Broadbent BH. The face of the normal child. Angle Orthod 1937;7:183-208.

38. Broadbent BH Sr. Ontogenic development of occlusion. Angle Orthod 1941;11:223-241.

39. Broadbent BH Sr, Broadbent BH Jr, Golden WH. Bolton Standards of Dentofacial Developmental Growth. St. Louis: Mosby, 1975.

40. Brodie AG. On the growth pattern of the human head from the third month to the eighth year of life. Am J Anat 1941;68:209-262.

41. Buschang PH, Shulman JD. Incisor crowding in untreated persons 15-50 years of age: United States, 1988-994. Angle Orthod 2003;73:502-508.

42. Clinch LM. An analysis of serial models between three and eight years of age. Dent Rec 1951;71:61-72.

43. Coffin WH. A generalized treatment of irregularities. Trans Int Congr Med (London) 1881, 7th Session. Vol. III:542-547.

44. Crefcoeur JM. Orthodontisch uitneembare apparaten met universele mogelijkheden. Ned Tijdschr Tandheelkd 1953;60:914-921.

45. Crosby DR, Alexander CG. The occurrence of tooth size discrepancies among different malocclusion groups. Am J Orthod Dentofacial Orthop 1989;95:457-461.

46. Czochrowska EW, Stenvik A, Album B, Zachrisson BU. Autotransplantation of premolars to replace maxillary incisors: A comparison with natural teeth. Am J Orthod Dentofacial Orthop 2000;118:592-600.

47. Dachi SF, Howell FV. A survey of 3,874 routine full-mouth radiographs. II. A study of impacted teeth. Oral Surg Oral Med Oral Pathol 1961;14:1165-1169.

48. Daskalogiannakis J. Glossary of Orthodontic Terms. Chicago: Quintessence, 2000.

49. Davey KW. Effect of premature loss of deciduous molars on the anteroposterior position of maxillary first first permanent molars and other maxillary teeth. J Can Dent Assoc 1966;32:406-416.

50. De Boer M. Aspekten van de gebitsontwikkeling bij kinderen tussen vijf en tien jaar [doctoral thesis]. Utrecht, The Netherlands: Utrecht Univ., 1970.

51. De Kanter RJAM. Prevalence and etiology of craniomandibular dysfunction [doctoral thesis]. Nijmegen, The Netherlands: Univ. of Nijmegen, 1990.

52. DeVincenzo JP. Changes in mandibular length before, during and after successful orthopedic correction of Class II malocclusions, using a functional appliance. Am J Orthod Dentofacial Orthop 1991;99:241-257.

53. Dewel BF. A critical analysis of serial extraction in orthodontic treatment. Am J Orthod 1959;45:424-455.

54. De Wijn JF, De Haas JH. Groeidiagrammen van 1-25 jarigen in Nederland. Leiden: Nederlands Instituut voor Praeventieve Geneeskunde, 1960.

55. Diedrich P, Rudzki-Janson I, Wehrbein H, Fritz U. Effects of orthodontic bands on marginal periodontal tissues. A histologic study on two human specimens. J Orofac Orthop 2001;62:146-156.

56. Du X, Hägg U, Rabie ABM. Effect of headgear Herbst and mandibular step-by-step advancement versus conventional Herbst appliance and maximal jumping of the mandible. Eur J Orthod 2002;24:167-174.

57. Duterloo HS. An Atlas of Dentition in Childhood. Orthodontic Diagnosis and Panoramic Radiology. London: Wolfe Publishing Ltd., 1991.

58. Duterloo HS. Development of the dentition under influence of functional factors. In: Hunter WS, Carlson DS (eds). Essays in Honor of Robert E. Moyers, monograph 24, Craniofacial Growth Series. Ann Arbor, MI: Center for Human Growth and Development, Univ. of Michigan, 1991:103-122.

59. Ehmer U, Tulloch CJ, Proffit WR, Phillips C. An international comparison of early treatment of Angle Class-II/1 cases. Skeletal effects of the first phase of a prospective clinical trial. J Orofac Orthop 1999;60:392-408.

60. Ericson S, Bjerklin K, Falahat B. Does the canine dental follicle cause resorption of permanent incisor roots? A computed tomographic study of erupting maxillary canines. Angle Orthod 2002;72:95-104.

61. Ericson S, Kurol J. Incisor resorption caused by maxillary cuspids. A radiographic study. Angle Orthod 1987;57:332-346.

62. Ericson S, Kurol J. Early treatment of palatally erupting maxillary canines by extraction of the primary canines. Eur J Orthod 1988;10:283-295.

63. Ericson S, Kurol J. Incisor root resorptions due to ectopic maxillary canines imaged by computerized tomography: A comparative study in extracted teeth. Angle Orthod 2000;70:276-283.

64. Ericson S, Kurol J. Resorption of incisors after ectopic eruption of maxillary canines: A CT study. Angle Orthod 2000;70:415-423.

65. Falck F, Fränkel R. Die labiale Alveolenwand unter dem Einfluss des durchbrechenden Schneidezahnes Fortschr Kieferorthop 1973;34:37-47.

66. Faltin RM, Arana-Chavez VE, Faltin K, Sander FG, Wichelhaus A. Root resorption in upper first premolars after application of continuous intrusive forces. Intra-individual study. J Orofac Orthop 1998;59:208-219.

67. Fanning EA. A longitudinal study of tooth calcification and root resorption. J Dent Res 1958;73:4.

68. Fernandez E, Bravo LA, Canteras M. Eruption of the permanent upper canine: A radiologic study. Am J Orthod Dentofacial Orthop 1998;113:414-420.

69. Fränkel R. Decrowding during eruption under the screening influence of vestibular shields. Am J Orthod 1974;65:372-406.

70. Fränkel R. Technik und Handhabung der Funktionsregler. ed 2. Berlin: VEB Verlag Volk und Gesundheit, 1976.

71. Fränkel R, Falck F. Zahndurchbruch und vererbung beim Deckbiss. Fortschr Kieferorthop 1967;28:175-182.

72. Frankenmolen FWA. Orale gezondheid en zelfzorg van Nederlandse adolescenten [doctoral thesis]. Nijmegen, The Netherlands: University of Nijmegen, 1990.

73. Fredriks AM, Van Buuren S, Burgmeijer RJ, et al. Continuing positive secular growth change in the Netherlands 1955-1997. Pediatr Res 2000;47:316-323.

74. Fredriks AM, Van Buuren S, Wit JM, Verloove-Vanhorick SP. Body index measurements in 1996-7 compared with 1980. Arch Dis Child 2000;82:107-112.

75. Freeman JE, Maskeroni AJ, Lorton L. Frequency of Bolton tooth size discrepancies among different orthodontic patients. Am J Orthod 1996;110:24-27.

76. Fujiki T, Inoue M, Miyawaki S, Nagasaki T, Tanimoto K, Takano-Yamamoto T. Relationship between maxillofacial morphology and deglutitive tongue movement in patients with anterior open bite. Am J Orthod Dentofacial Orthop 2004;125:160-167.

77. Ghafari J, Shofer FS, Jacobsson-Hunt U, Markowitz DL, Laster LL. Headgear versus functional regulator in the early treatment of Class II, division 1 malocclusion: A randomized clinical trial. Am J Orthod Dentofacial Orthop 1998;113:51-61.

78. Goldstein MS, Stanton FL. Various types of occlusion and amounts of overbite in normal and abnormal occlusion between two and twelve years. Int J Orthodont 1936;22:549-569.

79. Guerrero CA, Bell WH, Contasti GI, Rodriguez AM. Intraoral mandibular distraction osteogenesis. Semin Orthod 1999;5:35-40.

80. Haack DC, Weinstein S. The mechanics of centric and eccentric cervical traction. Am J Orthod Dentofacial Orthop 1958;44:346-357.

81. Harris EF, Baker WC. Loss of root length and crestal bone height before and during treatment in adolescent and adult orthodontic patients. Am J Orthod Dentofacial Orthop 1990;98:463-469.

82. Harris EF, Butler ML. Patterns of incisor root resorption before and after orthodontic correction in cases with anterior open bites. Am J Orthod Dentofacial Orthop 1992;101:112-119.

83. Harvold EP. The role of function in the etiology and treatment of maloclusion. Am J Orthod 1968;54:883-898.

84. Harvold EP. The Activator in Interceptive Orthodontics. St. Louis: Mosby, 1974.

85. Harvold EP, Vargervik K. Morphogenetic response to activator treatment. Am J Orthod 1971;60:478-490.

86. Helm S. Prevalence of malocclusion in relation to development of the dentition. An epidemiological study of Danish school children. Acta Odontol Scand 1970;28(suppl 58):1+.

87. Helm S, Siersbaek-Nielsen S. Crowding in the permanent dentition after early loss of deciduous molars or canines. Trans Eur Orthod Soc. 1973:137-149.

88. Herren P. The activator's mode of action. Am J Orthod 1959;45:512-527.

89. Hooymaayer J, Van der Linden FPGM, Boersma H. Post treatment facial development in corrected class II division 1-anomalies. J Dent Res 1989;68:632.

90. Hotz R. Orthodontie in der täglichen Praxis. Bern: Hans Huber, 1970.

91. Hrdlicka A. Shovel-shaped teeth. Am J Phys Anthrop 1920;3:429-465.

92. Hurme VO. Ranges of normalcy in the eruption of permanent teeth. J Dent Child 1949;16:11-15.

93. Ilizarov GA. The principles of the Ilizarov method. Bull Hosp Jt Dis Orthop Inst 1988;48:1-11.

94. Illing HM, Morris DO, Lee KT. A prospective evaluation of Bass, Bionator and Twin Block appliances. Part I – The hard tissues. Eur J Orthod 1998;20:501-516.

95. Ingram AH. Premolar enucleation. Angle Orthod 1976;46:219-231.

96. Janson GR, Metaxas A, Woodside DG, De Freitas MR, Pinzan A. Three-dimensional evaluation of skeletal and dental asymmetries in Class II subdivision malocclusions. Am J Orthod Dentofacial Orthop. 2001;119:406-418.

97. Johnston CD, Burden DJ, Stevenson MR. The influence of dental to facial midline discrepancies on dental attractiveness ratings. Eur J Orthod 1999;21:517-522.

98. Junkin JB, Andria LM. Comparative long term post-treatment changes in hyperdivergent Class II Division 1 patients with early cervical traction treatment. Angle Orthod 2002;72:5-14.

99. Karwetzky R. Die Anwendung des U-bügelaktivators in der zahnarztlichen Praxis. Dtsch Zahnarztl Z 1974;29:891-893.

100. King GJ, Wheeler SP, McGorray SP. Randomized prospective clinical trial evaluating early treatment of Class II malocclusions [abstract]. Eur J Orthod 1999;21:445.

101. Kjellgen B. Serial extraction as a corrective procedure in dental orthopedic therapy. Acta Odont Scand. 1948:17-43.

102. Klammt G. Der elastisch-offene Aktivator. Leipzig: Johann Ambrosius Barth, 1984.

103. Knott VB, Meredith MV. Statistics on eruption of the permanent dentition from serial data from North American white children. Angle Orthod 1966;36:68-79.

104. Kokich VG, Spear FM. Guidelines for managing the orthodontic-restorative patient. Semin Orthod 1997;3:3-20.

105. Kokich VO Jr, Kiyak HA, Shapiro PA. Comparing the perception of dentists and lay people to altered dental esthetics. J Esthet Dent 1999;11:311-324.

106. Kolf J. Le syndrome hypertonique antérieur ou propos sur la Classe II, div. 2. Rev Orthop Dento Faciale 1976;10:149-161.

107. Korkhaus G. Biomechanische Gebiss- und Kieferorthopädie. Handbuch der Zahnheilk. Bd. IV. München: J.F. Bergmann, 1939.

108. Korkhaus G. German methodologies in maxillary orthopedics. In: Kraus BS, Riedel RA (eds). Vistas in Orthodontics. Philadelphia: Lea & Febiger, 1962:259-286.

109. Kristerson L. Autotransplantation of human premolars. A clinical and radiographic study of 100 teeth. Int J Oral Surg 1985;14:200-213.

110. Kusters ST, Kuijpers-Jagtman AM, Maltha JC. An experimental study in dogs of transseptal fiber arrangement between teeth which have emerged in rotated or non-rotated positions. J Dent Res 1991;70:192-197.

111. Lagerström L, Kristerson L. Influence of orthodontic treatment on root development of autotransplanted premolars. Am J Orthod 1986;89:146-150.

112. Langford SR, Sims MR. Upper molar root resorption because of distal movement. Report of a case. Am J Orthod 1981;79:669-679.

113. Leighton BC, Adams CP. Incisor inclination in Class 2 division 2 malocclusions. Eur J Orthod 1986;8:98-105.

114. Linder-Aronson S. The effect of premature loss of deciduous teeth. A biometric study in 14- and 15-year olds. Acta Odont Scand 1960;18:101-122.

115. Linge L, Linge BO. Patient characteristics and treatment variables associated with apical root resorption during orthodontic treatment. Am J Orthod Dentofacial Orthop 1991;99:35-43.

116. Little RM. Stability and relapse of mandibular anterior alignment: University of Washington studies. Semin Orthod 1999;5:191-204.

117. Little RM, Riedel RA, Stein A. Mandibular arch length increase during the mixed dentition: Postretention evaluation of stability and relapse. Am J Orthod Dentofacial Orthop 1990;97:393-404.

118. Little RM, Wallen TR, Riedel RA. Stability and relapse of mandibular anterior alignment — first premolar extraction cases treated by traditional edgewise orthodontics. Am J Orthod 1981;80:349-365.

119. Lo RT, Moyers RE. Studies in the etiology and prevention of malocclusion. I. The sequence of eruption of the permanent dentition. Am J Orthod 1953;39:460-467.

120. Logan WHG, Kronfeld R. Development of the human jaws and surrounding structures from birth to the age of fifteen years. J Am Dent Assoc 1933;20:379-427.

121. Lupi JE, Handelman CS, Sadowsky C. Prevalence and severity of apical root resorption and alveolar bone loss in orthodontically treated adults. Am J Orthod Dentofacial Orthop 1996;109:28-37.

122. Magnusson TE. The effect of premature loss of deciduous teeth on the spacing of the permanent dentition. Eur J Orthod 1979;1:243-249.

123. Manke M, Miethke R-R. Die Grösse des anterioren Bolton-Index und die Häufigkeit von Bolton-diskrepanzen im Frontzahnsegment bei unbehandelten kieferorthopädischen patienten. Fortschr Kieferorthop 1983;44:59-65.

124. Mäntysaari R, Kantomaa T, Pirttiniemi P, Pykäläinen A. The effects of early headgear treatment on dental arches and craniofacial morphology: A report of a 2 year randomized study. Eur J Orthod 2004;26:59-64.

References

125. McCarthy JG, Stelnicki EJ, Grayson BH. Distraction osteogenesis of the mandible: A ten-year experience. Semin Orthod 1999;5:3-8.

126. McIntyre GT, Millett DT. Crown-root shape of the permanent maxillary central incisor. Angle Orthod 2003;73:710-715.

127. McNamara. JA Jr, Brudon WL. Orthodontics and Dentofacial Orthopedics. Ann Arbor, MI: Needham Press, 2001.

128. McNamara. JA Jr, Van der Linden FPGM. Unpublished data, 1970.

129. McNamara. JA Jr, Van der Linden FPGM. Vertical dimension. In: McNamara JA Jr, Brudon WL. Orthodontics and Dentofacial Orthopedics. Ann Arbor, MI: Needham Press, 2001:111-148.

130. McNeill RW, Joondeph DR. Congenitally absent maxillary lateral incisors: Treatment planning considerations. Angle Orthod 1973;43:24-29.

131. Melsen B. Effects of cervical anchorage during and after treatment: An implant study. Am J Orthod 1978;73:526-540.

132. Melsen B, Dalstra M. Distal molar movement with Kloehn headgear: Is it stable? Am J Orthod Dentofacial Orthop 2003;123:374-378.

133. Meng HP, Gebauer U, Ingervall B. Die Entwicklung des tertiären Engstandes der unteren Incisiven im Zusammenhang mit Veränderungen der Zahnbögen und des Gesichtsschädels bei Individuen mit guter Okklusion von der Pubertät bis zum Erwachsenenalter. Schweiz Monatsschr Zahnmed 1985;95:762-777.

134. Miller EL, Bodden WR Jr, Jamison HC. A study of the relationship of the dental midline to the facial median line. J Prosthet Dent 1979;41:657-660.

135. Mirabella AD, Årtun J. Risk factors for apical root resorption of maxillary anterior teeth in adult orthodontic patients. Am J Orthod Dentofacial Orthop. 1995;108:48-55.

136. Moore AW. The mechanism of adjustment to wear and accident in the dentition and periodontium. Angle Orthod 1956;26:50-58.

137. Moorrees CF. The Dentition of the Growing Child: A Longitudinal Study of Dental Development Ages 3-18. Cambridge, MA: Harvard University Press, 1959.

138. Moorrees CF. Normal variation in dental development determined with reference to tooth eruption status. J Dent Res 1965;44(suppl):161-173.

139. Moorrees CF, Chadha JM. Available space for the incisors during dental development—a growth study based on physiologic age. Angle Orthod 1965;35:12-22.

140. Moorrees CF, Reed RB. Correlations among crown diameters of human teeth. Arch Oral Biol 1964;115:685-697.

141. Morley J, Eubank J. Macroesthetic elements of smile design. J Am Dent Assoc 2001;132:39-45.

142. Moyers RE. Handbook of Orthodontics, ed 4. Chicago: Year Book Medical Publishing, 1988.

143. Moyers RE, Van der Linden FPGM, Riolo ML, McNamara JA Jr. Standards of Human Occlusal Development, monograph 5, Craniofacial Growth Series. Ann Arbor, MI: Center for Human Growth and Development, Univ. of Michigan, 1976.

144. Nanda RS, Meng H, Kapila S, Goorhuis J. Growth changes in the soft tissue facial profile. Angle Orthod 1990;60:177-190.

145. Nelson PA, Årtun J. Alveolar bone loss of maxillary anterior teeth in adult orthodontic patients. Am J Orthod Dentofacial Orthop 1997;111:328-334.

146. Nicol WA. The lower lip and the upper incisor teeth in Angle's Class II, division 2 malocclusion. Dent Pract Dent Rec (Bristol) 1963;14:179-182.

147. Nord CFL. Loose appliances in orthodontia. Dental Cosmos 1928;70:681-687.

148. Nord CFL. The advantage of removable appliances. Trans Eur Orthod Soc 1929.

149. Nordquist GG, McNeill RW. Orthodontic vs. restorative treatment of the congenitally absent lateral incisor—long term periodontal and occlusal evaluation. J Periodontol 1975:46:139-143.

150. Ochoa BK, Nanda RS. Comparison of maxillary and mandibular growth. Am J Orthod Dentofacial Orthop 2004;125:148-159.

151. Ömblus J, Malmgren O, Pancherz H, Hägg U, Hansen K. Long-term effects of Class II correction in Herbst and Bass therapy. Eur J Orthod 1997;19:185-193.

152. O'Neill J. Personal communication, 2002.

153. Pancherz H. The effects, limitations, and long-term dentofacial adaptations to treatment with the Herbst appliance. Semin Orthod 1997;3:232-243.

154. Pancherz H, Ruf S. The Herbst appliance: Research-based updated clinical possibilities. World J Orthod 2000;1:17-31.

155. Pancherz H, Zieber K, Hoyer B. Cephalometric characteristics of Class II division 1 and Class II division 2 malocclusions: A comparative study in children. Angle Orthod 1997;67:111-120.

156. Peck H, Peck S. An index for assessing tooth shape deviations as applied to the mandibular incisors. Am J Orthod 1972;60:384-401.

157. Peck S, Peck H. Orthodontic aspects of dental anthropology. Angle Orthod 1975;45:95-102.

158. Petrik L. Funktionelle Therapie – Spezieller Teil. In: Häupl K, ed. Die Zahn-, Mund- und Kieferheilkunde. 5. Band. München: Urban & Schwarzenberg, 1955:277-414.

159. Pfeiffer JP, Grobéty D. Simultaneous use of cervical appliance and activator: An orthopedic approach to fixed appliance therapy. Am J Orthod 1972;61:353-373.

160. Pfeiffer JP, Grobéty D. A philosophy of combined orthopedic-orthodontic treatment. Am J Orthod 1982;81:185-201.

161. Pollard LE, Manandras AH. Male postpuberal facial growth in Class II malocclusions. Am J Orthod Dentofacial Orthop 1995;108:62-68.

162. Popovich F. Thumb-, fingersucking and bruxism in children: Comments and critique. In: Bryant P, Gale E, Rugh J (eds). Oral Motor Behavior: Impact on Oral Conditions and Dental Treatment. Bethesda, MD: US Department of Health, Education, and Welfare, Public Health Service, National Institutes of Health, 1979:23-27.

163. Power SM, Short MBE. An investigation into the response of palatally displaced canines to the removal of deciduous canines and an assessment of factors contributing to favourable eruption. Br J Orthod 1993;20:215-223.

164. Prahl-Andersen B, Kowalski CW, Heydendael PHJ (eds). A Mixed-Longitudinal, Interdisciplinary Study of Growth and Development. New York: Academic Press, 1979.

165. Proffit WR. Equilibrium theory revisited: Factors influencing position of the teeth. Angle Orthod 1978;48:175-186.

166. Proffit WR, Fields HW. Contemporary Orthodontics, ed 3. St. Louis: Mosby Year Book, 2000.

167. Radlanski RJ. Personal communication, 1999.

168. Robertsson S, Mohlin B. The congenitally missing upper lateral incisor. A retrospective study of orthodontic space closure versus restorative treatment. Eur J Orthod 2000;22:697-710.

169. Roede MJ, Van Wieringen JC. Growth diagrams 1980: Netherlands third nation-wide survey. Tijdschr Soc Gezondheidsz 1985;63(suppl):1-34.

170. Roeters JM, Kloet HJ de. Handboek voor Esthetische Tandheelkdunde. Nijmegen: STI, 1998.

171. Rosa M. Sequential slicing of deciduous teeth. J Clin Orthod 2001;35:696-701.

172. Rosa M, Zachrisson BU. Integrating esthetic dentistry and space closure in patients with missing maxillary lateral incisors. J Clin Orthod 2001;35:221-234.

173. Rossi M, Ribeiro E, Smith R. Craniofacial asymmetry in development: An anatomical study. Angle Orthod 2003:73:381-385.

174. Rudzki-Janson I, Paschos E, Diedrich P. Orthodontic tooth movement in the mixed dentition. Histological study of a human specimen. J Orofac Orthop 2001;62:177-190.

175. Samuels RH, Jones ML. Orthodontic facebow injuries and safety equipment. Eur J Orthod 1994;16:385-394.

176. Samuels RH, Willner F, Knox J, Jones ML. A national survey of orthodontic facebow injuries in the UK and Eire. Br J Orthod 1996;23:11-20.

177. Santoro M, Ayoub ME, Pardi VA, Cangialosi TJ. Mesiodistal crown dimensions and tooth size discrepancy of the permanent dentition of Dominican Americans. Angle Orthod 2000;70:303-307.

178. Sarver DM. The importance of incisor positioning in the esthetic smile: The smile arc. Am J Orthod Dentofacial Orthop 2001;120:98-111.

179. Sarver DM, Ackerman MB. Dynamic smile visualization and quantification: Part 2. Smile analysis and treatment strategies. Am J Orthod Dentofacial Orthop 2003;124:116-127.

180. Savara BS, Steen JC. Timing and sequence of eruption of permanent teeth in a longitudinal sample of children from Oregon. J Am Dent Assoc 1978;97:209-214.

181. Seel D. Extra oral hazards of extra oral traction. Br J Orthod 1980;7:53.

182. Sergl HG, Klages U, Zentner A. Pain and discomfort during orthodontic treatment: Causative factors and effects on compliance. Am J Orthod Dentofacial Orthop 1998;114:684-691.

183. Sergl HG, Zentner A. A comparative assessment of acceptance of different types of functional appliances. Eur J Orthod 1998;20:517-524.

184. Sheridan JJ. Air-rotor stripping. J Clin Orthod 1985;19:43-59.

185. Sinclair PM. Maturation of untreated normal occlusions. Am J Orthod 1983;83:114-123.

186. Smeets HJL. A roentgenocephalometric study of the skeletal morphology of Class II, division 2 malocclusion in adult cases. Trans Eur Orthod Soc 1962;38:247-259.

187. Solow B. The dentoalveolar compensatory mechanism: Background and clinical implications. Br J Orthod 1980;7:145-161.

188. Sparks AL. Interproximal enamel reduction and its effect on the long-term stability of mandibular incisor position [abstract]. Am J Orthod Dentofacial Orthop 2001;120:224-225.

189. Stockfisch H. Der Kinetor in der Kieferorthopädie. Heidelberg: Hüthig Verlag, 1966.

190. Stöckli PW, Ingervall VB, Joho JP, Wieslander L. Myofunktionelle Therapie. Fortschr Kieferorthop 1987;48:460-463.

191. Tanner JM. Growth as a mirror of the condition of society: Secular trends and class distinctions. In: Demirjian A (ed). Human Growth: A Multidisciplinary Review. London: Taylor & Francis, 1986:3-34.

192. Tanner JM, Whitehouse RH, Marubini E, Resele LF. The adolescent growth spurt of boys and girls of the Harpender growth study. Ann Hum Biol 1976;3:109-126.

193. Tarnow DP, Magner AW, Fletcher P. The effect of the distance from the contact point to the crest of bone on the presence or absence of the interproximal dental papilla. J Periodontol 1992;63:995-996.

194. Teuscher U. A growth-related concept for skeletal class II treatment. Am J Orthod 1978;74:258-275.

195. Thilander B, Jakobsson SO. Local factors in impaction of maxillary canines. Acta Odontol Scand 1968;26:145-168.

196. Thilander B, Myrberg N. The prevalence of malocclusion in Swedish schoolchildren. Scand J Dent Res 1973;81:12-21.

197. Thilander B, Ödman J, Lekholm U. Orthodontic aspects of the use of oral implants in adolescents: A 10-year follow-up study. Eur J Orthod 2001;23:715-731.

198. Thordarson A, Zachrisson BU, Mjör IA. Remodeling of canines to the shape of lateral incisors by grinding: A long-term clinical and radiographic evaluation. Am J Orthod Dentofacial Orthop 1991;100:123-132.

199. Toth LR, McNamara JA Jr. Treatment effects produced by the twin-block appliance and the FR-2 appliance of Fränkel with an untreated Class II sample. Am J Orthod Dentofacial Orthop 1999;116:597-609.

200. Tränkmann J. Frühe, gleichzeitige, symmetrische, systematische Entfernung von Zähnen der 1. und 2. Dentition im Rahmen einer kieferorthopädischen Behandlung. Kieferorthop 1994;8:227-234.

201. Tulloch JC, Phillips C, Proffit WR. Benefit of early Class II treatment: Progress report of a two-phase randomized clinical trial. Am J Orthod Dentofacial Orthop 1998;113:62-72.

202. Üçüncü N, Türk T, Carels C. Comparison of modified Teuscher and Van Beek functional appliance therapies in high-angle cases. J Orofac Orthop 2001;62:224-237.

203. Van Beek H. Overjet correction by a combined headgear and activator. Eur J Orthod 1982;4:279-290.

204. Van Beek H. Failures in headgear-activator therapy. In: Studyweek 1990. Nederlandse Vereniging voor Orthodontische Studie, 1990:193-206.

205. Van Beek H. Personal communication, 2002.

206. Van der Linden FPGM. Genetic and environmental factors in dentofacial morphology. Am J Orthod 1966;52:576-583.

207. Van der Linden FPGM. The application of removable orthodontic appliances in multiband techniques. Angle Orthod 1969;39:114-117.

208. Van der Linden FPGM. The interpretation of incremental data and velocity growth curves. Growth 1970;34:221-224.

209. Van der Linden FPGM. A study of röentgenocephalometric bony landmarks. Am J Orthod 1971;59:111-125.

210. Van der Linden FPGM. Theoretical and practical aspects of crowding in the human dentition. J Am Dent Assoc 1974;89:139-153.

211. Van der Linden FPGM (ed). Transition of the Human Dentition, monograph 13, Craniofacial Growth Series. Ann Arbor, MI: Center for Human Growth and Development, Univ. of Michigan, 1982.

212. Van der Linden FPGM. Development of the Dentition. Chicago: Quintessence, 1983.

213. Van der Linden FPGM. Facial Growth and Facial Orthopedics. Chicago: Quintessence, 1986.

214. Van der Linden FPGM. Problems and Procedures in Dentofacial Orthopedics. Chicago: Quintessence, 1990.

215. Van der Linden FPGM. Practical Dentofacial Orthopedics. London: Quintessence, 1996.

216. Van der Linden FPGM. Orthodontics with Fixed Appliances. London: Quintessence, 1997.

217. Van der Linden FPGM. Simultaneous removal of first deciduous molars and first permanent premolars [abstract]. Eur J Orthod 1996;18:428.

218. Van der Linden FPGM. The future of orthodontics: Overview and discussion. In: Carels C, Willems G (eds). The Future of Orthodontics. Leuven, Belgium: Leuven University Press, 1998:273-281.

219. Van der Linden FPGM. The development of long and short faces, and their limitations in treatment. In: McNamara JA Jr (ed). The Enigma of the Vertical Dimension, monograph 36, Craniofacial Growth Series. Ann Arbor, MI: Center for Human Growth and Development, Univ. of Michigan, 2000:61-73.

220. Van der Linden FPGM. The Van der Linden retainer. J Clin Orthod 2003;37:260-267.

221. Van der Linden FPGM, Boersma H. Diagnosis and Treatment Planning in Dentofacial Orthopedics. London: Quintessence, 1987.

222. Van der Linden FPGM, Boersma H, Prahl-Andersen B. Development of the dentition. In: Prahl-Andersen B, Kowalski CJ, Heydendael PHJ (eds). A Mixed-Longitudinal Interdisciplinary Study of Growth and Development. New York: Academic Press, 1979:521-536.

223. Van der Linden FPGM, Duterloo HS. Development of the Human Dentition: An Atlas. Hagerstown: Harper & Row, 1976.

224. Van der Linden FPGM, Hirschfeld WJ, Miller RL. On the analysis and presentation of longitudinally collected growth data. Growth 1970;34:385-400.

225. Van der Linden FPGM, McNamara. JA Jr, Burdi AR. Tooth size and position before birth. J Dent Res 1972;51:71-74.

226. Van der Linden FPGM, Proffit WR, McNamara JA Jr, Miethke R-R (eds). Dynamics of Orthodontics [video series]. Chicago: Quintessence, 2000.

227. Van der Linden FPGM, Radlanski RJ, McNamara. JA Jr. Normal Development of the Dentition [videotape]. Chicago: Quintessence, 2000.

228. Van der Linden FPGM, Radlanski RJ, McNamara. JA Jr. Malocclusions and Interventions [videotape]. Chicago: Quintessence, 2000.

229. Van der Schueren GL, De Smit AA. Combined fixed-functional Class II treatment. J Clin Orthod 1994;28:15-20.

230. Van Limborgh J. The role of genetic and local environmental factors in the control of postnatal craniofacial morphogenesis. Acta Morphol Neerl Scand 1972;10:37-47.

231. Van Wieringen JC, Wafelbakker F, Verbrugge HP, De Haas JH (eds). Groeidiagrammen 1965 Nederland. Groningen: Wolters-Noordhoff, 1965.

232. Vig PS, Cohen AM. Vertical growth of the lips: A serial cephalometric study. Am J Orthod 1979;75:405-415.

233. Weber AD. A longitudinal analysis of premolar enucleation. Am J Orthod 1969;56:394-402.

234. Weinstein S, Haack DC, Morris LY, Snyder BB, Attaway HE. On an equilibrium theory of tooth position. Angle Orthod 1963;33:1-11.

235. Weise W. Kieferorthopädische Kombinationstherapie. München: Urban & Schwarzenberg, 1992.

236. Wheeler TT, McGorray SP, Dolce C, Taylor MG, King GJ. Effectiveness of early treatment of Class II malocclusion. Am J Orthod Dentofacial Orthop 2002;121:9-17.

237. Wieslander L. Long-term effects of treatment with headgear–Herbst appliance in the early mixed dentition. Stability or relapse? Am J Orthod Dentofacial Orthop 1993;104:319-329.

238. Williams BH. Diagnosis and prevention of maxillary cuspid impaction. Angle Orthod 1981;51:30-40.

239. Woodside DG. The activator. In: Graber TM, Neumann B (eds). Removable Orthodontic Appliances. Philadelphia: W.B. Saunders Co., 1977:269-336.

240. Yoshihara T, Matsumoto Y, Suzuki J, Sato N, Oguchi H. Effect of serial extraction alone on crowding: Spontaneous changes in dentition after serial extraction. Am J Orthod Dentofacial Orthop 2000;118:611-616.

241. Zachrisson BU. Improving orthodontic results in cases with maxillary incisors missing. Am J Orthod 1978;73:274-289.

242. Zachrisson BU. JCO/interviews Dr Björn U. Zachrisson on excellence in finishing. Part 2. J Clin Orthod 1986;20:536-556.

243. Zachrisson BU. Esthetic factors involved in anterior tooth display and the smile: Vertical dimension. J Clin Orthod 1998;32:432-445.

244. Zachrisson BU. Bonding in orthodontics. In: Graber TM, Vanarsdall RL Jr (eds). Orthodontics. Current Principles and Technique, ed 3. St. Louis: Mosby, 2000:557-645.

245. Zachrisson BU. Dental to facial midline positions. World J Orthod 2001;2:362-364.

Index

*Orthodontic Concepts
and Strategies*

Index

C

Canine(s)

distal movement of, 148, 157

extraction of, 163

extrusion of, 157

impacted maxillary

case study application of, 164-175

causes of, 162

in Class I malocclusion, 172

in Class II division 1 malocclusions, 167, 170-171

in Class II division 2 malocclusions, 168-169, 174-175

follow-up for, 176

prevalence of, 161

prognosis for, 162

spontaneous eruption of, 163

treatment of, 161-176

mandibular, 6

palatal movement of, 66, 151

partial fixed appliance impaction of, 133

resorption of, 5

surface grinding of, 18

uprighting of, 73, 133, 157

Canine bar, 277

Catch-up growth, 126

C-clasps, 36

Cervical headgear

asymmetric force exerted by, 208

deep bite treated with, 80

description of, 51-52

facial growth and, 55, 115-117

maxillary incisor intrusion using, 134

open bite treated with, 215

parietal headgear vs, 57

permanent maxillary first molar movement, 57

vertical facial height stimulated using, 53

Clasps

Adams, 35, 36, 48

arrow, 35, 36

ball, 35, 36

C-, 36

claw, 42, 43, 151, 189-191

retention of, 34-36

undercuts for, 34-35

Class I malocclusions

asymmetries in, 198-199, 203

coverbite in, 181-183, 187

crowding in, 238, 252

description of, 177

maxillary canine impaction in, 172

maxillary central incisor loss, 232

maxillary lateral incisor agenesis, 231

partial fixed appliances for, 129, 141-142

retention plate for, 282

Class II division 1 malocclusions

activators for, 88-96

asymmetries in, 197, 200, 202, 206-207

case study of, 11-13

coverbite, posttreatment development of, 185-186

with crowding, 22, 24-26

dental arch in

description of, 16

disto-occlusion, 67

widening of, 102

diastemata in, 82

disto-occlusion in, 246-248

etiology, 16

extraoral traction in, 55

headgear for. *See* Headgear.

headgear-activators for, 106-111

headgear-plates for, 69, 74-79

illustration of, 8, 10

incisor transitions in, 10-11

initiation of treatment for, 50

lip-incisor relationship, 69

maxillary anterior teeth in, 226, 236, 255

maxillary canine impaction in, 167, 170-171

maxillary incisors in, 11, 226, 236, 263-265

non-occlusions in, 215, 217-219

with open bite, 68

open bite in, 215, 217-219, 222-223, 239

primary factor, 10, 16

secondary aspects, 10, 16

simultaneous extraction procedure for, 22, 24-26, 28-29

with solid intercuspation, 68

solid intercuspations for, 127

Class II division 2 malocclusions

asymmetries in, 204-205

coverbite in, 181-182, 188-189

description of, 177

headgear-activators for, 102

maxillary canine impaction in, 168-169, 174-175

primary factor, 16, 90

removable appliance-fixed appliance combination for, 160

secondary aspects, 16, 68, 90, 106

Type A, 185

Type B, 185

Type C, 185

Class III malocclusions

open bite with, 224

plate-fixed appliance combination for, 154

Collum angle, 181

Condyles, 50-51

"Cone-funnel" mechanism, 241-242

Construction bite

for activators, 82-85

for Van Beek headgear-activator, 98-99

H

Headgear
  activating, 59, 64
  adjusting, 59, 73
  asymmetric, 66, 208
  with bite plate, 65–80
  case studies of, 60–63
  cervical
    asymmetric force exerted by, 208
    deep bite treated with, 80
    description of, 51–52
    facial growth and, 55, 115–117
    with Kahn spur, 134, 136
    maxillary incisor intrusion using, 134
    open bite treated with, 215
    parietal headgear vs, 57
    permanent maxillary first molar movement, 57
  vertical facial height stimulated using, 53
  controlling, 59, 64
  dental casts for, 59
  description of, 49
  elastics for, 64, 66
  follow-up evaluations, 64
  force exerted by, 49
  high pull. See Headgear, parietal.
  indications, 80
  injuries caused by, 64
  inner bow sizes for, 59
  lower lip positioning, 69
  maxillary anterior development restricted by, 53
  maxillary dental arch space increased using, 55
  maxillofacial skeletal growth affected by, 49
  molar bands
    description of, 49
    fitting of, 58
    placement of, 58
    size selection of, 58
  molar movement using, 80
  neutral, 51
  parietal
    with a Bass plate, 204
    cervical headgear vs, 57
    illustration of, 51
    maxillary incisor intrusion using, 134
    open bite treated with, 215
    permanent maxillary first molar movement, 57
    vertical facial height restricted using, 53, 118, 124
  patient instructions about, 64
  permanent maxillary first molar movement, 56–57
  placing, 59
  removal of, 64
  general, 49–64
  sleep positioning considerations, 64

  traction directions for, 51
  wearing of, 64
Headgear-activators
  acrylic resin trimming for, 98
  avoidance reflex, 98
  for anterior open bite, 101–102
  auxiliary devices in, 97
  bows for, 102
  case studies of, 104–111
  Class II division 2 malocclusions treated with, 102
  components of, 98
  construction bite for, 99
  crossbite treated with, 105
  design of, 97
  deep bite reduced using, 100
  description of, 97–98
  disadvantages of, 104
  elastics used with, 156
  fabrication of, 98
  fitting of, 98
  fixed appliance therapy with, 103
  forces of, 99, 102
  general, 27, 28, 97–112
  habituation period for, 99
  history of, 97
  indentations, 100
  indications for, 97, 98, 106, 112
  for lower anterior facial height, 101–102
  mandibular crowding caused by, 104
  maxillary anterior development inhibited by, 99
  maxillary posterior teeth changes using, 103, 112
  movement of teeth with, 103
  neutro-occlusion achieved using, 104
  open bite created by, 104
  overjet reduction using, 102
  patient instruction about, 99
  retention phase of, 103
  side effects of, 104
  trimming of, 100–103
  try-in, 99
Headgear-plates
  for anterior open bite, 70–71
  asymmetric, 66
  canine movement using, 66
  case studies of, 73–79
  Class II malocclusions treated with, 69, 74–79
  dental arch widening using
    mandibular, 67
    maxillary, 68
  description of, 65
  headgear placement, 70
  inner bow adjustments, 73
  labial arches, 71

N

Nasal passageway, 54, 81, 99, 124, 224
Neuromuscular control, 52
Neutral headgear, 51
Non-occlusions
    in adolescents, 211
    age-related changes in, 274
    anterior, 210
    case study treatment of, 216-223
    characteristics of, 210
    in Class II division 1 malocclusions, 215, 217-219
    description of, 209
    detection of, 214-215
    lateral cephalograms of, 215
    open bite vs, 211
    prevalence, 211
    teeth irregularities in, 274
    tongue movements in, 213-214
    total, 210, 275

O

Occlusal contacts
    anterior region, 251, 254
    open bite, 224
Occlusal disturbances, 44
Occlusal rests, 195
Occlusion. *See also* Disto-occlusion.
    in anterior region, 241, 256
    "cone-funnel" mechanism, 241-242
    dental arch continuity and, 256
    description of, 241
    in posterior region, 243, 256
    tooth size discrepancies, 252-254
Occlusograms, 103
One phase treatment, 128
Open activators, 87
Open bite
    in adolescents, 211
    age-related changes in, 274
    anterior, 70-71, 211, 213, 219, 239
    case study treatment of, 216-223
    characteristics of, 210
    in Class II division 1 malocclusions, 215, 217-219, 222-223
    in Class III malocclusions, 224
    dental, 212
    description of, 209
    digit sucking as cause of, 209
    headgear-activator, 104
    lateral cephalograms of, 215
    non-occlusions vs, 211
    occlusal contacts in, 224

    overjet and, 263
    posterior, 213, 274
    prevalence, 211
    skeletal, 212-213, 219
    teeth irregularities in, 274
    tongue interpositioning and, 209
    tongue movements during swallowing in, 213
Orthognathic surgery, 128
Overbite, reversed, 3
Overjet
    anterior open bite and, 263
    description of, 11-13
    headgear-activator for, 102
    posterior bite block for, 44
    relapse of, 104

P

Palatal arch. *See* Palatal bar.
Palatal bar, 57, 196, 205, 208
Palatal tipping of maxillary incisors
    description of, 30, 180
    plates for, 43
Papillae
    interdental, 131, 139, 226, 232, 240
    retraction of, 131, 271
Parietal headgear
    cervical headgear vs, 57
    illustration of, 51
    large anterior facial height treated using, 128
    maxillary incisor intrusion using, 134
    open bite treated with, 215
    permanent maxillary first molar movement, 57
    vertical facial height restricted using, 53, 118
Partial fixed appliances
    bands, 130
    brackets for, 132
    case study applications of, 135-143
    Class I malocclusions treated with, 129, 141-142
    Class II malocclusions treated with, 136-140
    incisor rotations treated with, 133
    indications for, 129
    maxillary anterior teeth alignment using
        archwire for, 133
        description of, 132
        preformed arches for, 132-134
    maxillary incisors treated with, 133-134
Passive lingual arch, 20
Periodontium
    general, 259
    initial therapy, 260
    periodontal spaces, 285
    supra-alveolar fiber cutting. *See* Fibrectomy.
    loss of, 258